MULTIPLE SCLEROSIS

Contemporary Neurology Series

MULTIPLE SCLEROSIS

Moses Rodriguez, M.D.
Professor of Neurology
Mayo Clinic College of Medicine
Rochester, Minnesota

Orhun H. Kantarci, M.D.
Assistant Professor of Neurology
Mayo Clinic College of Medicine
Rochester, Minnesota

Istvan Pirko, M.D.
Associate Professor of Neurology
Mayo Clinic College of Medicine
Rochester, Minnesota

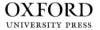
OXFORD
UNIVERSITY PRESS

OXFORD
UNIVERSITY PRESS

Oxford University Press is a department of the University of Oxford.
It furthers the University's objective of excellence in research, scholarship,
and education by publishing worldwide.

Oxford   New York
Auckland   Cape Town   Dar es Salaam   Hong Kong   Karachi
Kuala Lumpur   Madrid   Melbourne   Mexico City   Nairobi
New Delhi   Shanghai   Taipei   Toronto

With offices in
Argentina   Austria   Brazil   Chile   Czech Republic   France   Greece
Guatemala   Hungary   Italy   Japan   Poland   Portugal   Singapore
South Korea   Switzerland   Thailand   Turkey   Ukraine   Vietnam

Oxford is a registered trademark of Oxford University Press in the UK and certain other
countries.

Published in the United States of America by
Oxford University Press
198 Madison Avenue, New York, NY 10016

Library of Congress Cataloging-in-Publication Data
Rodriguez, Moses.
Multiple sclerosis / Moses Rodriguez, Orhun H. Kantarci, Istvan Pirko.
    p. ; cm. — (Contemporary neurology series ; 84)
Includes bibliographical references and index.
ISBN 978–0–19–974046–8 (alk. paper)—ISBN 978–0–19–997019–3 (alk. paper)
I. Kantarci, Orhun H.   II. Pirko, Istvan.   III. Title.   IV. Series: Contemporary neurology series ; 84. 0069-9446
[DNLM: 1. Multiple Sclerosis. W1 CO769N v.84 2013 / WL 360]
LC Classification not assigned
616.8′34—dc23
2012051007

9 8 7 6 5 4 3 2
Printed in China
on acid-free paper

Preface

During the past 25 years, there has been tremendous advancement in our knowledge of the pathophysiology and, more importantly, the treatment of the most common demyelinating disease of the central nervous system, multiple sclerosis (MS). Traditionally, MS has been considered a primary demyelinating disease in which the immune system mainly injures the myelin sheath. However, increasing data suggest that the disease is much more complex and is likely a much more heterogeneous process. In some cases, the disease attacks the myelin sheath, but in other situations, the oligodendrocytes appear to be the primary site of injury. There have been increasing data regarding the differential role of the immune response in the generation of the disease process.

Traditionally, MS has been considered an autoimmune disease; that is, immune cells such as CD4$^+$ T cells or immunoglobulins are directed against self antigens on the myelin sheath. However, this hypothesis has proven difficult to substantiate. Clearly, we know that the disease is immune-mediated. However, whether the disease is directed against an endogenous antigen or is induced by an exogenous antigen that is acquired in the environment is yet unproven. Even without this critical knowledge, the advancement of the treatment of the disease has been remarkable. At the time of the writing of this book, the U.S. Food & Drug Administration has approved eight new treatments to prevent relapses. All of them target some aspect of the immune response. A group of slightly different drugs are the interferons, which were primarily designed to stop viral infections but in MS may also regulate some aspects of the immune repertoire that induces destruction of the myelin or the oligodendrocytes. Interferons continue to be the mainstay of treatment. Because viruses from multiple family members can induce demyelination both in human diseases and animal models, there is considerable support for the hypothesis that virus infection either initiates the disease process or persists in the central nervous system to recruit the inflammatory response.

In this book, we attempt to provide the practicing clinician with a careful understanding of the pathophysiology of the disease process. Specifically, we highlight some of the newer concepts from the standpoint of pathology, immunology, genetics, epidemiology, and imaging. In addition, we provide the rationale for treatment protocols for the currently available drugs that prevent relapses and give an accurate presentation of their utility and potential side effects. We devote some effort to discussing the newer drugs entering phase II and phase III clinical trials; these will likely add to the armamentarium for the practicing clinician caring for MS patients. All of these drugs appear to target the inflammatory phase of the disease; that is, the phase characterized by relapses and remissions. Most patients begin with a relapsing–remitting course; therefore, it is reasonable to focus on this aspect of the disease process. Unfortunately, none of the established drugs and none of the newer drugs are likely to be curative even if begun at the earliest stage of disease. There is at present very little evidence that stopping relapses or the inflammatory response prevents patients from entering the progressive phase of the disease.

There is a critical need to prevent patients from entering the progressive phase or to help patients with already established, persistent neurological deficits. Newer approaches, such as neuroprotective agents and remyelinating agents, are reviewed as possible means of achieving these therapeutic goals.

It has become apparent that MS is not merely a disease of myelin but also affects axons and neurons. There is increasing evidence that cortical demyelination may be a critical feature of the disease and may actually correlate better with long-term disability. In addition, loss of neurons in the gray matter as well as axons, as seen frequently in degenerative diseases, has now been well documented both by MRI and in pathological specimens. These findings widen our thinking regarding the pathogenesis of the disease and force investigators to look at it from a new perspective. As a result, future drugs will need to prevent neuronal death, axonal destruction, and cortical lesions. In other words, these drugs will need to address targets of the disease process; that is, neurons, astrocytes, microglia, axons, and oligodendrocytes. Delivery systems via monoclonal antibodies will need to be devised to target specific structures within the central nervous system. Already, antibodies have proven effective in several animal models of MS in which either oligodendrocytes or neurons are the primary targets of the drug. These drugs are designed to promote remyelination (when targeting oligodendrocytes) or neuronal preservation (when targeting neurons or axons). These are just two examples of new approaches that may be available to the clinician in the future.

This book also provides a novel approach to the concept of symptomatic therapy in MS. It proposes an integrative approach to symptom management and recognizes the interaction between fatigue, depression, pain, cognitive impairment, bladder dysfunction, and infections. By approaching the illness in an integrative way, instead of just addressing specific symptoms, it may be possible to chose medications that target multiple symptoms so that the patient ultimately uses fewer drugs and experiences fewer side effects.

Many books written about MS and demyelination focus primarily on the basic science aspects of the disease and are therefore less useful for the practicing clinician. Others are overly simplistic in their approach to management and do not provide the underlying scientific rationale for treatment. We hope this new book will offer a bench-to-bedside explanation of the link between pathophysiology and effective treatment. Ultimately, rather than treating patients in the established clinical categories of relapsing–remitting disease, secondary progressive disease, and primary progressive disease, we need to treat patients by addressing the basic pathophysiological processes occurring in their central nervous systems. For patients in whom antibodies play a primary role in injury, we hope that future approaches will target depletion of pathogenic immunoglobulins by plasma exchange or drugs that target B cells or plasma cells. In the cases of microglial cell-mediated demyelinating disease, it may be necessary to target those cells in the central nervous system. In disease characterized by dying-back oligodendrogliopathy, it may be necessary to design drugs that prevent apoptosis of oligodendrocytes. Treating patients based on pathophysiology and the immunopathology that characterizes the lesions will ultimately result in an "individualized-medicine" approach to MS treatment.

In the following section, we acknowledge a number of individuals who have helped conceptually in the generation of this book. However, at this point, we would like to acknowledge the specific contributions of Dr. Bharath Wootla, who created many of the figures dealing with the immunology of MS, and Mrs. Lea Dacy, who transcribed and edited all of the chapters so that all three authors spoke as one voice. At Oxford University Press, we appreciate the assistance of Mr. Craig Panner and Ms. Kathryn Winder. We also thank the following individuals and foundations that made this work possible: the National Multiple Sclerosis Society, the Hilton Foundation, Mr. and Mrs. Eugene Applebaum, Dr. and Mrs. Moon Park, Ms. Kathryn Peterson and the McNeilus family.

Acknowledgments

We thank the members of the Division of Multiple Sclerosis and Autoimmune Neurology, who have been our colleagues. Through informal conferences and sharing cases, they have helped to formulate our conceptual thinking of the treatment of this disorder:

Jonathan L. Carter, M.D.
Ralitza H. Gavrilova, M.D.
B. Mark Keegan, M.D.
Daniel H. LaChance, M.D.
Claudia F. Lucchinetti, M.D.
Marc C. Patterson, M.D.
Andrew McKeon, M.B., B.Ch.

John H. Noseworthy, M.D.
Sean M. Pittock, M.D.
Elizabeth A. Shuster, M.D.
Jan-Mendelt Tillema, M.D.
Brian G. Weinshenker, M.D.
Dean M. Wingerchuk, M.D.

In addition, we thank members of our basic science laboratories who have contributed to our understanding of the pathophysiology of the disorder:

Kathleen S. Allen
Pascal Aliihnui Atanga
Jennifer Ayers-Ringler
Michael P. Bell
Allan J. Bieber, Ph.D
Daniel D. Billadeau, Ph.D.
William A. Carey, M.D.
Chella S. David, Ph.D.
Aleksandar Denic, M.D., Ph.D.
Sara J. Felts, Ph.D.
Jeffrey D. Gamez
Shailendra Giri, Ph.D.
Spencer Gladis
Yong Guo, M.D., Ph.D.
Michael J. Hansen
Karen E. Hedin, Ph.D.
John R. Henley, Ph.D.
Charles L. Howe, Ph.D.
Aaron J. Johnson, Ph.D.
Tatiana Kaptzan, Ph.D.
Jason Kerkvliet
Vanda A. Lennon, M.D., Ph.D.
Linda K. Linbo, R.N.
Slobodan I. Macura, Ph.D.

Louis J. Maher, III, Ph.D.
Ashutosh K. Mangalam, Ph.D.
Marcelo Matiello, M.D.
Meghan M. Painter
Louisa M. Papke
Kevin D. Pavelko, Ph.D.
M. Mateo Paz Soldan, M.D., Ph.D.
Larry R. Pease, Ph.D.
Tobias M. Peikert, M.D.
Jodi C. Picasso, M.D.
Mabel L. Pierce
Janet L. Schaefer Klein
Isobel A. Scarisbrick, Ph.D.
Diane M. Sneve, R.N.
Jaime R. Sorum
David X. Sun
Virginia P. Van Keulen
Arthur E. Warrington, Ph.D.
Jens O. Watzlawik, Ph.D.
Delana M. Weis
Bharath Wootla, Ph.D.
Xiaohua Xu, Ph.D.
Patricia Ziemer
Laurie J. Zoecklein

Contents

SECTION 2   TREATMENT

MULTIPLE SCLEROSIS

PATHOGENESIS

Chapter 1

The Spectrum and Diagnosis of Multiple Sclerosis

Abstract

This chapter introduces our major goal of arriving at an accurate diagnosis of MS and accurate placement of the patient in the evolution of the disease. Achieving this goal leads to valid treatment decisions, including recruitment in epidemiological studies and clinical trials, and enables the treating physician to provide the patient with an understanding of his or her prognosis. This chapter will discuss the diagnosis of prototypical MS, including the different phases of MS and the predictors of conversion from one phase to another, as well as predictors of more severe phenotypes within each phase.

We will introduce the clinical concepts behind treatment approaches for each phase discussed in later chapters. We will discuss the other idiopathic inflammatory demyelinating diseases briefly in the context of early phases of MS.

THE SPECTRUM OF IDIOPATHIC INFLAMMATORY DEMYELINATING DISEASES

Multiple sclerosis (MS) is an idiopathic inflammatory demyelinating disease (IIDD) of the central nervous system (CNS). IIDDs differ

3

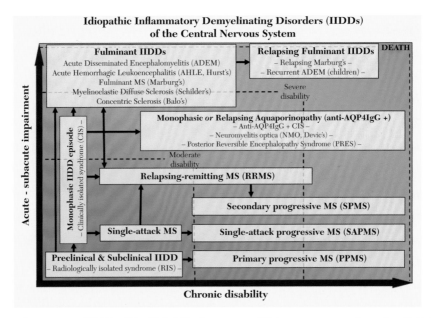

Figure 1–1. The spectrum of IIDDs of the CNS defined in two axes: (1) the acute extent and severity of initial pathology and (2) the chronic impact on disability of the patient. Also refer to Chapter 2 for further discussion on IIDDs. (Updated and modified from Kantarci & Weinshenker, Neurol Clin 2005.[47])

from each other both clinically and pathologically, although many can evolve into another IIDD in a continuum. MS is the "prototypical" form of IIDD. IIDDs fall into a spectrum with two axes: (1) the acuity and severity of initial pathology and (2) the chronic impact on disability of the patient (Fig. 1.1).

IIDDs with the relatively severe acute presentation of diffuse or tumorlike involvement of the CNS include acute disseminated encephalomyelitis (ADEM), acute hemorrhagic leukoencephalitis (AHLE or Hurst's disease), fulminant MS (Marburg's variant), myelinoclastic diffuse sclerosis (Schilder's disease), and concentric sclerosis (Balo's disease) (Fig. 1.1).

IIDDs with more restricted CNS involvement associated with the presence of antibodies against aquaporin-4 are referred to as aquaporinopathies. The prototypical form of this type of IIDD is neuromyelitis optica (NMO or Devic's disease) (Fig. 1.1).

Some IIDDs actually represent different phases of prototypical MS and are associated with more chronic disability. These include radiologically isolated syndrome (RIS), clinically isolated syndrome (CIS), single-attack MS (SAMS), relapsing–remitting MS (RRMS), single-attack progressive

MS (SAPMS), secondary progressive MS (SPMS), and primary progressive MS (PPMS) (Fig. 1.1).

Most IIDDs initially present with an acute monophasic episode, which is characterized by a degree of inflammation and demyelination arising from a baseline preclinical disease activity and followed by a subacute stage of remyelination and repair. These episodes are known as attacks, relapses, or exacerbations. PPMS is an exception to the rule because there is no presenting attack, and patients are recognized during a phase of insidious worsening.

In this first chapter, we will discuss the diagnosis of prototypical MS. We will then focus on different phases of MS and emphasize predictors of conversion from one phase to another as well as predictors of more severe phenotypes within each phase. We will introduce the clinical concepts behind treatment approaches for each phase discussed in later chapters. We will discuss the other IIDDs briefly in the context of early phases of MS. However, due to the clinically and biologically distinct nature of IIDDs other than MS, we will defer extensive discussions of these syndromes to the chapter on differential diagnosis of MS.

THE DIAGNOSIS OF PROTOTYPICAL MULTIPLE SCLEROSIS

The diagnosis of "definite MS" requires the dissemination in time and space of independent inflammatory–demyelinating attacks. These attacks could be symptomatic or asymptomatic. Asymptomatic attacks are recognized during clinical or subclinical examinations (radiological or electrophysiological examinations).

Evolution of Modern Diagnostic Criteria for Multiple Sclerosis

The widely accepted original criteria for the diagnosis of MS known as the Poser criteria required that these independent attacks be defined clinically.[1] The main problem with this definition is that it ignored subclinical disease activity, which is more common than clinical activity, and slowly worsening neurological function, such as in PPMS, when making a definite diagnosis of MS. Therefore, imaging changes (e.g., new nonenhancing or enhancing lesions that develop on magnetic resonance imaging [MRI]) did not play a role in the diagnosis of the disease. Until a second relapse occurred, most of these patients were categorized as having CIS.

Many MS patients demonstrate multiple new subclinical (asymptomatic) lesions in the brain or spinal cord subsequent to their first clinical attack and, hence, qualify for dissemination in time and space. However, by the Poser criteria, they had to wait for a second clinical attack to receive a definite diagnosis. Although the Poser criteria ensured accurate and conservative recruitment for multicenter clinical trials, many clinical neurologists found them too restricting to use in practice.

The next iteration of diagnostic criteria for MS is known as the McDonald criteria.[2,3] In Table 1.1, we point out the initial differences in the two sets of criteria for diagnosis of MS. The McDonald criteria de-emphasized electrophysiological evidence of a subclinical attack to define different categories such as possible or probable MS, except in the diagnosis of PPMS. The McDonald criteria allowed for the diagnosis of definite MS by demonstrating dissemination in time and space by MRI even in the absence of a clinical relapse. Allowing for MRI evidence of dissemination in time and space led to a two to fourfold increase in the diagnosis of definite MS in the first 12 months following a CIS.[4,5] However, the 2005 revision of these criteria still had major pitfalls for the practicing clinician. For example, if a patient presented with both enhancing and nonenhancing lesions at the time of his or her initial clinical event, most experienced clinicians would still consider the patient to have MS because the different lesion ages would prove dissemination in time and space.

In 2010 the McDonald criteria were further revised to account for subclinical MRI activity at the initial presentation in addition to clinical activity.[6] Dissemination in time could therefore be defined by new T2 and/or gadolinium-enhancing lesion(s) on follow-up MRI, or the simultaneous presence of an asymptomatic gadolinium-enhancing lesion and nonenhancing lesion at the time of the initial clinical event (Table 1.2). The current criteria allow for dissemination in space to be defined by at least one lesion in two out of four locations typical of MS in the MRI (periventricular, juxtacortical, infratentorial, and spinal cord) (Table 1.2). The current criteria do not consider purely cortical lesions given the current limitations of MRI technology available (as of 2010) in detecting these lesions. We envision that cortical lesions will be considered in future diagnostic criteria, when better MRI detection of these lesions becomes available outside the specialized centers.

Using MRI criteria to make the diagnosis of MS requires discernment and accuracy in describing the location and orientation of lesions to differentiate them from T2 hyperintense lesions due to other factors. Aging, hypertension, smoking, migraine, and small vessel ischemic disease commonly cause T2 hyperintense lesions that may coexist with demyelinating disease or may solely explain the observed lesions. Our later chapters, which discuss MRI in MS, show some of the differentiating factors of a "relatively specific" MS lesion. However, the diagnostic criteria for MS in its current form do not specify the lesion characteristics other than T2 hyperintensity. Therefore, extreme caution is needed in interpreting any white

Table 1–1 **Comparison of Poser and McDonald (2005) Diagnostic Criteria for MS**

Poser criteria[1]					McDonald criteria (2005)[82]		
Category	Relapses	Clinical	Paraclinical*	CSF	Clinical (attacks)	Objective clinical lesion	Additionally
Clinically definite					≥2	≥2	None
A1	2	2	NA	NA	≥2	1	Dissemination in space by MRI **OR** (+) CSF and ≥2 MRI lesions **OR** further attack involving a different site
A2	2	1	1	NA			
Laboratory-supported definite					1	≥2	Dissemination in time by MRI **OR** 2nd clinical attack
B1	2	1	1	+	1°°	1	Dissemination in space by MRI *or* (+) CSF and ≥2 MRI lesions **AND** Dissemination in time by MRI *or* 2nd clinical attack
B2	1	2	NA	+			
B3	1	1	1	+			
Clinically probable					0°°°	1	Positive CSF **AND** Dissemination in space by ≥9 T2 brain lesions *or* ≥2 cord lesions *or* 4–8 brain and 1 cord lesion *or* 4–8 brain lesions and + VEP *or* <4 brain lesions and 1 cord lesion and + VEP **AND** Dissemination in time by MRI *or* continued progression for one year
C1	2	1	–	–			
C2	1	2	–	–			
C3	1	1	1	–			
Laboratory-supported probable							
D1	2	–	–	+			

NA, not applicable; VEP, visual evoked potential
° MRI or evoked potential
°° Monosymptomatic
°°° Progression from onset—PPMS

matter lesion as a possible MS lesion. Overly liberal use of these criteria can result in an overdiagnosis of MS and unnecessary anxiety for the patient. Moreover, even in the setting of a correct diagnosis of MS, a strict dogmatic interpretation may lead to overly aggressive, potentially dangerous treatment initiation or changes.

Table 1–2 Dissemination in Time and Space Criteria by MRI, Modified from 2010 McDonald Criteria for MS[6]

Dissemination in space by MRI[82,83]	Dissemination in time by MRI[84]
• ≥1 T2 hyperintense lesion (with or without gadolinium enhancement) in 2 of the 4 following typical locations for demyelinating lesions: periventricular, juxtacortical, infratentorial, spinal cord	• Simultaneous presence of asymptomatic gadolinium-enhancing and nonenhancing lesions at any time ***OR*** • A new T2 and or gadolinium-enhancing lesion(s) on follow-up MRI irrespective of timing of the baseline MRI from the time of initial clinical attack

Caution: If a subject has a brainstem or spinal cord syndrome, the symptomatic lesion is excluded from the total lesion count.
Caution: Sound judgment is needed in describing lesion location and orientation to differentiate T2 hyperintense lesions due to other factors such as aging, hypertension, smoking, migraine, and small vessel ischemic disease, which may coexist with demyelinating disease or solely explain the observed lesions.
Caution: With evolution of MRI technology and better resolution of cortical lesions, they may routinely be considered in the future. Currently only specialized centers with experience with such technologies should use them to help support a diagnosis of MS.

Diagnostic Approach to Multiple Sclerosis

Table 1.3 shows the diagnostic criteria used in our daily practice, modified from the 2010 McDonald criteria published in the original article.[6] Based on our clinical experience, we have added (and discuss below) several additional layers of requirements to secure a diagnosis of MS rather than strictly adhering to the original criteria. This slightly more conservative approach aims to minimize an overdiagnosis of MS.

Even in the setting of an objective clinical examination finding during an attack and historical evidence of other attacks, MS diagnosis should remain suspicious if MRI, evoked potentials, and cerebrospinal fluid studies are negative. The clinician should continue to rule out mimickers and not commit to the diagnosis of MS unless a future attack offers objective findings or follow-up MRIs fulfill dissemination in time and space criteria. We generally recommend a 6- to 18-month interval between MRIs, with the actual interval determined by the severity of the patient's presentation. Positive paraclinical studies and, especially, CSF findings increase the chance of a future attack in the setting of CIS. We discuss the predictive value of CSF in further detail in the section on CIS. Given the predictive value of CSF, an initial presentation that partially fulfills the criteria, accompanied by supportive evidence from CSF and evoked potential studies, indicates MS as the most likely diagnosis,

if alternative diagnoses are ruled out. In most cases, however, we would still wait for a future clinical attack and/or follow-up MRIs to fulfill dissemination in time and space criteria before initiating treatment.

In addition to the McDonald criteria,[6] in the setting of progressive symptoms, we recommend objective documentation by neurological examination, evoked potentials, or MRI of a lesion consistent with demyelination in the area of the CNS indicated by progressive symptoms. Other explanations should be pursued for progressive symptoms that cannot be objectively assigned to a CNS lesion, and the neurologist should first rule out other possible causes for symptoms such as progressive fatigue or progressive pain in the absence of evolving MRI or clinical examination findings. A lack of caution (or excessive zeal) can lead to inappropriate diagnosis of progressive MS or delayed diagnosis of another disease. For example, patients might present with progressively worsening chronic fatigue syndrome and fibromyalgia, and it would be most unfortunate if the treating neurologist tried to arrest these with aggressive MS treatments. Often, these syndromes are not directly secondary to MS; the explanation may be another common problem, such as obstructive sleep apnea or anxiety. In some other instances, disease-modifying, injectable MS medications cause patients to present with flulike side effects that may indeed give the appearance of progressive fatigue. Many additional neurological problems, such

Table 1–3 Practical Diagnostic Criteria for Diagnosis of MS, Modified from 2010 McDonald Criteria[6]

Presenting clinical scenario	Dissemination in time and space criteria for a diagnosis of MS at the time of presentation
≥2 attacks° with appropriate time course of onset, stabilization and recovery suggestive of distinct demyelinating episodes°°	*1 of 3 of the following are needed* (**relapsing–remitting MS**): • Objective examination findings°° for ≥2 lesions in separate CNS sites in all attacks • Objective examination findings°° for a single lesion in one attack **and** strong historical evidence for other lesion(s) in separate CNS site(s) in other attack(s) • Objective examination findings°° for a single lesion in one attack **and** dissemination in space by MRI criteria in **Table-1.2**
1 attack° with appropriate time course of onset, stabilization and recovery suggestive of distinct demyelinating episode (**clinically isolated syndrome**)	*1 of 2 of the following are needed* (**single-attack MS**): • Objective examination findings°° for ≥2 lesions in separate CNS sites **and** dissemination in time by MRI criteria in **Table-1.2** • Objective examination findings°° for one lesion **and** dissemination in space and time by MRI criteria in **Table-1.2**
Progressive neurological dysfunction of ≥1 year (retrospectively or prospectively determined) suggestive of demyelinating disease	*Objective examination findings°°° **and** 2 of 3 of the following are needed* (**progressive MS**): • Dissemination in space by MRI criteria in **Table-1.2** • Dissemination in time by MRI criteria in **Table-1.2** • Positive CSF (isoelectric focusing evidence of oligoclonal bands **and/or** elevated IgG index)

° From the McDonald criteria[6]: *"An attack (relapse, exacerbation) is defined as patient reported or objectively observed events typical of an acute inflammatory demyelinating event in the CNS, current or historical, with duration of at least 24 hours, in the absence of fever or infection. It should be documented by contemporaneous neurological examination, but some historical events with symptoms and evolution characteristics for MS, but for which no objective neurological findings are documented, can provide reasonable evidence of a prior demyelinating event. Reports of paroxysmal symptoms should, however, consist of multiple episodes occurring over at least 24 hours"*
°° From the McDonald criteria[6]: *"Before a definite diagnosis of MS can be made, at least one attack must be corroborated by findings on neurological examination, visual evoked potential response in patients reporting prior visual disturbance, or MRI consistent with demyelination in the area of the CNS indicated in the historical report of neurological symptoms."*
°°° In our opinion in addition to the McDonald criteria,[6] in the setting of progressive symptoms one needs objective documentation by neurological examination, evoked potentials, or MRI consistent with demyelination in the area of the CNS indicated by progressive symptoms. Other explanations should be pursued for progressive symptoms that cannot be objectively assigned to a lesion, and they should not be used as the sole basis of making a diagnosis of progressive MS.
Caution: Even in the setting of an objective clinical examination, if MRI, evoked potentials, and CSF studies are all negative, MS is suspicious during the first presentation and alternative diagnoses should be considered.[6] In the setting of partially fulfilling the above criteria, MS is possible during the first presentation *(especially with further supportive evidence from CSF and evoked potential studies)* if alternative diagnoses are ruled out. Wait for a future clinical attack **and/or** follow-up MRIs *(reasonable intervals determined by the level of suspicion; our recommendation is 6–18 months)* to fulfill dissemination in time and space criteria before a definite diagnosis of MS is made.

as an independent peripheral neuropathy or even motor neuron disease, can contribute to an apparent progression of MS.[7]

The latest diagnostic criteria do not include patients with RIS. However, this group fulfills both dissemination in time and space by the McDonald MRI criteria, as illustrated in Table 1.2. Our adapted diagnostic algorithm utilizes the most recent McDonald diagnostic criteria (Fig. 1.2).[6] We discuss individual phases of this algorithm in the following section.

THE PHASES AND EVOLUTION OF PROTOTYPICAL MULTIPLE SCLEROSIS

Clearly, the contemporary diagnosis of MS has evolved from the earlier diagnostic criteria based solely on disseminated clinical relapses to include subclinical disease activity. As mentioned earlier, MS is a continuum starting in a preclinical stage of unknown age and duration. From there, it evolves in an age-dependent fashion initially to attacks (symptomatic or asymptomatic) and

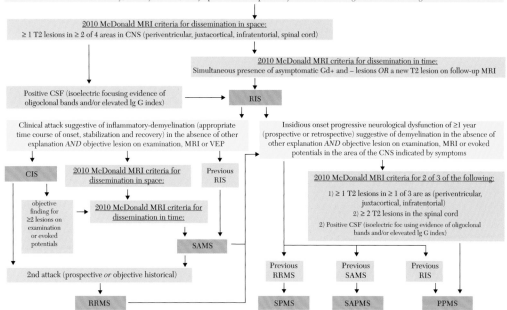

Figure 1–2. Diagnostic algorithm for MS and its different phases, adapted from the most recent McDonald diagnostic criteria[6] to practical daily use.

then to progressive disease course.[8] While most patients experience all of these phases of the disease, some remain asymptomatic and are discovered to have MS during autopsy.[9,10] Some patients will only develop one or more symptomatic or asymptomatic attacks and not experience progression.[8] Some patients will reach the typical age of progression without symptomatic attacks but then develop insidiously worsening PPMS.

In practice, depending on when an individual is clinically recognized within the continuum of MS, he or she is labeled as having RIS, CIS, SAMS, RRMS, SAPMS, SPMS, or PPMS. These phases of MS are illustrated in Figure 1.3 scaled against the disability axis with a rough estimate of the percentage of patients recognized and remaining in each category. We discuss the individual phases of MS in detail below.

Radiologically Isolated Syndrome

RIS describes patients in the preclinical stages of MS with incidental white matter changes

that suggest demyelinating disease observed in an MRI obtained for reasons unrelated to MS symptoms. Alternatively, the presenting symptoms may be nonspecific and not objectively localized to a CNS lesion suggestive of a typical episode of demyelination, or symptoms that can be explained by alternative neurological and nonneurological disorders.[6,9,10] This represents the earliest "subclinical relapsing" phase of MS (Fig. 1.3). However, in the absence of definite symptoms to attribute to MS, these patients fall outside the latest McDonald diagnostic criteria.[5]

When they develop the first symptom attributed to the lesions, these patients actually fulfill the dissemination in time and space criteria, since their lesions had been discovered prior to their symptomatic presentation. At this point, we can reliably diagnose these patients as having MS, although technically they would have already been diagnosed with CIS if they were recognized during their first symptom. This concept is reflected in the diagnostic algorithm (Fig. 1.2).

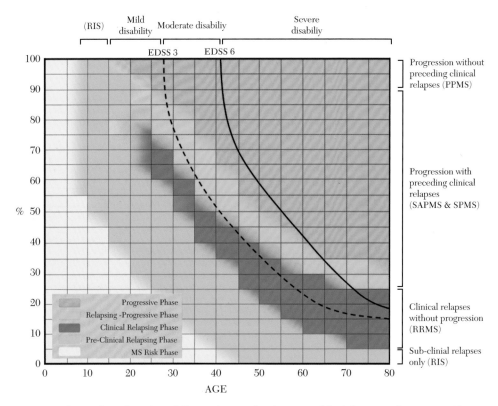

Figure 1–3. Evolution of MS through its different phases indexed to age and disability. A rough estimate of the percentage of patients recognized in each category and those who remain in each category are shown as well. RIS, radiologically isolated syndrome; CIS, clinically isolated syndrome; RRMS, relapsing–remitting MS; SAPMS, single-attack progressive MS; SPMS, secondary progressive MS; PPMS, primary progressive MS.

A diagnosis of RIS, although it does not carry a clear risk of conversion to clinical MS, can be a significant source of anxiety for patients. The natural history of RIS has been difficult to assess, since these patients are randomly recognized. Unlike CIS, it has no official beginning of the preclinical phase of MS to establish a time course. However, it is clear that even during a CIS or at the onset of PPMS, the multiple established lesions would indicate a preclinical relapsing phase of unknown duration. Studies have unequivocally shown, though, that some patients have prolonged time courses, where multiple new T2 hyperintense lesions can appear, enhance, lose enhancement, disappear, or persist without any associated symptom.[6,9,10] This is not surprising, since similar lesion evolution can occur even in the absence of associated symptoms in patients with established MS and their relatives. Up to 4% of asymptomatic relatives of sporadic MS patients have evidence of MRI lesions. This increases to 10% in families with multiple affected members, and the rate of detection of silent MRI lesions in the non-MS discordant monozygotic twin is about 20%.[11–18]

The conversion rate from RIS to MS (development of first symptom attributable to MS) is ~20% at 2 years and ~30% at 3 years from the first MRI diagnosis of MS lesions.[6,9,10] Oligoclonal bands in CSF and the presence of cervical lesions on MRI are useful to stratify patients for increased risk of conversion to MS.[19,20] Patients with RIS seemingly convert to MS at a slower rate than CIS patients in the placebo arms of CIS trials and no faster than the CIS patients in the treatment arms of the same trials.[6,9,10,21–24] Therefore, until a specific treatment trial proves effective in RIS, there is no reason to initiate disease-modifying therapy. However, one could argue that if the treatment goal is to prevent lesion burden in MS, these patients represent the earliest opportunity for benefit. A properly designed clinical trial is clearly needed.

Clinically Isolated Syndrome and Single-Attack Multiple Sclerosis

When a patient is first seen during an isolated IIDD episode (optic neuritis, transverse myelitis, brainstem-cerebellar syndrome, cortical or subcortical syndrome) in the absence of a previous history of demyelinating disease, we refer to him or her as having a monophasic IIDD or CIS. There are several possibilities for clinical evolution of a patient with CIS (Fig. 1.1).

A patient with CIS may present with lesions in limited locations in the CNS that may be positive for a specific serological marker, namely an anti-aquaporin-4 antibody (anti-AQP4IgG)[25] (Fig. 1.1). These syndromes are aquaporinopathies that can be monophasic or relapsing. They are prototypically characterized by Devic's disease (NMO), as discussed in a later chapter.[26] Differentiating these syndromes from other CISs early on by their telltale imaging findings and/or positive anti-AQP4IgG serology has a significant impact on early treatment choices and prognosis.[26] Generally patients with NMO have fewer but more severe relapses than patients with MS. NMO patients rarely have progressive syndromes. The current diagnostic criteria for MS also emphasize the need for serology and imaging criteria to differentiate aquaporinopathies that are otherwise clinically similar to other CISs.[6]

A patient with CIS may also present with a fulminant, diffuse, or tumorlike syndrome such as ADEM, AHLE (Hurst's disease), Marburg's variant of MS, Schilder's myelinoclastic diffuse sclerosis, or Balo's concentric sclerosis. Many of these syndromes have more severe attacks than prototypical MS. They can occur as a single episode or multiple recurrences. In some cases, these syndromes convert to prototypical MS at a later date. Although they are mentioned here, they merit separate, detailed discussion in the following chapters (Fig. 1.1).

Of all CIS patients without differentiating aquaporinopathies, 88% with an initial brain MRI suggestive of MS at presentation develop clinically definite MS by the Poser criteria within 14 years of onset, compared to only 19% with a normal MRI.[27] As mentioned earlier, the original McDonald criteria, which include MRI criteria, led to a two- to fourfold increase in the diagnosis of definite MS in the first 12 months following a CIS.[4,5] In the current iteration of diagnostic criteria for MS,[6] some previous CIS patients actually fulfill dissemination in time and space criteria by MRI at the time of presentation, and they are defined as having MS. We refer to this group of patients as having single attack MS (SAMS) (Table 1.3 and Fig. 1.2). As discussed later in the chapter, patients with SAMS who develop progressive MS are labeled as having SAPMS.

The separation of SAMS from CIS, as it occurs in the most recent diagnostic criteria for MS, is significant to help understand the context of earlier clinical trials that labeled both syndromes as CIS. For example, the primary outcome measure in earlier clinical trials in CIS was the development of a second clinical event (or clinically definite MS by the Poser criteria).[28,29] However, 72% of these patients actually fulfilled the radiological criteria for MS during enrollment, and 30% actually had enhancing lesions.[30] Therefore, one third of these patients would qualify as having SAMS today, while the others would qualify as having CIS. Given the effect size and the relationship of effect size to higher lesion loads from the original CIS trials, it is logical to predict that the responders to disease-modifying treatments in these trials had SAMS. It is unclear whether CIS, as defined by modern MS criteria, would actually respond as positively to MS drugs. The impact of future modifications to diagnostic criteria on practice paradigms should always be considered in interpreting past studies.

Predictors of conversion from CIS to MS are well studied, albeit using different diagnostic criteria. For example, long intracanalicular lesions of the optic nerve on MRI correlate with poor recovery from an optic neuritis attack.[31,32] Recent studies suggest that these lesions indeed represent an aquaporinopathy rather than MS.[26] The 10-year risk of developing MS after any acute episode of optic neuritis in adults is 56% with one or more lesions suggestive of MS on MRI and 22% if the MRI is normal.[33] The MRI predictors of conversion from CIS to MS are further discussed in Chapter 4. In the latter group, male gender, absence of pain, and presence of optic disk swelling, peripapillary hemorrhages, or retinal exudates carry a lower risk of conversion to MS. The risk of conversion to MS is lower in children: 13% in 10 years and 26% in 40 years.[34] Recurrent or bilateral sequential optic neuritis increases the risk of conversion to MS.[34] The presence

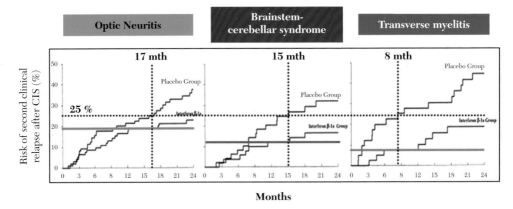

Figure 1–4. Risk of second demyelinating attack (clinically definite MS by Poser criteria) following a clinically isolated syndrome in patients treated with interferon beta-1a versus patients who have received placebo.[39] It takes about 17 months for 25% of patients with isolated optic neuritis to develop a new relapse, while it takes 15 months for patients with an isolated brainstem syndrome and 8 months for patients with an isolated transverse myelitis to reach the same target. Benefit is most prominent in the transverse myelitis group.

of oligoclonal bands in the CSF, in addition to three or more lesions suggestive of MS, predicts conversion 63% of the time within about 2 years after an isolated attack of optic neuritis, while the absence of either invariably predicts no conversion to MS (negative predictive value of 100%).[35] Although not routinely tested in clinical practice, the presence of HLA-DR2 (DR15) genotype has a positive predictive value of 44% and a negative predictive value of 71% in determining conversion to definite MS.[35] Sensory symptoms, posterolateral location of the lesion in the spinal cord, abnormal brain MRI, and oligoclonal bands in the CSF all independently predict conversion to MS after an acute transverse myelitis attack.[36,37] On the other hand, longitudinal, centralized lesions extending through multiple spinal segments predict an aquaporinopathy or other explanations such as viral myelitis, sarcoidosis, or lymphoma.[26,38] As previously discussed, the current diagnostic criteria for MS do not sufficiently emphasize CSF. We envision future iterations of the diagnostic criteria that will utilize CSF changes early in the diagnosis of MS.

Not all CIS groups behave the same. Phenotypically, optic neuritis is more benign from the standpoint of conversion to MS than transverse myelitis or brainstem-cerebellar syndromes. According to the data from the placebo arms of the subgroup analyses of the IFNβ1a in CIS trial, it takes ~17 months for 25% of patients with isolated optic neuritis to

develop a new relapse, while it takes 15 months for patients with an isolated brainstem syndrome and 8 months for patients with an isolated transverse myelitis to reach the same target (Fig. 1.4).[39] Notably, treatment has the least effect on the optic neuritis group. One should exercise caution in opting for long-term prophylactic treatment in these patients because optic neuritis has a relatively benign course compared to other isolated syndromes, especially in the absence of any of the predictors of conversion to MS discussed above.

Relapsing–Remitting Multiple Sclerosis

The most common form of IIDD is RRMS. RRMS is the evolution from CIS or SAMS by development of additional symptomatic attacks or relapses (Fig. 1.2). It is important to differentiate true symptomatic relapses (attacks, exacerbations) from pseudo-relapses (pseudo-attacks, pseudo-exacerbations). Pseudo-relapses are generally recurrences of existing symptoms, usually in the setting of infections or other reasons for increased body temperature, fatigue, and stress without accompanying objective lesion development. They last generally less than 24 hours (although exceptions exist), are self-limited (disappear with treatment of infection or cooling down after exercise), and require only reassurance of the patient. Unfortunately, misdiagnosing these as true relapses leads to unnecessary requests for steroid infusions and premature changes to disease-modifying treatments. Please refer to Chapter 8 for differentiation of a relapse from a pseudo-relapse. It should be noted, however, that some pseudo-relapses help to identify a previously asymptomatic lesion. If the lesion was previously not documented on imaging or electrophysiological studies, one could, arguably, consider this as a true relapse to justify a short course of steroids. Any future recurrence of the pseudo-relapse (without clear identification of a newly formed lesion), however, should not be treated as a relapse (Chapter 8).

RRMS is characterized by a multifocal inflammatory demyelination and variable degrees of accompanying axonal injury leading to a significant heterogeneity among patients.[40] The pathological heterogeneity of RRMS is also notable in its evolution. Most patients will continue to have symptomatic or asymptomatic relapses at a highly variable rate, some with complete remission and others with a stepwise accumulation of deficits that clearly add to long-term disability (Fig. 1.3). Whereas about one third of patients remain indefinitely in the RRMS phase, most patients will develop progression after SAMS or RRMS.[8] Identifying the underlying biology and predictors of non-progression will improve patient counseling, help better stratify patients for clinical trials, and help design novel therapeutics to prevent progression. This is highly important because the disease-modifying treatments available for MS at time of this writing seem to work only during RRMS. If we were to prevent all lesion formation and induce complete repair in all lesions, we would hypothetically prevent disability accumulation and the potential for progressive MS. To date, there is no known treatment to prevent the development of progressive MS itself except by preventing additional relapse-induced disability during the early stages of progressive MS.[41] We refer to this overlapping period at the end of the relapsing phase (symptomatic or asymptomatic) and the early progressive phase of MS as the relapsing progressive phase (Fig. 1.3).

The heterogeneity in relapse behavior is reflected in the cumulative severity that results from RRMS, likely determined by the number and recovery potential of patients from individual relapses. This has led to differentiation of a subgroup of patients with "benign MS."[42]

Benign MS is not really a phase of MS such as RRMS or SPMS but rather a phenotypic subgroup of predominantly RRMS (although rare, relatively benign cases of PPMS also exist). The consensus definition of benign MS is a patient who remains fully functional in all neurological systems 15 years after disease onset.[43] However, in practice, it has not been easy to identify an all-encompassing cutoff for all neurological systems.

Most natural history studies before the availability of modern disease-modifying medications used the Expanded Disability Status Scale (EDSS) to assess disability accumulating over time as an outcome measure.[43–51] EDSS is very sensitive to ambulatory disability, but as an ordinal measure (0–10), it is insensitive to cognitive dysfunction, which affects attention and fluency in 54% of patients even before a diagnosis of definite MS.[52] Cognitive dysfunction seems to correlate better with the volume of MS lesions in the brain.[53] A more contemporary clinical assessment tool, the Multiple Sclerosis Functional Composite (MSFC) addresses concerns about the sensitivity, reproducibility, and detection of cognitive impairment in MS.[54] MSFC also correlates better than EDSS with hypointense T1-weighted and hyperintense T2-weighted lesion volume, brain parenchymal fraction, and ventricular fraction volumes on MRI.[55–57]

Nevertheless, historically, most studies have used EDSS cutoffs to define benign versus non-benign MS, and therefore "benign MS" actually refers to "ambulatory–benign MS." Hence, a patient with benign MS may have significant cognitive disability, although this is rare. By 15 years after disease onset, one in three patients still has an EDSS score below 3.[46] Almost half the patients still have an EDSS score below 6 (needing one-sided support to walk) after 25 years.[46,49,58] In the longitudinally followed population-based cohort from Olmsted County, 10 years after initial ascertainment, 68% of the patients with an EDSS score below 3 in the initial cohort remained fully functional at an EDSS score below 3, while only 17% had an EDSS score of 6 or more.[25,59,60] Therefore, about one in five patients with MS has an "ambulatory–benign" disease phenotype in the Western world even without any treatment. The largest exception is the Icelandic population, where, curiously, a large population of benign MS patients has been identified. In an untreated, prospective 50-year ascertainment of all MS patients in Iceland, 76% still had an EDSS score of 3.5 or less 15 years after onset, and 69% still had an EDSS score of 3.5 or less after 25 years.[61]

There are several predictors of nonbenign MS phenotypes.[47] Ultimately, symptomatic attacks alone only lead to moderate to low levels of sustained long-term disability (as opposed to the peak deficit during an attack).[8] The impact of symptomatic attacks on disability also seems to decrease with time.[62] The clinical predictors of a nonbenign MS phenotype during the relapsing phase of MS are male sex; older age at onset (>40); motor, cerebellar, or sphincter symptoms at initial presentation; multifocal (polysymptomatic) disease at onset; relatively frequent attacks within the first 5 years; a short interval between the first two attacks; and a relatively short time to reach an EDSS score of 4.[44,46,49,58,59,63–68] All the factors that apparently determine progression or accumulating disability over time seem to be operative until a disability level of EDSS 4 is reached. After this point, the course is usually independent of baseline predictive factors.[69] However, seemingly benign cases may develop into progressive disease,[70] and the progressive course is the strongest determinant of severe disability in the progressive phase measured by EDSS.[43–47,49–51] In the following section, we discuss the progressive phase of MS in further detail. We highlight the importance of differentiating progressive disability accumulation from progressive MS.

Progressive Multiple Sclerosis

Progressive disease course in MS is defined as insidious and irreversible worsening of neurological function. Progression is widely attributed to the superimposition of a degenerative phenotype of progressive axonal injury exceeding the "clinical threshold." Progressive MS is the phase of MS that starts with the onset of progression that cannot be explained by other neurological or nonneurological causes or attacks. The term *progressive disease* should not be confused with *disability progression*, a term commonly used in MS clinical trials. Disability progression in MS can result from insufficient recovery from relapses and/or progressive disease course in MS. An intervention, such as use of steroids or plasma-exchange treatment, enhances recovery after a relapse, and disease-modifying agents decrease the number of relapses. Therefore, these interventions may dampen or prevent disability progression but may not prevent a progressive disease course.[41]

The diagnosis of progressive MS requires objective documentation of a progressive disease course of at least 1 year's duration. Unlike relapses, patients often do not immediately recognize the insidious decline in neurological function and may postpone seeking medical attention. Detailed, rigorous historical documentation and clinical examination closest in time to symptom presentation are required to determine the onset of progressive MS. Progressive axonal injury can happen in any neurological pathway, but progressive weakness, ataxia, or bladder dysfunction is generally easier to document objectively than exclusively sensory progression.

PPMS is defined as progression without previous symptomatic attacks, although certainly patients have MRI lesions that suggest the presence of previous asymptomatic attacks. SAPMS is defined as progression following a CIS or SAMS.[71] SPMS is defined as progression following RRMS. Alternatively, SAPMS and SPMS are also categorized together as bout-onset progressive MS in some studies. Relapsing progressive MS defines ongoing relapses superimposed on progressive MS. However, we consider ongoing relapses after the onset of progression as part of a continuum of the symptomatic (i.e., SPMS, SAPMS) or asymptomatic (i.e., PPMS) relapsing phase as it evolves into the progressive phase of MS (Fig. 1.3).[72,73]

The onset of progression in MS is dependent on age rather than preprogression disease duration.[8,74,75] The age at progression onset is almost identical between the subcategories of PPMS, SAPMS, and SPMS.[8,45,71] The age at last symptomatic relapse is also almost identical between the subcategories of PPMS, SAPMS, and SPMS.[8] Similar to the age-related resolution of the relapsing phase, progression rates slow down and plateau with advancing age. This suggests that the biological mechanisms determining progression are also age-dependent. PPMS occurs only infrequently in children, further supporting progression as an age-dependent process.[76,77]

PPMS represents 20% of all cases of MS in a population-based study from Ontario.[73]

PPMS appears to be a different phenotype of progression from SPMS due to the lack of female preponderance, the predilection to chronic progressive myelopathy, the lack of preceding symptomatic relapses, the paucity of gadolinium-enhancing lesions on MRI, and the paucity of brain lesions in many patients.[78] However, PPMS patients may have brain MRIs that look identical to those from SPMS or SAPMS patients, and the female-to-male ratio is identical in PPMS, SAPMS, and SPMS.[8] Therefore, the difference between PPMS and other groups may not be due to a difference in the biology of progression itself. Indeed, patients matched for the number of lesions, SPMS, and PPMS mainly differ by the presence of previous and ongoing inflammatory demyelination and the recovery potential of individual lesions; they clearly share a similar spectrum of slowly expanding demyelination and axonal injury (see Chapter 5). Progressive forms of MS may share a unified neurodegenerative mechanism of progression and differ only in the extent to which inflammatory–demyelinating activity manifests as a symptomatic relapse.[45,71]

Only 2% of patients reach a sustained disability level of EDSS 6 (needing unilateral support to walk) or above in the RRMS phase.[8] The onset of the progressive phase of MS is the most important predictor of ambulatory disability levels of EDSS 6 and high rates of unemployment with financial dependence.[43–47,49–51,79] This is not surprising, since EDSS 6 and higher levels of the scale are biased toward the longest corticospinal tracts, making it especially suitable for measuring progression-related disability.[45,71] However, as expected, patients with multiple attacks before the onset of progressive MS (SPMS) are more likely to accumulate disability than patients with a single attack before the onset of progressive MS (SAPMS), who, in turn, accumulate more disability than patients with only asymptomatic attacks before the onset of progression (PPMS).[50,51] Therefore, the definitions of PPMS, SAPMS, and SPMS actually predict the amount of and how fast a patient will accumulate MS-related, long-term disability.

SUMMARY

An accurate diagnosis of MS and accurate placement of the patient in the evolution of MS is critical for patient recruitment in epidemiological studies and clinical trials. However, more importantly, a diagnosis of MS leads to considerable anxiety in patients, who may be acquainted with other, significantly disabled MS patients. It is, therefore, crucial to provide patients with early, comprehensive information about the evolution of phases of MS and requirements for diagnosis of each phase. Albeit time-consuming, this approach provides the patient and treating physician with an understanding of what to expect from future treatment decisions. Furthermore, early, ongoing sharing of the diagnostic and prognostic approach with patients decreases their initial frustration and anxiety associated with the unknown while preparing them to become educated partners in their care. The information presented in this chapter shapes all of our treatment decisions in MS, as discussed in the following chapters of this book.

REFERENCES

1. Poser CM, Paty DW, Scheinberg L, et al. New diagnostic criteria for multiple sclerosis: guidelines for research protocols. Ann Neurol; 13:227–231, 1983.
2. McDonald WI, Compston A, Edan G, et al. Recommended diagnostic criteria for multiple sclerosis: guidelines from the International Panel on the diagnosis of multiple sclerosis. Ann Neurol; 50:121–127, 2001.
3. Polman CH, Reingold SC, Edan G, et al. Diagnostic criteria for multiple sclerosis: 2005 revisions to the "McDonald Criteria." Ann Neurol; 58:840–846, 2005.
4. Dalton CM, Brex PA, Miszkiel KA, et al. Application of the new McDonald criteria to patients with clinically isolated syndromes suggestive of multiple sclerosis. Ann Neurol; 52:47–53, 2002.
5. Tintore M, Rovira A, Rio J, et al. New diagnostic criteria for multiple sclerosis: application in first demyelinating episode. Neurology; 60:27–30, 2003.
6. Polman CH, Reingold SC, Banwell B, et al. Diagnostic criteria for multiple sclerosis: 2010 revisions to the McDonald criteria. Ann Neurol; 69:292–302, 2011.
7. Rahmlow M, Sorenson EBC, Lucchinetti C, Kantarci O, Carter J. The co-occurrence of MS and ALS: chance or shared biology? Neurology; 78, 2012.
8. Tutuncu M, Tang J, Zeid NA, et al. Onset of progressive phase is an age-dependent clinical milestone in multiple sclerosis. Mult Scler, 2012 Jun 26. [Epub ahead of print]
9. Engell T. A clinical patho-anatomical study of clinically silent multiple sclerosis. Acta Neurol Scand; 79:428–430, 1989.
10. Mews I, Bergmann M, Bunkowski S, Gullotta F, Bruck W. Oligodendrocyte and axon pathology in clinically

silent multiple sclerosis lesions. Mult Scler; 4:55–62, 1998.

11. De Stefano N, Cocco E, Lai M, et al. Imaging brain damage in first-degree relatives of sporadic and familial multiple sclerosis. Ann Neurol; 59:634–639, 2006.

12. Lebrun C, Bensa C, Debouverie M, et al. Unexpected multiple sclerosis: follow-up of 30 patients with magnetic resonance imaging and clinical conversion profile. J Neurol Neurosurg Psychiatry; 79:195–198, 2008.

13. Lynch SG, Rose JW, Smoker W, Petajan JH. MRI in familial multiple sclerosis. Neurology; 40:900–903, 1990.

14. Okuda DT, Mowry EM, Beheshtian A, et al. Incidental MRI anomalies suggestive of multiple sclerosis: the radiologically isolated syndrome. Neurology; 72:800–805, 2009.

15. Siger-Zajdel M, Selmaj K. Proton magnetic resonance spectroscopy of normal appearing white matter in asymptomatic relatives of multiple sclerosis patients. Eur J Neurol; 13:296–298, 2006.

16. Siva A, Saip S, Altintas A, Jacob A, Keegan BM, Kantarci OH. Multiple sclerosis risk in radiologically uncovered asymptomatic possible inflammatory-demyelinating disease. Mult Scler; 15:918–927, 2009.

17. Tienari PJ, Salonen O, Wikstrom J, Valanne L, Palo J. Familial multiple sclerosis: MRI findings in clinically affected and unaffected siblings. J Neurol Neurosurg Psychiatry; 55:883–886, 1992.

18. Uitdehaag BM, Polman CH, Valk J, Koetsier JC, Lucas CJ. Magnetic resonance imaging studies in multiple sclerosis twins. J Neurol Neurosurg Psychiatry; 52:1417–1419, 1989.

19. Constantinescu CS, Grossman RI, Finelli PF, Kamoun M, Zmijewski C, Cohen JA. Clinical and subclinical neurological involvement in children of conjugal multiple sclerosis patients. Mult Scler; 1:170–172, 1995.

20. Sadovnick AD, Armstrong H, Rice GP, et al. A population-based study of multiple sclerosis in twins: update. Ann Neurol; 33:281–285, 1993.

21. Fulton JC, Grossman RI, Mannon LJ, Udupa J, Kolson DL. Familial multiple sclerosis: volumetric assessment in clinically symptomatic and asymptomatic individuals. Mult Scler; 5:74–77, 1999.

22. Jacobs LD, Beck RW, Simon JH, et al. Intramuscular interferon beta-1a therapy initiated during a first demyelinating event in multiple sclerosis. CHAMPS Study Group. N Engl J Med; 343:898–904, 2000.

23. Lebrun C, Bensa C, Debouverie M, et al. Association between clinical conversion to multiple sclerosis in radiologically isolated syndrome and magnetic resonance imaging, cerebrospinal fluid, and visual evoked potential: follow-up of 70 patients. Arch Neurol; 66:841–846, 2009.

24. Okuda DT, Mowry EM, Cree BA, et al. Asymptomatic spinal cord lesions predict disease progression in radiologically isolated syndrome. Neurology; 76:686–692, 2011.

25. Lennon VA, Wingerchuk DM, Kryzer TJ, et al. A serum autoantibody marker of neuromyelitis optica: distinction from multiple sclerosis. Lancet; 364:2106–2112, 2004.

26. Weinshenker BG, Wingerchuk DM. Neuromyelitis optica: clinical syndrome and the NMO-IgG autoantibody marker. Curr Top Microbiol Immunol; 318:343–356, 2008.

27. Brex PA, Ciccarelli O, O'Riordan JI, Sailer M, Thompson AJ, Miller DH. A longitudinal study of abnormalities on MRI and disability from multiple sclerosis. N Engl J Med; 346:158–164, 2002.

28. Champs Study Group. Interferon beta-1a for optic neuritis patients at high risk for multiple sclerosis. Am J Ophthalmol; 132:463–471, 2001.

29. Champs Study Group. Predictors of short-term disease activity following a first clinical demyelinating event: analysis of the CHAMPS placebo group. Mult Scler; 8:405–409, 2002.

30. Champs Study Group. Baseline MRI characteristics of patients at high risk for multiple sclerosis: results from the CHAMPS trial. Controlled High-Risk Subjects Avonex Multiple Sclerosis Prevention Study. Mult Scler; 8:330–338, 2002.

31. Miller DH, Newton MR, van der Poel JC, et al. Magnetic resonance imaging of the optic nerve in optic neuritis. Neurology; 38:175–179, 1988.

32. Miller DH, Ormerod IE, McDonald WI, et al. The early risk of multiple sclerosis after optic neuritis. J Neurol Neurosurg Psychiatry; 51:1569–1571, 1988.

33. Beck RW, Trobe JD, Moke PS, et al. High- and low-risk profiles for the development of multiple sclerosis within 10 years after optic neuritis: experience of the optic neuritis treatment trial. Arch Ophthalmol; 121:944–949, 2003.

34. Lucchinetti CF, Kiers L, O'Duffy A, et al. Risk factors for developing multiple sclerosis after childhood optic neuritis. Neurology; 49:1413–1418, 1997.

35. Soderstrom M, Ya-Ping J, Hillert J, Link H. Optic neuritis: prognosis for multiple sclerosis from MRI, CSF, and HLA findings. Neurology; 50:708–714, 1998.

36. Cordonnier C, de Seze J, Breteau G, et al. Prospective study of patients presenting with acute partial transverse myelopathy. J Neurol; 250:1447–1452, 2003.

37. Ford B, Tampieri D, Francis G. Long-term follow-up of acute partial transverse myelopathy. Neurology; 42:250–252, 1992.

38. Kumar N, Keegan BM, Rodriguez FJ, Hammack JE, Kantarci OH. Intravascular lymphoma presenting as a longitudinally-extensive myelitis: diagnostic challenges and etiologic clues. J Neurol Sci; 303:146–149, 2011.

39. Beck RW, Chandler DL, Cole SR, et al. Interferon beta-1a for early multiple sclerosis: CHAMPS trial subgroup analyses. Ann Neurol; 51:481–490, 2002.

40. Lucchinetti C, Bruck W, Parisi J, Scheithauer B, Rodriguez M, Lassmann H. Heterogeneity of multiple sclerosis lesions: implications for the pathogenesis of demyelination. Ann Neurol; 47:707–717, 2000.

41. Kappos L, Weinshenker B, Pozzilli C, et al. Interferon beta-1b in secondary progressive MS: a combined analysis of the two trials. Neurology; 63:1779–1787, 2004.

42. Pittock SJ, McClelland RL, Mayr WT, et al. Clinical implications of benign multiple sclerosis: a 20-year population-based follow-up study. Ann Neurol; 56:303–306, 2004.

43. Lublin FD, Reingold SC. Defining the clinical course of multiple sclerosis: results of an international survey. National Multiple Sclerosis Society (USA) Advisory Committee on Clinical Trials of New

Agents in Multiple Sclerosis. Neurology; 46:907–911, 1996.

44. Confavreux C, Aimard G, Devic M. Course and prognosis of multiple sclerosis assessed by the computerized data processing of 349 patients. Brain; 103:281–300, 1980.

45. Confavreux C, Vukusic S. Natural history of multiple sclerosis: a unifying concept. Brain; 129:606–616, 2006.

46. Kantarci O, Siva A, Eraksoy M, et al. Survival and predictors of disability in Turkish MS patients. Turkish Multiple Sclerosis Study Group (TUMSSG). Neurology; 51:765–772, 1998.

47. Kantarci OH, Weinshenker BG. Natural history of multiple sclerosis. Neurol Clin; 23:17–38, 2005.

48. Kurtzke JF: Rating neurologic impairment in multiple sclerosis: an Expanded Disability Status Scale (EDSS). Neurology; 33:1444–1452, 1983.

49. Runmarker B, Andersen O. Prognostic factors in a multiple sclerosis incidence cohort with twenty-five years of follow-up. Brain; 116 (Pt 1):117–134, 1993.

50. Weinshenker BG, Bass B, Rice GP, et al. The natural history of multiple sclerosis: a geographically based study. I. Clinical course and disability. Brain; 112 (Pt 1):133–146, 1989.

51. Wolinsky JS. The diagnosis of primary progressive multiple sclerosis. J Neurol Sci; 206:145–152, 2003.

52. Achiron A, Barak Y. Cognitive impairment in probable multiple sclerosis. J Neurol Neurosurg Psychiatry; 74:443–446, 2003.

53. Hohol MJ, Guttmann CR, Orav J, et al. Serial neuropsychological assessment and magnetic resonance imaging analysis in multiple sclerosis. Arch Neurol; 54:1018–1025, 1997.

54. Rudick R, Antel J, Confavreux C, et al. Clinical outcomes assessment in multiple sclerosis. Ann Neurol; 40:469–479, 1996.

55. Kalkers NF, Bergers E, Castelijns JA, et al. Optimizing the association between disability and biological markers in MS. Neurology; 57:1253–1258, 2001.

56. Kalkers NF, Bergers L, de Groot V, et al. Concurrent validity of the MS Functional Composite using MRI as a biological disease marker. Neurology; 56:215–219, 2001.

57. Rudick RA, Cutter G, Baier M, et al. Use of the Multiple Sclerosis Functional Composite to predict disability in relapsing MS. Neurology; 56:1324–1330, 2001.

58. Weinshenker BG, Rice GP, Noseworthy JH, Carriere W, Baskerville J, Ebers GC. The natural history of multiple sclerosis: a geographically based study. 3. Multivariate analysis of predictive factors and models of outcome. Brain; 114 (Pt 2):1045–1056, 1991.

59. Rodriguez M, Siva A, Ward J, Stolp-Smith K, O'Brien P, Kurland L. Impairment, disability, and handicap in multiple sclerosis: a population-based study in Olmsted County, Minnesota. Neurology; 44:28–33, 1994.

60. Pittock SJ, Mayr WT, McClelland RL, et al. Change in MS-related disability in a population-based cohort: a 10-year follow-up study. Neurology; 62:51–59, 2004.

61. Benedikz J, Stefansson M, Guomundsson J, et al. The natural history of untreated multiple sclerosis in Iceland. A total population-based 50 year prospective study. Clin Neurol Neurosurg; 104:208–210, 2002.

62. Tremlett H, Yousefi M, Devonshire V, Rieckmann P, Zhao Y. Impact of multiple sclerosis relapses on progression diminishes with time. Neurology; 73:1616–1623, 2009.

63. Kurtzke JF, Beebe GW, Nagler B, Auth TL, Kurland LT, Nefzger MD. Studies on the natural history of multiple sclerosis. 6. Clinical and laboratory findings at first diagnosis. Acta Neurol Scand; 48:19–46, 1972.

64. Levic ZM, Dujmovic I, Pekmezovic T, et al. Prognostic factors for survival in multiple sclerosis. Mult Scler; 5:171–178, 1999.

65. Myhr KM, Riise T, Vedeler C, et al. Disability and prognosis in multiple sclerosis: demographic and clinical variables important for the ability to walk and awarding of disability pension. Mult Scler; 7:59–65, 2001.

66. Phadke JG: Clinical aspects of multiple sclerosis in north-east Scotland with particular reference to its course and prognosis. Brain; 113 (Pt 6):1597–1628, 1990.

67. Riise T, Gronning M, Fernandez O, et al. Early prognostic factors for disability in multiple sclerosis, a European multicenter study. Acta Neurol Scand; 85:212–218, 1992.

68. Scott TF, Schramke CJ, Novero J, Chieffe C. Short-term prognosis in early relapsing-remitting multiple sclerosis. Neurology; 55:689–693, 2000.

69. Confavreux C, Vukusic S, Moreau T, Adeleine P. Relapses and progression of disability in multiple sclerosis. N Engl J Med; 343:1430–1438, 2000.

70. Thompson AJ. Benign multiple sclerosis. J Neurol Neurosurg Psychiatry; 67:138, 1999.

71. Kremenchutzky M, Rice GP, Baskerville J, Wingerchuk DM, Ebers GC. The natural history of multiple sclerosis: a geographically based study 9: observations on the progressive phase of the disease. Brain; 129:584–594, 2006.

72. Andersson PB, Waubant E, Gee L, Goodkin DE. Multiple sclerosis that is progressive from the time of onset: clinical characteristics and progression of disability. Arch Neurol; 56:1138–1142, 1999.

73. Cottrell DA, Kremenchutzky M, Rice GP, Hader W, Baskerville J, Ebers GC. The natural history of multiple sclerosis: a geographically based study. 6. Applications to planning and interpretation of clinical therapeutic trials in primary progressive multiple sclerosis. Brain; 122 (Pt 4):641–647, 1999.

74. Koch M, Mostert J, Heersema D, De Keyser J. Progression in multiple sclerosis: further evidence of an age-dependent process. J Neurol Sci; 255:35–41, 2007.

75. Scalfari A, Neuhaus A, Daumer M, Ebers GC, Muraro PA. Age and disability accumulation in multiple sclerosis. Neurology; 77:1246–1252, 2011.

76. Renoux C, Vukusic S, Mikaeloff Y, et al. Natural history of multiple sclerosis with childhood onset. N Engl J Med; 356:2603–2613, 2007.

77. Yeh EA, Chitnis T, Krupp L, et al. Pediatric multiple sclerosis. Nat Rev Neurol; 5:621–631, 2009.

78. Revesz T, Kidd D, Thompson AJ, Barnard RO, McDonald WI. A comparison of the pathology of primary and secondary progressive multiple sclerosis. Brain; 117 (Pt 4):759–765, 1994.

79. McDonnell GV, Hawkins SA. Clinical study of primary progressive multiple sclerosis in Northern Ireland, UK. J Neurol Neurosurg Psychiatry; 64:451–454, 1998.

80. Abou Zeid N, Kale N, Atkinson E, Kantarci O. Secondary progression is associated with worse

long-term outcome than primary progression in multiple sclerosis. Multiple Sclerosis; 15, 2009.

81. Kale N, Abou Zeid N, Atkinson E, Kantarci O. Determinants of long-term outcome in clinical subtypes of progressive multiple sclerosis. Multiple Sclerosis; 15, 2009.

82. Montalban X, Tintore M, Swanton J, et al. MRI criteria for MS in patients with clinically isolated syndromes. Neurology; 74:427–434, 2010.

83. Swanton JK, Fernando K, Dalton CM, et al. Modification of MRI criteria for multiple sclerosis in patients with clinically isolated syndromes. J Neurol Neurosurg Psychiatry; 77:830–833, 2006.

84. Kappos L, Polman CH, Freedman MS, et al. Treatment with interferon beta-1b delays conversion to clinically definite and McDonald MS in patients with clinically isolated syndromes. Neurology; 67:1242–1249, 2006.

Chapter 2

The Differential Diagnosis of Multiple Sclerosis

OTHER IDIOPATHIC INFLAMMATORY DEMYELINATING DISEASES
Diffuse Idiopathic Inflammatory Demyelinating Diseases
Tumorlike Idiopathic Inflammatory Demyelinating Diseases

NEURO-MYELITIS OPTICA SPECTRUM DISORDERS (AQUAPORINOPATHIES)

NON-IDIOPATHIC INFLAMMATORY DEMYELINATING DISEASES CNS SYNDROMES THAT MIMIC MULTIPLE SCLEROSIS

SUMMARY

Abstract

The differential diagnosis of MS includes conditions well within the spectrum of IIDDs as MS as well as other non-IIDD inflammatory syndromes of the CNS. IIDDs fall into a spectrum with two axes: (1) the acuity and severity of initial pathology and (2) the chronic impact on disability of the patient. These entities are generally rare, with distinct pathological features, and have a more fulminant course than MS. Prompt identification and treatment are essential. Fulminant IIDDs have a relatively severe, acute presentation of diffuse or tumorlike involvement of the CNS and respond to plasma-exchange treatment. IIDDs with more restricted CNS involvement associated with the presence of antibodies against aquaporin-4 are referred to as aquaporinopathies.

OTHER IDIOPATHIC INFLAMMATORY DEMYELINATING DISEASES

The differential diagnosis of MS includes conditions well within the spectrum of IIDDs as MS as well as other non-IIDD inflammatory syndromes of the CNS (e.g., sarcoidosis or lymphoma). In this chapter, we will further discuss these differential diagnostic entities.

In the first chapter, we introduced the concept of MS as an IIDD. We also discussed how IIDDs differ from each other both clinically and pathologically, although many can evolve into another IIDD in a continuum. IIDDs fall into a spectrum with two axes: (1) the acuity and severity of initial pathology and (2) the chronic impact on disability of the patient (Fig. 2.1). These entities are generally rare, with distinct pathological features (Fig. 2.2).[1] Despite their uncommon nature, these entities have a more fulminant course than MS and, therefore, require prompt identification and treatment. These fulminant IIDDs often respond positively to plasma-exchange treatment when steroids fail.[2] IIDDs with a relatively severe, acute presentation of diffuse or tumorlike involvement of the CNS include acute disseminated encephalomyelitis (ADEM), acute hemorrhagic leukoencephalitis (AHLE or Hurst's disease), fulminant MS (Marburg's variant), myelinoclastic diffuse sclerosis (Schilder's disease), and concentric sclerosis (Balo's disease) (Fig. 2.1). IIDDs with more restricted CNS involvement associated with the presence of antibodies against aquaporin-4 are referred to as aquaporinopathies. The prototypical form of this type of IIDD is neuromyelitis optica (NMO or Devic's disease) (Fig. 2.1).

Diffuse Idiopathic Inflammatory Demyelinating Diseases

ADEM AND AHLE

ADEM is typically a monophasic IIDD. Although commonly considered in the differential diagnosis of MS, it is more appropriate to consider ADEM in the differential diagnosis of clinically isolated syndrome (CIS), since recurrences in children are rare and are unlikely, even controversial in adults. Therefore, it is no surprise that the consensus diagnostic criteria for ADEM have been established in children (Table 2.1).[3] However, MS can happen in young children and ADEM can happen in adults, so age should not be the sole criterion for diagnosing ADEM. In the absence of specific criteria for adults, it is appropriate at this time to use the criteria established for children regardless of age.

As seen in the consensus criteria, the definition of ADEM is operational but requires the presence of encephalopathy as a cardinal symptom to differentiate most ADEM cases from

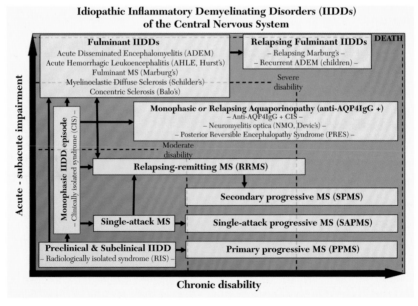

Figure 2–1. The spectrum of IIDDs of the CNS defined in two axes: (1) the acuity and severity of initial pathology and (2) the chronic impact on disability of the patient. (Updated and modified from Kantarci OH, Weinshenker BG. Natural history of multiple sclerosis. Neurol Clin; 23:17–38, v, 2005.[42])

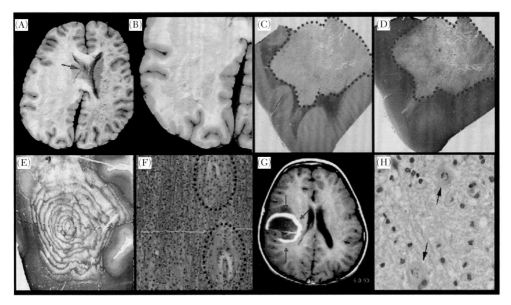

Figure 2–2. Pathologic spectrum of IIDDs. (**A, B**) Gross specimens of Marburg-type MS. Large confluent lesions lead to mass effect and herniation. (**C, D**) Microscopy of the lesion shown in **A** and **B** with extensive demyelination (LFB-PAS) and axonal loss (Bielschowsky's silver impregnation). (**E**) Balo's concentric sclerosis showing the characteristic alternating bands of demyelination and preserved myelin. (**F**) ADEM lesions are characterized by perivascular inflammation and only minimal, mainly perivenular demyelination (*circles*). (**G**) Tumefactive lesion with severe edema and mass effect. (**H**) Hypertrophic astrocyte (Creutzfeld-Peters cell) in an acute demyelinating lesion. (Reprinted from Lucchinetti CF, Parisi J, Bruck W. The pathology of multiple sclerosis. Neurol Clin; 23:77–105, vi, 2005.[1])

Table 2–1 Diagnostic Criteria for ADEM Modified for Practical Use[3]

Monophasic ADEM	• In the absence of a clinical history of a previous demyelinating event, new-onset encephalopathy consisting of behavioral changes or alteration in consciousness with additional evidence for multifocal/diffuse (polysymptomatic) CNS involvement that cannot be explained by anything other than an IIDD and that improves with or without residual deficits
	• New or fluctuating symptoms, signs, or MRI findings occurring within 3 months of the inciting ADEM event are considered part of the acute event.
	• In the absence of evidence for previous destructive white matter changes, brain MRI with FLAIR or T2-weighted images reveals large (>1–2 cm) lesions that are multifocal, hyperintense, and located predominantly in the supratentorial or infratentorial white matter regions. Gray matter, especially basal ganglia and thalamus, is frequently involved. In rare cases, brain MR images show a large single lesion (1–2 cm), predominantly affecting white matter.
	• Spinal cord MRI may show confluent intramedullary lesion(s) with variable enhancement, in addition to abnormal brain MRI findings specified previously.
Recurrent ADEM	• In the absence of any other explanation, recurrence of the initial ADEM symptoms and signs at least 3 months after the first ADEM attack without involvement of new clinical areas by history, examination, or neuroimaging (MRI shows no new lesions; original lesions may have enlarged) occurring at least 1 month after completing steroid therapy
Multiphasic ADEM	• In the absence of any other explanation, recurrence of a new ADEM event fulfilling monophasic ADEM criteria above at least 3 months after the first ADEM attack with involvement of new clinical areas by history, examination, or neuroimaging (MRI shows new lesions; original lesions should be resolving) occurring at least 1 month after completing steroid therapy

Modified from Krupp LB, Banwell B, Tenembaum S. Consensus definitions proposed for pediatric multiple sclerosis and related disorders. Neurology; 68:S7–12, 2007.

CIS. In the clinical setting, headache, although omitted from the original criteria, often accompanies the acute presentation.

The pathology of ADEM consists of rather limited regions of perivenular demyelination as opposed to the more confluent demyelination seen in association with reactive astrocytes and the completely demyelinated regions observed in MS (Fig. 2.3).[4] In pathologically confirmed cases, several factors support ADEM over MS: depressed level of consciousness; headache with meningismus and CSF pleocytosis (lymphocytic meningitis), generally without the presence of oligoclonal bands; and multifocal, enhancing MRI lesions.[4] Behavioral changes are more common in ADEM, but the presence of behavioral symptoms also can lead to overdiagnosis of ADEM.[4] The consensus criteria seem to be 80% sensitive and 91% specific for pathologically defined ADEM.[4] The presence of oligoclonal

bands in the CSF should lead to consideration of other etiologies, but it could also indicate a future risk of developing MS. In our experience, patients may present with transiently elevated oligoclonal bands that resolve in repeat taps. This may represent an association with acute infection that precedes some ADEM cases, but no systematic study has been undertaken since the establishment of new criteria.

ADEM typically demonstrates multiple, diffusely enhancing, subcortical, perivenous white matter lesions on MRI. However, MRI presentations can also be large, multifocal lesions with indistinct borders that involve gray matter structures more readily than MS.[5] It is also not uncommon to see diffuse, punctate T2 hyperintense lesions with limited enhancement in T1-weighted images (Fig. 2.4). Please see Chapter 4 for further discussion of MRI in ADEM.

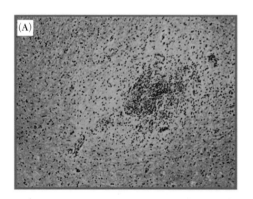
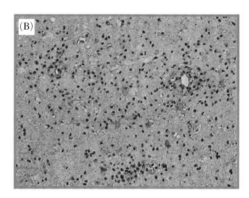
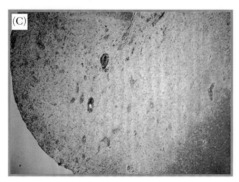

Figure 2–3. Pathological features of ADEM. A Luxol fast blue periodic acid-Schiff myelin stain illustrates (**A**) perivenous sleeve of inflammation and demyelination, (**B**) three coalescing perivenous lesions, and (**C**) extensive region of confluent demyelination with areas of perivenous demyelination in the periplaque white matter. (Reproduced from Young NP, Weinshenker BG, Parisi JE, et al. Perivenous demyelination: association with clinically defined acute disseminated encephalomyelitis and comparison with pathologically confirmed multiple sclerosis. Brain; 133:333–348, 2010.[4])

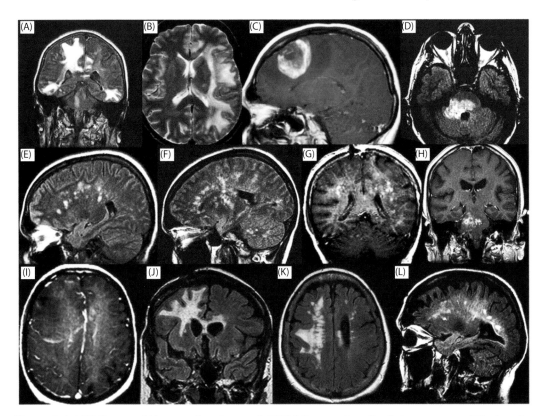

Figure 2–4. MRI features of biopsy-confirmed cases of ADEM illustrate the rather heterogeneous, multifocal, confluent, and, at times, ill-defined lesions of ADEM. (**A**) Coronal fluid attenuated inversion recovery (FLAIR): multifocal large ill-defined supratentorial and brainstem lesions without enhancement; (**B**) axial T2: large ill-defined nonenhancing unihemispheric lesion; (**C**) T1 with gadolinium: single large open ring enhancing mass with surrounding edema; (**D**) axial FLAIR: large brainstem lesion with (**H**) punctate central and peripheral rim of enhancement; (**E**, **F**) sagittal FLAIR: numerous multifocal bilateral nonenhancing T2 lesions in subcortical white matter, basal ganglion, cerebellum; (**G**) coronal T1 with gadolinium: numerous bilateral enhancing subcortical white matter lesions; (**I**) T1 with gadolinium: faint rim of enhancement of large ill-defined lesion with mass effect; (**J**) coronal FLAIR: residual confluent signal change crossing the corpus callosum; (**K**) axial FLAIR: residual signal change oriented perpendicular to corpus callosum becoming confluent; (**L**) new nonenhancing periventricular white matter lesions in patient with both perivenous demyelination and confluent demyelination. (Reproduced from Young NP, Weinshenker BG, Parisi JE, et al. Perivenous demyelination: association with clinically defined acute disseminated encephalomyelitis and comparison with pathologically confirmed multiple sclerosis. Brain; 133:333–348, 2010.[4])

Other clinical features support a diagnosis of ADEM over CIS. These include the higher incidence of seizures and antecedent infection or vaccination compared to CIS.[6] Even though the criteria in Table 2.1 do not include recent exposure to a vaccine or infection in the diagnostic requirement, this information can aid diagnosis. However, patients often do not recall incidents of overt exposure. The seasonal peaking of ADEM supports an infectious trigger.[7] However, similar events can precede MS relapses as well.[8] Therefore, caution should be exercised in using antecedent infection or vaccine exposure as sole evidence for ADEM.

Most of the studies looking at the prognosis of ADEM predate current consensus criteria, which makes it hard to interpret the results. The extensive history of ADEM is reviewed elsewhere.[9] We suggest using current criteria as outlined in Table 2.1 to diagnose ADEM with the additional considerations suggested above. When doubt exists, a diagnosis of "undifferentiated demyelinating disease" is appropriate because a diagnosis of ADEM suggests a relatively benign long-term course with no recurrence. Less clear-cut cases may require a brain biopsy for the ultimate diagnosis.

AHLE (Hurst's disease) is a clinically hyperacute fulminant monophasic IIDD with hemorrhagic, demyelinating lesions that are pathologically similar to ADEM with the additional findings of petechial hemorrhage and perivenular necrosis.[10] Overt hemorrhages do not show on MRI, but this could improve with increased sensitivity of MRI techniques for detecting hemorrhage.[11] The prognosis is somewhat grim given the rapidity at which the disease progresses. Usually viral encephalitis (i.e., herpes) is entertained in the differential diagnosis.[12] Lesions can appear anywhere in the CNS and, at times, are suggestive of a mass lesion (Fig. 2.5).[10–13] Pure brainstem presentations mimicking other space-occupying lesions have also been reported.[13]

Treatment of ADEM or AHLE first requires exclusion of an infectious etiology, followed by consideration of intravenous methylprednisolone (children, 30 mg/kg daily; adults, 1,000 mg daily) for 3 to 5 days, although the evidence is mostly anecdotal with no proper trial. Plasma exchange and intravenous immunoglobulin are viable alternatives for patients who fail to respond to the previous treatment approach.[14–16] Given the rapidity of the AHLE disease course, management is usually done in the intensive care unit. Prompt recognition of AHLE is important in utilizing plasma exchange as a timely, potentially life-saving intervention.[17]

MARBURG'S VARIANT

Marburg's variant of MS is also known as fulminant MS. This is somewhat of a misnomer, since many other IIDDs also can have a fulminant presentation. It is, therefore, common to classify

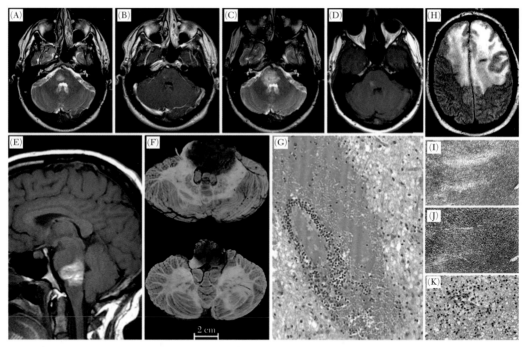

Figure 2–5. MRI and pathological features of AHLE. (**A, B**) MRI head axial T2 and T1 with gadolinium demonstrating brainstem lesion at presentation. (**C, D**) At 2 weeks, axial T2 and T1 without gadolinium demonstrates progression of the brainstem lesion and early hemorrhage. (**E**) At 4 weeks sagittal T1 without gadolinium demonstrates extension of the lesion, with marked edema and gross hemorrhage. (**F**) Gross pathology of brainstem demonstrating hemorrhage and necrosis. (**G**) Microscopy shows perivascular inflammation associated with hemorrhage. (**H**) In a separate patient, frontal lesion is shown on MRI. (**I**) Biopsied brain sections from the cerebral white matter on the day after admission show perivascular loss of myelin (Kluver-Barrera stain). (**J**) There is relative sparing of axons (Bielschowsky stain). (**K**) Perivascular neutrophils and macrophages (hematoxylin–eosin stain). (**A–G** reproduced with permission from Abou Zeid NE, Burns JD, Wijdicks EF, Giannini C, Keegan BM. Atypical acute hemorrhagic leukoencephalitis (Hurst's disease) presenting with focal hemorrhagic brainstem lesion. Neurocrit Care; 12:95–97, 2010.[13] **H–K** reproduced with permission from Gibbs WN, Kreidie MA, Kim RC, Hasso AN. Acute hemorrhagic leukoencephalitis: neuroimaging features and neuropathologic diagnosis. J Comput Assist Tomogr; 29:689–693, 2005.[12])

patients as having Marburg's variant when they may, in fact, have any of the other IIDDs that present with a severe onset of diffuse or multifocal brain lesions and associated symptoms.

Patients with Marburg's variant of MS may die or recover with significant morbidity. Patients with relapsing Marburg's presentation may also evolve into a typical relapsing–remitting MS (RRMS) course after recovering from the initial attack.[18] This disease-course heterogeneity suggests that Marburg's designation, when used clinically, may refer to a fulminant relapse of an otherwise typical ADEM or MS pathology. We reserve this designation for patients with confluent areas of typically asymmetric, enhancing hemispheric demyelination on MRI in the absence of oligoclonal bands, who have demyelination with associated necrosis (Fig. 2.2).[19,20] The lesions may also be associated with vasculitis.[21]

Figure 2.6 shows two separate fulminant presentations. MRI may not be sufficient to differentiate patients with ADEM from Marburg's variant of MS, and even pathological features of this disease are not well defined at this time.[21,22] If pathology is not available and a patient recovers from a fulminant attack, it is more appropriate to refer to the clinical presentation with a conservative and generic designation of "fulminant IIDD attack." The treatment of Marburg's variant is similar to ADEM.

Tumorlike Idiopathic Inflammatory Demyelinating Diseases

This section covers presentations of demyelinating disease in which the lesion may behave like a mass lesion, both clinically and in how it presents in imaging studies. For clarification, in the setting of Marburg's variant, ADEM, and MS, an individual lesion may be larger than the others, resembling a tumor. Although in most cases these lesions are not separate entities, primary and secondary CNS tumors must, nevertheless, be included in the differential diagnosis of this group of IIDDs. Sometimes a biopsy, partly due to sampling, may be nondiagnostic. However, the presence of large numbers of infiltrating macrophages in the setting of myelin loss and relative axonal preservation is more indicative of an IIDD rather than a tumor. Misdiagnosis of a malignancy in a young patient resulting from sampling issues can lead to whole-brain

radiation that, in return, can provoke significant acute worsening of IIDDs, with associated severe morbidity and mortality. Therefore, it is of utmost importance for the practicing clinician to consider a diagnosis of IIDDs in a tumorlike presentation. When doubt exists, a biopsy should be attempted, followed by a trial of steroids afterwards and, if necessary, plasma exchange.

TUMEFACTIVE MS

The prototypical form of tumorlike presentation in IIDDs is known as tumefactive MS. While pathologically indistinguishable from other manifestations of MS, the initial presentation may, on occasion, have the clinical and radiographic appearance of a brain tumor, and often these patients undergo a brain biopsy.[23,24] The size of the lesion (>20 mm) can be used to define tumorlike lesions.[24] Lesion size clearly correlates with more mass effect and edema in these patients.[24] Lesion size, however, does not determine the long-term prognosis.[24,25] Patients whose IIDD onset presents as a tumorlike lesion can remain monophasic (e.g., CIS) with complete recovery or evolve into typical MS, while similar lesions can also be observed during the typical course of MS.[24,25]

Tumefactive lesions appear anywhere typical of MS lesions, following the white matter tracts.[24] Multiple tumorlike lesions may form at the same time. While open- or closed-ring enhancement is present, many different patterns of enhancement can be observed in these patients (Fig. 2.7).[24,25] In some but not all patients, the ring enhancement colocalizes to a hypointense rim on T2-weighted images.[24] Occasionally, the timing of the MRI in regard to the evolution of the lesion, rather than a different phenotype, may account for the lack of a T2-weighted hypointense rim in some patients. In select cases, diffusion-weighted imaging studies and MR spectroscopy can differentiate demyelinating lesions from tumors.

It is intriguing that patients who present with these lesions tend to have a better overall prognosis than typical MS patients.[24] Biologically, it suggests that either the extent or the type of inflammatory response (and/or the rather rapidly expanding demyelination associated with these lesions) leads to a potential protective effect or better recovery in regards to future relapses. This aspect of tumefactive presentation in MS is mostly unexplored; future study

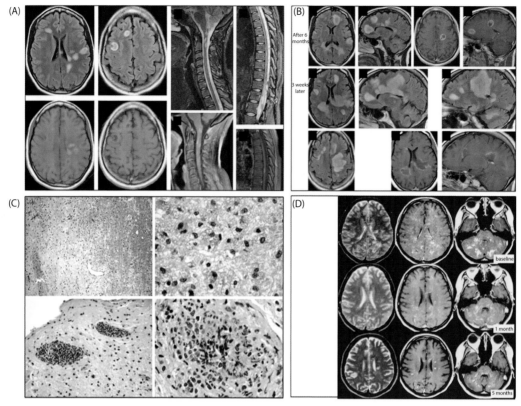

Figure 2–6. MRI and pathological features of two separate patients with fulminant presentation diagnosed as having Marburg's variant of MS. (**A**) MRI at the time of initial fulminant presentation of a patient with spinal cord and brain involvement with lesions that could otherwise be considered typical of MS. (**B**) Follow-up MRIs during a more typical MS-like disease course show enlargement of lesions. (**C**) Brain biopsy is deemed consistent with Marburg's variant with unexpected findings of vasculitis associated with extensive demyelination. (**D**) Marburg disease with serial MR images of the brain shows contrast-enhanced focal lesions multifocally/diffusely involving the cerebral and cerebellar hemispheres and the brainstem. As some lesions persist, others evolve. The patient died 5 months after symptom onset. In contrast to the previous case, this one has more of an appearance by MRI that could have also been considered ADEM at presentation. (**A–C** reproduced with permission from Elenein RG, Sharer LR, Cook SD, Pachner AR, Michaels J, Hillen ME. A second case of Marburg's variant of multiple sclerosis with vasculitis and extensive demyelination. Mult Scler; 17:1531–1538, 2011.[21]; **D** reproduced with permission from Canellas AR, Gols AR, Izquierdo JR, Subirana MT, Gairin XM. Idiopathic inflammatory-demyelinating diseases of the central nervous system. Neuroradiology; 49:393–409, 2007.[22])

in this area might provide clues for patient management during initial presentation.

BALO'S CONCENTRIC SCLEROSIS

Balo's concentric sclerosis is a rare but fulminant and tumorlike IIDD with a subacute course of weeks to months and high rates of mortality. However, lesions typical of Balo's concentric sclerosis are present in otherwise prototypical MS without the grave course.

The name "concentric sclerosis" derives from the onion ring-like appearance of demyelinating rings alternating with preserved myelin (Fig. 2.2). The pattern of demyelination also trends toward complete rings. Interestingly, the active components of the rings resemble hypoxia-like injury, and the active edge of lesions apparently expresses neuroprotective molecules, which could account for the preserved myelin immediately outside the active demyelination.[26] Vascular injury documented in high-resolution MRI studies further supports the hypoxic injury hypothesis.[27] Concentric lesions have also been reported in patients with fulminant transverse myelitis typical of the longitudinally extensive lesions observed in NMO, the

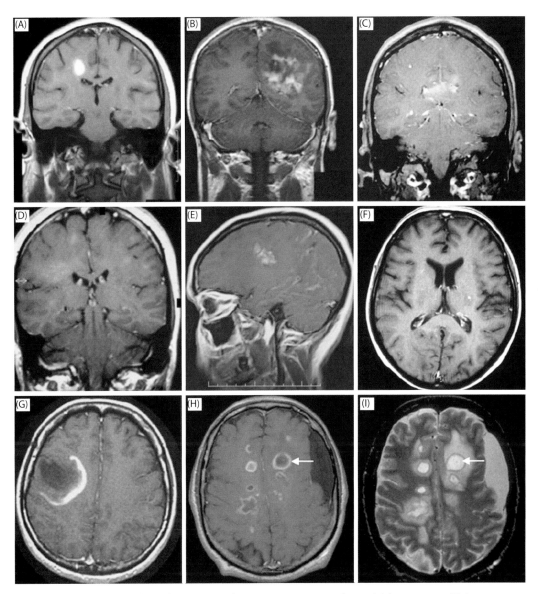

Figure 2–7. MRI features of tumefactive MS. Enhancement patterns are shown: (**A**) homogenous; (**B**) heterogeneous; (**C**) patchy and diffuse; (**D**) cotton-ball; (**E**) nodular; (**F**) punctate; (**G**) open ring; (**H**) multiple closed rings indicated by the arrow; (**I**) multiple T2 hypointense rims colocalize with ring enhancement (*arrow*; T2-weighted MRI). (**A–H**) T1-weighted MRI with gadolinium. (Reproduced with permission from Lucchinetti CF, Gavrilova RH, Metz I, et al. Clinical and radiographic spectrum of pathologically confirmed tumefactive multiple sclerosis. Brain; 131:1759–1775, 2008.[24])

prototypical aquaporinopathy.[28] Of note, a recent study reported extensive loss of connexins and aquaporin-4, which suggests that some concentric lesions may be aquaporinopathies unrelated to MS (discussed later in this chapter) but also lacking the characteristic antibodies against aquaporin-4.[29] Hence, not all concentric lesions indicate an independent diagnosis of Balo's concentric sclerosis.

The demyelinated and gliotic rings correspond to hypointense rings on T2-weighted images with colocalized enhancing rings and decreased diffusivity, identical to T2 hypointense rings with enhancement observed at the edge of expanding active MS lesions (Fig. 2.8).[30–32] Biopsied cases typically show pattern III MS (distal oligodendrogliopathy) (see Chapter 5 for a discussion of lesion patterns). This lesion pattern can be the

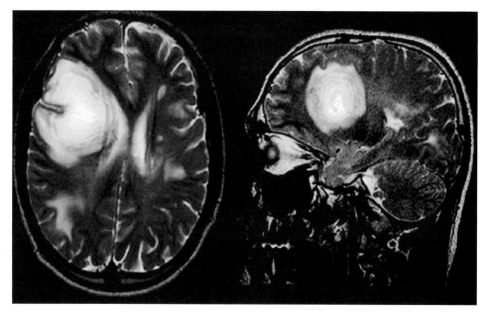

Figure 2–8. MRI in Balo's concentric sclerosis. (Reproduced with permission from Wengert O, Siebert E. Images in clinical medicine. Balo's concentric sclerosis. N Engl J Med; 365:742,2011.[32])

first presentation of MS but has also been pathologically confirmed during established MS.[26] Treatment can follow protocols similar to ADEM or fulminant MS attack, but timely administration of plasma exchange might also be appropriate. Medication options for long-term stability are ambiguous, but clinicians have reported good results with mitoxantrone and natalizumab.[27,28] This preference is most likely due to these medications' rapid response to the aggressive onset of the disease rather than a consensus about their superiority to other disease-modifying agents in MS. Additionally, since concentric lesions also occur in aquaporinopathies, long-term medication choices may need to be tailored to this possible etiology.

MYELINOCLASTIC DIFFUSE SCLEROSIS (SCHILDER'S DISEASE)

Schilder's disease is a rare, acute or subacute IIDD affecting children and young adults.[33] The clinical presentation may be indistinguishable from ADEM, with a predominance of behavioral and cognitive symptoms with acute intracranial hypertension and recurrences. The imaging may demonstrate tumorlike presentation and posterior-dominant, rather symmetric lesions suggestive of other disorders such as adrenoleukodystrophy, given the age group. However, the enhancement pattern can be typical of MS-like lesions, and a Schilder's-like onset may evolve into prototypical MS.[34,35] Except for cavitary lesions, the pathology seems indistinguishable from MS or ADEM.[36,37] In the absence of a pathological hallmark and given its great response to steroids, Schilder's disease may not stand the test of time as an independent disease.[38] It is more likely that patients with this diagnosis will be classified as having either ADEM or MS in the future.

NEURO-MYELITIS OPTICA SPECTRUM DISORDERS (AQUAPORINOPATHIES)

In this section we will discuss the spectrum of disorders identified by the prototypical NMO (Devic's disease).[39] This spectrum is distinct from the other IIDDs because its pathological hallmark is the absence of aquaporin-4 (AQP4) immunoreactivity in associated lesions.[40] The pathology of this entry is discussed extensively in Chapter 5.

NMO spectrum disorders have a relapsing–remitting disease course; a secondary slowly progressive disease course is extremely unlikely.[41] Table 2.2 reviews the distinguishing features of NMO spectrum disorders compared to

Table 2–2 Practical Distinguishing Diagnostic Features of NMO Spectrum Disorders (Aquaporinopathies) from MS

	NMO (Devic's disease) spectrum[39]	MS spectrum
Demographics	• *Ethnicity:* Non-whites > whites • *HLA-DRB1°1501:* 1.75× decreased risk of NMO[69] • *Female/Male:* 2–3/1 • *Mean age at onset:* 3rd decade	• *Ethnicity:* Whites > non-whites • *HLA-DRB1°1501:* 3.9× increased risk of MS[69] • *Female/Male:* 9/1 • *Mean age at onset:* 4th decade
Clinical & imaging features	• *Transverse myelitis:* cigar-shaped centrally located lesions ≥3 spinal cord segments long. (*Caveat: After resolution of the attack, lesions may break down into individual segments that may have multiple short lesion appearance.*) • *Optic neuritis:* long lesions that can involve the chiasm with poor recovery • *Brainstem syndrome:* characteristic intractable hiccups or vomiting with periaqueductal location of lesions • *Posterior reversible encephalopathy syndrome (PRES)*[50,51]: can happen • Near-simultaneous optic neuritis and transverse myelitis can happen. • Brain lesions can happen predominantly in AQP4-rich locations of hypothalamus, corpus callosum, periventricular areas, and periaqueductal brainstem.	• *Transverse myelitis:* short peripheral lesions with relatively good recovery • *Optic neuritis:* focal lesions with relatively good recovery • *Brainstem syndrome:* cerebellar, nuclear and long-tract signs common without typical intractable hiccups or vomiting • *Posterior reversible encephalopathy syndrome (PRES):* not described • Near-simultaneous optic neuritis and transverse myelitis is exceedingly rare. • Imaging criteria as described in **Chapter 1**
Disease course	• Monophasic (15%); relapsing–remitting (85%); rare cases with bout-onset progressive course[41]; none with primary progressive disease course • Infrequent relapses with poor recovery from most	• Relapsing–remitting (25%); Bout-onset progressive (55%); Primary progressive (15%) • Frequent and early relapses with significant recovery from most
CSF	• *Pleocytosis:* prominent with polymorpho-nuclear cells & mononuclear cells • *Oligoclonal bands:* 85%	• *Pleocytosis:* mild with mononuclear cells • *Oligoclonal bands:* <30%
Anti-AQP4 antibody (NMO-IgG) in serum[46,47]	• 73% sensitive, 91–100% specific for NMO • <25% seronegative	• Absent
Other autoimmune diseases or autoantibodies	• Common in family history and the patient[70]	• Uncommon
Pathology (acute lesions)	• *Eosinophil & neutrophil infiltration:* common[52] • *AQP4 immunoreactivity:* absent[40] • Characteristic vasculocentric complement activation around thickened blood vessels • Prominent axonal injury and necrosis with cavitation	• *Eosinophil & neutrophil infiltration:* unlikely • *AQP4 immunoreactivity:* increased

prototypical MS. The natural history of untreated NMO is quite severe compared to MS: the 5-year survival rate is a grim 68%, with most deaths due to respiratory failure. MS is a significantly less severe disease.[42–44] The common disease-modifying agents used for relapse prevention in MS do not seem to work for NMO, but conventional immunosuppressants seem to work better for NMO than MS. Because NMO has more severe attacks with a lesser degree of recovery than MS, the early clinical distinction is of the utmost importance.

The presence of the following symptoms justifies a clinical diagnosis of NMO: optic neuritis, transverse myelitis, or both, in the absence of another explanation (e.g., sarcoidosis, mass lesions, lymphoma, or infectious etiology such as VZV). In addition, patients should meet two of the three following criteria:[45] (a) a central, cigar-shaped, longitudinally extensive spinal cord lesion of three or more spinal cord segments (Fig. 2.9); (b) seropositivity for NMO-IgG[46,47]; and (c) brain lesions not fulfilling the criteria for MS (see Chapter 1). Brain lesions in NMO have a characteristic distribution that follows AQP4-rich areas of the CNS (Fig. 2.10), whereas more widespread lesions are observed in MS.

As with every relapsing–remitting IIDD, the initial presentation of NMO can be monophasic until the next recurrence. The discovery of anti-AQP4 antibodies (NMO-IgG) as a diagnostic and pathogenic hallmark of NMO,[46,47] together with the imaging features of longitudinally extensive lesions in the CNS, has made it possible to predict evolution into NMO during the initial CIS presentation. If transverse myelitis patients have a cigar-shaped central spinal cord lesion of three or more spinal segments, the presence of NMO-IgG predicts a 40% chance of recurrence within a year as opposed to those who were seronegative.[48] In patients with recurrent optic neuritis, the presence of NMO-IgG predicts both a poor visual outcome and a future, longitudinally extensive transverse myelitis fulfilling NMO diagnostic criteria.[49] In some patients, NMO-IgG may present as posterior reversible encephalopathy syndrome (PRES).[50,51] The spectrum of NMO may expand further as more atypical IIDD patients become recognized as having an aquaporinopathy through rather typical serology and pathology findings (Fig. 2.11).[40,52]

Acute management of NMO spectrum disorders follows a similar protocol to other fulminant IIDDs with high-dose steroid infusion followed by plasma exchange.[2] However, in our experience, individual NMO relapses require the use of plasma exchange more frequently than do relapses of MS. The immediate effect of steroids may be due to closing of

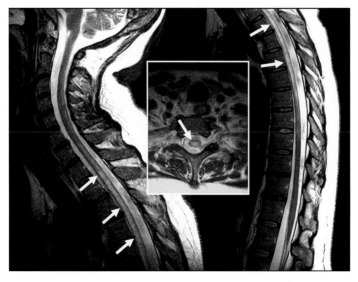

Figure 2–9. Typical centrally located, longitudinally extensive spinal cord lesion in a patient with neuromyelitis optica indicated by the arrows. (From Mayo Clinic archives.)

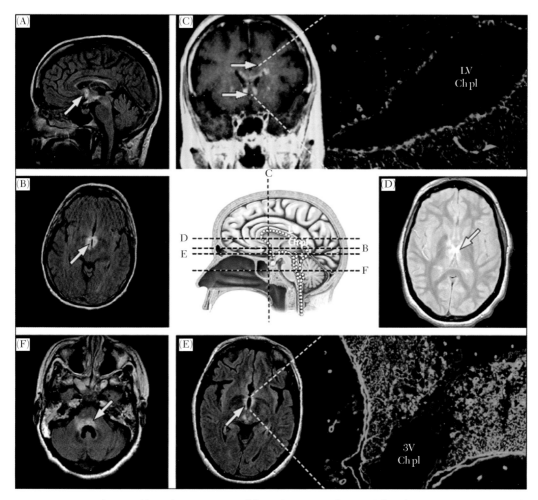

Figure 2–10. Distribution of brain lesions in NMO follows the AQP4-rich areas (*white dots* in center picture). In the center picture the *dashed black lines* show the anatomical level of MRI in the diagram; *arrows* show abnormality on fluid-attenuated inversion recovery (FLAIR), T2-weighted signal or after being given gadolinium. Patient 1: Image **A** (sagittal) and image **B** (axial) have FLAIR-signal abnormality around the third ventricle, with extension into the hypothalamus. Patient 2 (image **C**; coronal, postcontrast T1-weighted image) has subependymal enhancement along the frontal horns bilaterally and in the adjacent white matter. The immunofluorescence photomicrograph linked to image **C** shows the binding pattern of the serum IgG from a patient with NMO in a mouse brain (400×). Intense immunoreactivity of basolateral ependymal cell membranes lining the lateral ventricle (LV) and extending into the subependymal astrocytic mesh coincides with aquaporin-4 immunoreactivity; the choroid plexus (Ch pl) is unstained. Patient 3 has contiguous signal abnormality throughout the periventricular tissues: diencephalon (image **D**; axial T2-weighted), third ventricle (image **E**; axial, FLAIR), and fourth ventricle (image **F**; axial FLAIR). Immunofluorescence photomicrograph linked to image **E** shows the binding pattern of the serum IgG from a patient with NMO in a mouse brain (400×), with intense staining of periventricular tissues (third ventricle, 3V); choroid plexus (Ch pl) is unstained. (Reproduced with permission from Wingerchuk DM, Lennon VA, Lucchinetti CF, Pittock SJ, Weinshenker BG. The spectrum of neuromyelitis optica. Lancet Neurol; 6:805–815, 2007.[39])

the blood–brain barrier, followed by immuno-suppressive effects. As an antibody-mediated, organ-specific autoimmune disorder, NMO is likely to respond quickly to removal of antibodies through plasma exchange. Additionally, given the severity of relapses and more limited recovery in NMO, we do not wait more than a week to 10 days after the initial round of steroids to start plasma exchange. In the future, with better correlation between serological marker titers and acute disease severity, plasma exchange could replace steroids as the first-line treatment of NMO in some patients.

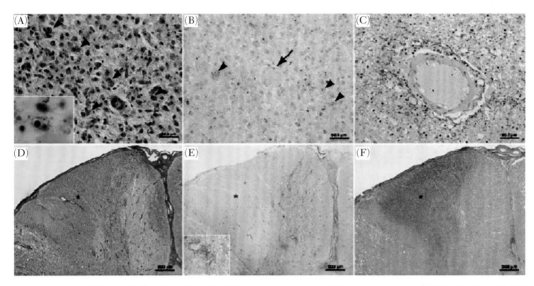

Figure 2–11. Pathological hallmarks of NMO. AQP4 immunoreactivity (IR) in acute pattern II MS (**A–C**) and NMO (**D–F**) lesions. (**A**) Numerous macrophages containing myelin debris are dispersed throughout the active lesion (*arrowheads* and inset; Luxol fast blue/periodic acid–Schiff). (**B**) C9neo antigen is present within macrophages (*arrowheads*) but absent around blood vessels (*arrow*). (**C**) Higher magnification reveals AQP4 IR is prominent in a rosette pattern surrounding a penetrating blood vessel in the lesion. (**D**) In NMO, there is extensive demyelination involving both gray and white matter (Luxol fast blue/periodic acid–Schiff); °indicates preserved myelin in the periplaque white matter. (**E**) C9neo is deposited in a vasculocentric rim and rosette pattern (inset) within the active lesions but not in the peri-plaque white matter. (**F**) The lesions lack AQP4, which is retained in the peri-plaque white matter (°) and gray matter. **A, D,** Luxol fast blue/periodic acid–Schiff; **B, E,** C9neo IHC; **C, F,** AQP4 IHC. (Reproduced with permission from Roemer SF, Parisi JE, Lennon VA, et al. Pattern-specific loss of aquaporin-4 immunoreactivity distinguishes neuromyelitis optica from multiple sclerosis. Brain; 130:1194–1205, 2007.[40])

Given the severity of individual relapses, we recommend that patients be considered for long-term immunotherapy even after the first presentation in clinically definite cases. Experience suggests that immunomodulatory agents typically used for RRMS are not beneficial for NMO patients.[53,54] Interferon preparations in particular may result in a higher relapse rate and an increased NMO-IgG antibody titer.[55–59] We usually start the patient on oral steroids (1 mg/kg) and introduce a steroid-sparing immunosuppressive agent. To date, no placebo-controlled trial has been undertaken in NMO management, so the choice of immunosuppressive treatment is based on familiarity with the agent used. Our first-line choice is generally azathioprine (2.5–3.0 mg/kg) or mycophenolate mofetil with rituximab in more severe presentations. All of these agents seem to decrease relapse frequency and minimize cumulative long-term disability while mean corpuscular volume changes during treatment seem to correlate with response to mediations such as azathioprine.[60–65] Mitoxantrone and intravenous immunoglobulin also seem to decrease relapse frequency in NMO.[66,67] Future therapies may involve more specific interventions directed at peptide epitopes of anti-AQP4 antibody.[68]

NON-IDIOPATHIC INFLAMMATORY DEMYELINATING DISEASES CNS SYNDROMES THAT MIMIC MULTIPLE SCLEROSIS

This book is dedicated to MS and related disorders. Chapter 1 reviewed the specifics of MS diagnosis. In clinical practice, the disorders already covered in this chapter are the main contenders in the biology and differential diagnosis of MS. However, many diseases should be included as part of the differential diagnosis, especially during the first presentation of a patient with IIDD. Once a disease course typical of MS is established, it is unlikely to be confused with any other disease.

These non-IIDD MS mimickers include paraneoplastic or nonparaneoplastic autoimmune disorders, such as CRMP5- or GAD65-related autoimmunity; connective tissue disorders, including systemic lupus erythematosus, antiphospholipid antibody syndrome, Sjögren's disease, or Behçet's disease; systemic vasculitides; sarcoidosis; B- and T-cell lymphomas; infections such as HIV, herpes, syphilis and Lyme disease; neurodegenerative disorders, including motor neuron disease, spinocerebellar ataxias, amyloidoma, and polyglucosan body disease; toxic, metabolic, or congenital dysmyelinating disorders (Marchiafava-Bignami disease, central and noncentral pontine myelinolysis, pernicious anemia, copper deficiency, adrenomyeloneuropathy, metachromatic leukoencephalopathy, mitochondrial disorders); and infections such as progressive multifocal leukoencephalopathy (PML) especially in the setting of natalizumab and other immunosuppressant use. Certainly, not all of the above disorders need to be considered in every patient. Indeed, the time course and typical clinical or laboratory findings of these disorders are generally so different from the IIDD spectrum that only in few instances and early on do they pose a differential diagnostic challenge. The discussion of these individual entities and the clinical circumstances in which each should be considered is beyond the scope of this book, but some of these disorders are further discussed as related to pathology in Chapter 5.

SUMMARY

IIDDs differ from each other both clinically and pathologically, although many can evolve into another IIDD in a continuum. The disorders covered in this chapter are the most common in the differential diagnosis of MS. Many diseases should be included as part of the differential diagnosis during the first presentation of a patient with IIDD.

REFERENCES

1. Lucchinetti CF, Parisi J, Bruck W. The pathology of multiple sclerosis. Neurol Clin; 23:77–105, 2005.
2. Weinshenker BG, O'Brien PC, Petterson TM, et al. A randomized trial of plasma exchange in acute central nervous system inflammatory demyelinating disease. Ann Neurol; 46:878–886, 1999.
3. Krupp LB, Banwell B, Tenembaum S. Consensus definitions proposed for pediatric multiple sclerosis and related disorders. Neurology; 68:S7–S12, 2007.
4. Young NP, Weinshenker BG, Parisi JE, et al. Perivenous demyelination: association with clinically defined acute disseminated encephalomyelitis and comparison with pathologically confirmed multiple sclerosis. Brain; 133:333–348, 2010.
5. Dale RC, Branson JA. Acute disseminated encephalomyelitis or multiple sclerosis: can the initial presentation help in establishing a correct diagnosis? Arch Dis Child; 90:636–639, 2005.
6. Dale RC, de Sousa C, Chong WK, Cox TC, Harding B, Neville BG. Acute disseminated encephalomyelitis, multiphasic disseminated encephalomyelitis and multiple sclerosis in children. Brain; 123 Pt 12:2407–2422, 2000.
7. Hynson JL, Kornberg AJ, Coleman LT, Shield L, Harvey AS, Kean MJ. Clinical and neuroradiologic features of acute disseminated encephalomyelitis in children. Neurology; 56:1308–1312, 2001.
8. Marrie RA, Wolfson C, Sturkenboom MC, et al. Multiple sclerosis and antecedent infections: a case-control study. Neurology; 54:2307–2310, 2000.
9. Young NP, Weinshenker BG, Lucchinetti CF. Acute disseminated encephalomyelitis: current understanding and controversies. Semin Neurol; 28:84–94, 2008.
10. Hart MN, Earle KM. Haemorrhagic and perivenous encephalitis: a clinical-pathological review of 38 cases. J Neurol Neurosurg Psychiatry; 38:585–591, 1975.
11. Kuperan S, Ostrow P, Landi MK, Bakshi R. Acute hemorrhagic leukoencephalitis vs ADEM: FLAIR MRI and neuropathology findings. Neurology; 60:721–722, 2003.
12. Gibbs WN, Kreidie MA, Kim RC, Hasso AN. Acute hemorrhagic leukoencephalitis: neuroimaging features and neuropathologic diagnosis. J Comput Assist Tomogr; 29:689–693, 2005.
13. Abou Zeid NE, Burns JD, Wijdicks EF, Giannini C, Keegan BM. Atypical acute hemorrhagic leukoencephalitis (Hurst's disease) presenting with focal hemorrhagic brainstem lesion. Neurocrit Care; 12:95–97, 2010.
14. Keegan M, Pineda AA, McClelland RL, Darby CH, Rodriguez M, Weinshenker BG. Plasma exchange for severe attacks of CNS demyelination: predictors of response. Neurology; 58:143–146, 2002.
15. Marchioni E, Marinou-Aktipi K, Uggetti C, et al. Effectiveness of intravenous immunoglobulin treatment in adult patients with steroid-resistant monophasic or recurrent acute disseminated encephalomyelitis. J Neurol; 249:100–104, 2002.
16. Sahlas DJ, Miller SP, Guerin M, Veilleux M, Francis G. Treatment of acute disseminated encephalomyelitis with intravenous immunoglobulin. Neurology; 54:1370–1372, 2000.
17. Ryan LJ, Bowman R, Zantek ND, et al. Use of therapeutic plasma exchange in the management of acute hemorrhagic leukoencephalitis: a case report and review of the literature. Transfusion; 47:981–986, 2007.
18. Giubilei F, Sarrantonio A, Tisei P, Gasperini C, Salvetti M. Four-year follow-up of a case of acute multiple sclerosis of the Marburg type. Ital J Neurol Sci; 18:163–166, 1997.
19. Johnson MD, Lavin P, Whetsell WO, Jr. Fulminant monophasic multiple sclerosis, Marburg's type. J Neurol Neurosurg Psychiatry; 53:918–921, 1990.
20. Bitsch A, Wegener C, da Costa C, et al. Lesion development in Marburg's type of acute multiple sclerosis: from inflammation to demyelination. Mult Scler; 5:138–146, 1999.

21. Elenein RG, Sharer LR, Cook SD, Pachner AR, Michaels J, Hillen ME. A second case of Marburg's variant of multiple sclerosis with vasculitis and extensive demyelination. Mult Scler; 17:1531–1538, 2011.

22. Canellas AR, Gols AR, Izquierdo JR, Subirana MT, Gairin XM. Idiopathic inflammatory-demyelinating diseases of the central nervous system. Neuroradiology; 49:393–409, 2007.

23. Kepes JJ. Large focal tumor-like demyelinating lesions of the brain: intermediate entity between multiple sclerosis and acute disseminated encephalomyelitis? A study of 31 patients. Ann Neurol; 33:18–27, 1993.

24. Lucchinetti CF, Gavrilova RH, Metz I, et al. Clinical and radiographic spectrum of pathologically confirmed tumefactive multiple sclerosis. Brain; 131:1759–1775, 2008.

25. Altintas A, Petek B, Isik N, et al. Clinical and radiological characteristics of tumefactive demyelinating lesions: follow-up study. Mult Scler; 18(10):1448-53, 2012.

26. Stadelmann C, Ludwin S, Tabira T, et al. Tissue preconditioning may explain concentric lesions in Balo's type of multiple sclerosis. Brain; 128:979–987, 2005.

27. Berghoff M, Schlamann M, Maderwald S, et al. 7 Tesla MRI demonstrates vascular pathology in Balo's concentric sclerosis. Mult Scler; May 28. [Epub ahead of print] 2012.

28. Kreft KL, Mellema SJ, Hintzen RQ. Spinal cord involvement in Balo's concentric sclerosis. J Neurol Sci; 279:114–117, 2009.

29. Masaki K, Suzuki SO, Matsushita T, et al. Extensive loss of connexins in Balo's disease: evidence for an auto-antibody-independent astrocytopathy via impaired astrocyte-oligodendrocyte/myelin interaction. Acta Neuropathologica; 123:887–900; 2012.

30. Wiendl H, Weissert R, Herrlinger U, Krapf H, Kuker W. Diffusion abnormality in Balo's concentric sclerosis: clues for the pathogenesis. Eur Neurol; 53:42–44, 2005.

31. Korte JH, Bom EP, Vos LD, Breuer TJ, Wondergem JH. Balo concentric sclerosis: MR diagnosis. AJNR Am J Neuroradiol; 15:1284–1285, 1994.

32. Wengert O, Siebert E. Images in clinical medicine. Balo's concentric sclerosis. N Engl J Med; 365:742, 2011.

33. Garell PC, Menezes AH, Baumbach G, et al. Presentation, management and follow-up of Schilder's disease. Pediatr Neurosurg; 29:86–91, 1998.

34. Mehler MF, Rabinowich L. Inflammatory myelinoclastic diffuse sclerosis (Schilder's disease): neuroradiologic findings. AJNR Am J Neuroradiol; 10:176–180, 1989.

35. Sastre-Garriga J, Rovira A, Rio J, Tintore M, Grive E, Montalban X. Clinically definite multiple sclerosis after radiological Schilder-like onset. J Neurol; 250:871–873, 2003.

36. Eblen F, Poremba M, Grodd W, Opitz H, Roggendorf W, Dichgans J. Myelinoclastic diffuse sclerosis (Schilder's disease): cliniconeuroradiologic correlations. Neurology; 41:589–591, 1991.

37. Dresser LP, Tourian AY, Anthony DC. A case of myelinoclastic diffuse sclerosis in an adult. Neurology; 41:316–318, 1991.

38. Pretorius ML, Loock DB, Ravenscroft A, Schoeman JF. Demyelinating disease of Schilder type in three young South African children: dramatic response to corticosteroids. J Child Neurol; 13:197–201, 1998.

39. Wingerchuk DM, Lennon VA, Lucchinetti CF, Pittock SJ, Weinshenker BG. The spectrum of neuromyelitis optica. Lancet Neurol; 6:805–815, 2007.

40. Roemer SF, Parisi JE, Lennon VA, et al. Pattern-specific loss of aquaporin-4 immunoreactivity distinguishes neuromyelitis optica from multiple sclerosis. Brain; 130:1194–1205, 2007.

41. Wingerchuk DM, Pittock SJ, Lucchinetti CF, Lennon VA, Weinshenker BG. A secondary progressive clinical course is uncommon in neuromyelitis optica. Neurology; 68:603–605, 2007.

42. Kantarci OH, Weinshenker BG. Natural history of multiple sclerosis. Neurol Clin; 23:17–38, 2005.

43. Wingerchuk DM, Weinshenker BG. Neuromyelitis optica: clinical predictors of a relapsing course and survival. Neurology; 60:848–853, 2003.

44. Ghezzi A, Bergamaschi R, Martinelli V, et al. Clinical characteristics, course and prognosis of relapsing Devic's neuromyelitis optica. J Neurol; 251:47–52, 2004.

45. Wingerchuk DM, Lennon VA, Pittock SJ, Lucchinetti CF, Weinshenker BG. Revised diagnostic criteria for neuromyelitis optica. Neurology; 66:1485–1489, 2006.

46. Lennon VA, Wingerchuk DM, Kryzer TJ, et al. A serum autoantibody marker of neuromyelitis optica: distinction from multiple sclerosis. Lancet; 364:2106–2112, 2004.

47. Lennon VA, Kryzer TJ, Pittock SJ, Verkman AS, Hinson SR. IgG marker of optic-spinal multiple sclerosis binds to the aquaporin-4 water channel. J Exp Med; 202:473–477, 2005.

48. Weinshenker BG, Wingerchuk DM, Vukusic S, et al. Neuromyelitis optica IgG predicts relapse after longitudinally extensive transverse myelitis. Ann Neurol; 59:566–569, 2006.

49. Matiello M, Lennon VA, Jacob A, et al. NMO-IgG predicts the outcome of recurrent optic neuritis. Neurology; 70:2197–2200, 2008.

50. Magana SM, Matiello M, Pittock SJ, et al. Posterior reversible encephalopathy syndrome in neuromyelitis optica spectrum disorders. Neurology; 72:712–717, 2009.

51. Matiello M, Magana SM, Weinshenker BG. Asymptomatic spinal cord involvement in posterior reversible encephalopathy syndrome. Neurology; 74:1478–1479.

52. Lucchinetti CF, Mandler RN, McGavern D, et al. A role for humoral mechanisms in the pathogenesis of Devic's neuromyelitis optica. Brain; 125:1450–1461, 2002.

53. Papeix C, Vidal JS, de Seze J, et al. Immunosuppressive therapy is more effective than interferon in neuromyelitis optica. Mult Scler; 13:256–259, 2007.

54. Warabi Y, Matsumoto Y, Hayashi H. Interferon beta-1b exacerbates multiple sclerosis with severe optic nerve and spinal cord demyelination. J Neurol Sci; 252:57–61, 2007.

55. Palace J, Leite MI, Nairne A, Vincent A. Interferon beta treatment in neuromyelitis optica: increase in relapses and aquaporin 4 antibody titers. Arch Neurol; 67:1016–1017, 2010.

56. Shimizu J, Hatanaka Y, Hasegawa M, et al. IFNbeta-1b may severely exacerbate Japanese optic-spinal MS in neuromyelitis optica spectrum. Neurology; 75:1423–1427, 2010.

57. Kim SH, Kim W, Li XF, Jung IJ, Kim HJ. Does interferon beta treatment exacerbate neuromyelitis optica spectrum disorder? Mult Scler; 18:1480–1483, 2012.
58. Shimizu Y, Yokoyama K, Misu T, et al. Development of extensive brain lesions following interferon beta therapy in relapsing neuromyelitis optica and longitudinally extensive myelitis. J Neurol; 255:305–307, 2008.
59. Warabi Y, Matsumoto Y, Hayashi H. Interferon beta-1b exacerbates multiple sclerosis with severe optic nerve and spinal cord demyelination. J Neurol Sci; 252:57–61, 2007.
60. Jacob A, Matiello M, Weinshenker BG, et al. Treatment of neuromyelitis optica with mycophenolate mofetil: retrospective analysis of 24 patients. Arch Neurol; 66:1128–1133, 2009.
61. Jacob A, Weinshenker BG, Violich I, et al. Treatment of neuromyelitis optica with rituximab: retrospective analysis of 25 patients. Arch Neurol; 65:1443–1448, 2008.
62. Mandler RN, Ahmed W, Dencoff JE. Devic's neuromyelitis optica: a prospective study of seven patients treated with prednisone and azathioprine. Neurology; 51:1219–1220, 1998.
63. Cree BA, Lamb S, Morgan K, Chen A, Waubant E, Genain C. An open-label study of the effects of rituximab in neuromyelitis optica. Neurology; 64:1270–1272, 2005.
64. Costanzi C, Matiello M, Lucchinetti CF, et al. Azathioprine: tolerability, efficacy, and predictors of benefit in neuromyelitis optica. Neurology; 77:659–666, 2011.
65. Wingerchuk DM, Weinshenker BG. Neuromyelitis optica. Curr Treat Options Neurol; 10:55–66, 2008.
66. Weinstock-Guttman B, Ramanathan M, Lincoff N, et al. Study of mitoxantrone for the treatment of recurrent neuromyelitis optica (Devic disease). Arch Neurol; 63:957–963, 2006.
67. Bakker J, Metz L. Devic's neuromyelitis optica treated with intravenous gamma globulin (IVIG). Can J Neurol Sci; 31:265–267, 2004.
68. Yu X, Green M, Gilden D, Lam C, Bautista K, Bennett JL. Identification of peptide targets in neuromyelitis optica. J Neuroimmunol; 236:65–71, 2011.
69. Matiello M, Schaefer-Klein J, Brum DG, Atkinson EJ, Kantarci OH, Weinshenker BG. HLA-DRB1*1501 tagging rs3135388 polymorphism is not associated with neuromyelitis optica. Mult Scler; 16:981–984, 2010.
70. Wingerchuk DM, Weinshenker BG. The emerging relationship between neuromyelitis optica and systemic rheumatologic autoimmune disease. Mult Scler; 18:5–10, 2012.

Chapter 3

The Epidemiology of Multiple Sclerosis, Genetics, and Environment

**EPIDEMIOLOGY OF MULTIPLE
    SCLEROSIS: A COMPLEX DISEASE**

GENETICS OF MULTIPLE SCLEROSIS
Inheritance of Multiple Sclerosis
Genes of Multiple Sclerosis

**ENVIRONMENTAL RISK FACTORS IN
    MULTIPLE SCLEROSIS**
Epstein–Barr Virus Infection and Multiple
    Sclerosis Risk
Inadequate Vitamin D Intake and Lack of
    Sun Exposure and Multiple Sclerosis Risk
Smoking and Multiple Sclerosis Risk

SUMMARY

Abstract

MS is a complex disease with both environmental and genetic risk factors implicated in its etiology. Furthermore, the complex interaction between the environment and genetic risk factors is also responsible for the pathological and clinical heterogeneity in the disease course. The most important risk factor for MS is being a woman, which is reflected in the increasing incidence of MS in women. This does not seem to be due to classic risk factors that can be associated with hormones, X chromosome, or mitochondrial genome alone. There is a complex interaction between gender and inheritance of MS, leading to a parent-of-origin effect highly suspicious for an epigenetic inheritance of MS. Many genomic regions, the strongest of which is the HLADR15, and many environmental factors, the strongest of which are inadequate vitamin D, UV exposure, Epstein-Barr virus exposure, and smoking, have been associated with risk of MS as well as modifying the phenotype of MS. In this chapter we discuss the genetic and environmental epidemiology of MS.

EPIDEMIOLOGY OF MULTIPLE SCLEROSIS: A COMPLEX DISEASE

In 2000, the projected prevalence rate of MS for the white U.S. population was 191/100,000 and the incidence rate was 7.3/100,000 person-years at risk.[1] Given the prolonged survival, the prevalence of MS is increasing as well. As far back as 1994, the annual cost of MS in the United States in terms of direct care and lost productivity was estimated at $6.8 billion, and total lifetime cost per patient was $2.2 million.[2] This calculation was made around the time of introduction of disease-modifying treatments.[3,4] In Europe, MS accounts for 0.003% of all patients with any brain disease per 2004 calculations.[5] Although an apparently small percentage, this accounts for about 400,000 patients with MS in all of Europe, with a mean annual cost per person estimated around 23,695 Euros.[5] These are conservative calculations; actual current costs may be much higher due to the cost of disease-modifying medications themselves and MS-associated job loss. Except in its most benign forms, MS is a lifelong disease with significant socioeconomic impact.

As discussed in Chapters 1 and 2, MS is an idiopathic inflammatory demyelinating disease of the central nervous system defined by consensus clinical diagnostic criteria with pathological heterogeneity. The etiology of MS is complex and results from interaction of multiple environmental and genetic factors.[6] This interaction likely happens at several levels. Genetically determined susceptibility to as-yet-indeterminate environmental insults,

autoimmunity, myelin or axonal injury, environmental influences on gene expression in immune activation, myelin or axonal development and repair pathways all seem to be important.

As illustrated in Figure 3.1, genetics may play a strong role for some patients, while others may be affected by the environment. While genetics may increase the risk of MS through gene-expression modification, the environment can also modify genetic risk through epigenetic mechanisms. This latter field needs additional study.

Evidence supporting a genetic susceptibility to MS (Fig. 3.1) includes excess occurrence in Northern Europeans relative to indigenous populations from the same geographic location and familial aggregation. MS is 20 to 40 times more common in first-degree relatives and drops off rapidly with more distant relationships. The incidence of MS is not increased in adopted relatives of MS patients. The high concordance rate for MS (25–30%) in monozygotic twins rapidly drops to 3% to 5% in dizygotic twins (Table 3.1).[7–9]

Evidence in support of environmental susceptibility to MS (Fig. 3.1) includes variation in disease incidence and prevalence according to geography (including distance from the Equator), mutable risk of developing MS with migration from both low-to-high-prevalence and high-to-low-prevalence areas, the presence of rare clusters and epidemics of MS

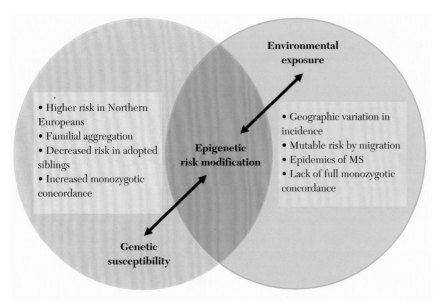

Figure 3–1. Potential mechanisms of interaction between genes and environment in complex diseases such as MS.

Table 3–1 **Risk of Developing MS According to the Relationship to an MS Patient**[7-9]

Relative with MS	Chance of Developing MS
Monozygotic twin	25–30%
Dizygotic twin	3–5%
First-degree relative (child or full sibling)	2–4%

(e.g., Faeroe Islands and Iceland), and incomplete concordance in monozygotic twins.[7-9]

The paradigm of complex etiology shown in Figure 3.1 likely reflects the pathological heterogeneity (discussed in later chapters) and highly variable natural history (discussed in earlier chapters) observed among patients with MS. We still do not fully understand why MS develops and behaves differently in different individuals.

MS is more common in women than in men. Some regions of the world have witnessed a relatively rapid increase in the incidence of MS in women.[10,11] Men have a tendency for later disease onset with worse prognosis, supporting gender-dependent factors in etiology and phenotypic variability.[12] Although MS incidence peaks in the late third decade, MS can manifest clinically as early as the first decade and as late as the eighth decade, although these extremes are rare. The progressive MS phenotype is highly age dependent, with incidence peaking in the fifth decade.[13] This chapter reviews the practical aspects of genetic and environmental epidemiology of MS.

GENETICS OF MULTIPLE SCLEROSIS

Inheritance of Multiple Sclerosis

The 2% to 4% risk of MS in a first-degree relative of a patient with established MS, corrected for the population risk, varies with incidence/prevalence figures for the population at large from which the individual is drawn. Recent studies have highlighted a complex inheritance of the disease significantly influenced by the gender of the affected parent, or a parent-of-origin effect (Fig. 3.2).[14] Whenever affected parent–child pairs are left out of the

model, expected maternal transmission of MS is increased due to the increased incidence of MS in women. Curiously, however, when affected parent–child pairs are directly studied at the nuclear family level, paternal transmission attains and even exceeds the rate of maternal transmission (Fig. 3.2).[15-19] Therefore, mechanisms beyond an enriched genetic load in a given family are required to inherit MS directly from an affected parent.

Existence of a parent-of-origin effect suggests several nongenetic inheritance mechanisms. There could be a dose-threshold effect due to an increased number of penetrant susceptibility genes in a given parent or parental lineage, or different epigenetic mechanisms may be operational in different families. In complex neurological disorders such as MS, both of these mechanisms may determine susceptibility to disease, and the importance of each may depend on the environmental exposure and the interacting genetic risk. The lack of full concordance for MS between monozygotic twins, who share a genetic code and most early-life environmental exposures, suggests that potential epigenetic mechanisms operate even before birth.[9] However, environmental influences can reach well beyond *in utero*. For example, exposures of the father, and even the paternal grandfather, seem to modify the multigenerational risk of complex traits such as obesity.[20]

Phenotypic heterogeneity in MS also has a genetic basis: relative pairs with MS in family studies have greater similarity of clinical course than expected by chance.[21] While affected sibling pairs are concordant for age and year of disease onset and disease course, they do not behave similarly when it comes to disease severity.[22] Concordance between affected parent and affected child is present only for age of onset.[22] Affected sibling pairs differ from their parents by also sharing a relatively similar environment when compared to their parents. Therefore, both similar genetic and similar environmental backgrounds contribute to the development of a similar MS clinical phenotype. Concordance in year of disease onset in affected sibling pairs suggests that shared exposure to environmental factor(s) at a critical period may also be necessary to develop a similar clinical phenotype.

As highlighted in Figures 3.1 and 3.2, inheritance of MS results from a complex interaction between environment and genetics and is

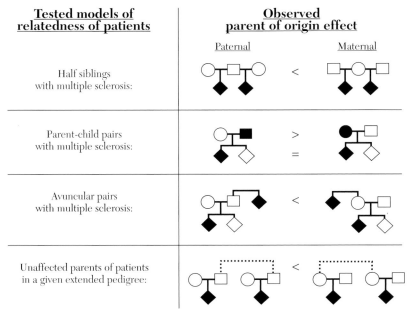

Tested models of relatedness of patients	Observed parent of origin effect	
	Paternal	Maternal
Half siblings with multiple sclerosis:		<	
Parent-child pairs with multiple sclerosis:		> =	
Avuncular pairs with multiple sclerosis:		<	
Unaffected parents of patients in a given extended pedigree:		<	

Figure 3–2. Parent-of-origin studies in MS. Half-sibling pairs with MS with unaffected parents are more likely to be related through their mothers than their fathers.[16] Mother–child pairs with MS are less frequent than expected for the higher and increasing incidence of MS in women, while father–child pairs with MS were more frequent than expected for the lower incidence of MS in men.[17,18] Where there is a very strong founder effect in a very large pedigree, patients with MS were more likely to be related to each other through a maternal lineage than a paternal lineage.[19] Full circles, diamonds, and squares indicate individuals with clinical diagnosis of MS. Empty circles, diamonds, and squares indicate individuals without MS. Solid lines indicate relatedness. (Reproduced and modified with permission from Kantarci OH, Spurkland A. Parent of origin in multiple sclerosis: understanding inheritance in complex neurologic diseases. Neurology; 71:786–787, 2008.[14])

significantly influenced by gender-dependent mechanisms, which suggests an epigenetic modification of risk. Further discussion of potential epigenetic mechanisms operating in complex neurological disorders is beyond the scope of this text. It is, however, important to note that identification of modifiable epigenetic mechanisms may lead to preventive treatment approaches.

Genes of Multiple Sclerosis

A discussion of all the genetic studies in MS as well as genetic epidemiology methods involved in detecting them is beyond the scope of this textbook. We will highlight some of the recent discoveries in this area.

The *HLA-DRB1*1501-DQB1*0602* haplotype on chromosome 6p21 is the strongest susceptibility locus for MS.[21,23–25] This association is further defined as being due to a stronger effect exerted by *HLA-DRB1* rather than the *DQ* allele.[26,27] While the presence of the

*HLA-DRB1*15* allele increases MS risk dominantly (about 3.5 fold), *HLA-DRB1*03* contributes to a smaller increased MS risk recessively, and *HLA-DRB1*14* decreases MS risk.[28] The inheritance of the HLA region is complex. Recent studies indicate a gender-specific parent-of-origin effect in the highly polymorphic MHC region, suggesting epigenetic modification of risk in this region.[29,30] In Figure 3.3 we summarize this inheritance pattern.[31] Although initial studies had suggested that HLA region had no impact on disease severity in MS, when an extremes-of-severity approach was taken as we had proposed, HLA-DRB1*01, previously implicated in disease resistance, was found to act as an independent modifier of disability progression in MS.[21,32]

There has been an extensive increase in the number of MS susceptibility loci identified by large international genome-wide efforts. Most recently, several non-HLA loci were identified from a meta-analysis of 2,529,394 unique single-nucleotide polymorphisms in 5,545 cases and 12,153 controls from seven large datasets

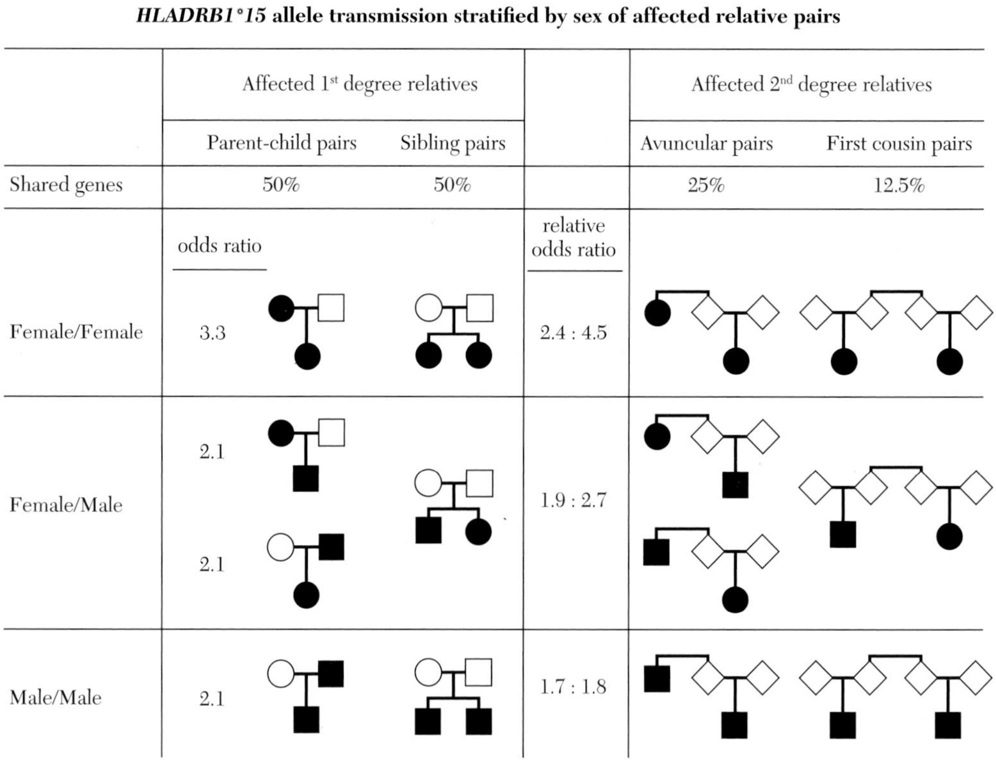

HLADRB1°15 allele transmission stratified by sex of affected relative pairs

Shared genes	Affected 1st degree relatives			Affected 2nd degree relatives	
	Parent-child pairs	Sibling pairs		Avuncular pairs	First cousin pairs
	50%	50%		25%	12.5%
	odds ratio		relative odds ratio		
Female/Female	3.3		2.4 : 4.5		
Female/Male	2.1 / 2.1		1.9 : 2.7		
Male/Male	2.1		1.7 : 1.8		

Figure 3–3. Parent-of-origin and sex-stratified inheritance of *HLA-DRB1°15* in MS. Odds ratios of transmission distortion for *HLA-DRB1°15* are shown for both second-degree relatives with MS and first-degree relatives with MS stratified by the sex of the affected pairs.[29] The lesser the genetic sharing between individuals, the higher is the interaction between female sex and inheritance of the *HLA-DRB1°15* risk allele. Odds ratios of transmission distortion for *HLA-DRB1°15* are also shown within nuclear families for parent–child trios stratified by the sex of the affected pairs.[30] A maternal parent-of-origin effect for *HLA-DRB1°15* transmission exists only when the affected is a daughter. Full circles, diamonds, and squares indicate individuals with a clinical diagnosis of MS. Empty circles, diamonds, and squares indicate individuals without MS. Solid lines indicate direct relationship. (Reproduced and modified with permission from Kantarci OH. Sex-stratified inheritance of MS: new horizons from studies in MHC region. Neurology; 76:210–212, 2010.[31])

to date.[33–36] These loci are *EOMES, MLANA, THADA, KIF1B, CD58, RGS1, KIF21B, CBLB, TMEM39A,IL12A, IL7RA, HLA-B, HLA-DRB1, IL2RA, CD6, TNFRSF1A, METTL1, MPHOSPH9, IRF8, CLEC16A, STAT3, CD226, CD40, IL12B, KPNB1/ TBKBP1/TBX21, EPS15L1, ILDR1/CD86, PLEK/FBXO48/C2of13, TAGAP, ZMIZ1,* and *TNP2/PRM3/PRM2/PRM1/C16orf75.* Some of these loci await replication. Because more genes will certainly be identified in the future, we refrain from committing to a definitive list of all final associations in MS.

Several of the "relatively strong" gene effects identified in these large efforts, such as the *IL7RA* located on chromosome 5p13, a region with some linkage to MS,[37] were previously associated with MS as a candidate gene.[38]

Then these gene effects, like the HLA region, were confirmed in independent populations of patients with MS, including a whole genomic association study.[34,38,39] We and others were able to confirm this locus in our own efforts.[40] However, in the same population, we failed to confirm the association with *IL2RA*, another relatively strong association identified in the genome-wide efforts.[41]

Many other genetic studies have yielded controversial results. An example is interferon-gamma, a cytokine with key regulatory, immunomodulatory, and effector roles both in autoimmunity and MS. Polymorphisms of *IFNG* are associated with MS susceptibility, likely in a gender-dependent fashion.[42–45] While this association has not been confirmed in all studied populations,[46–49] there is an observed association with *IFNG* polymorphisms that also affect the expression of the gene. At this time, population- and gender-specific effects of this gene cannot be ruled out.

Such examples of failure to replicate results are abundant and usually are assumed to be due to lack of power, but many genes with regional and population-specific influences may also not be observed in large samples, where a larger pool of patients without the genetic risk factor dilutes the otherwise population-specific modest associations. Therefore, caution should be exercised in interpreting only the large efforts as definitive. One Web effort has been monitoring such studies and replication efforts; we refer the reader to their site (http://www.msgene.org).

Most genes identified outside the HLA region, however, have very small odds ratios, which require very large datasets to find any association and make the importance of an individual gene in susceptibility to MS less likely. More importantly, together with the large international whole-genome screening efforts, recent gene-expression studies have identified several candidate molecular pathways associated with MS.[50] These pathways involve DNA-dependent transcription, regulation of cell proliferation, positive regulation of apoptosis, response to abiotic stimulus, release of cytochrome c from mitochondria, leukocyte differentiation, T-cell activation, macromolecular complex subunit organization, inflammatory response, cytokine–cytokine receptor interaction, transmembrane receptor protein serine/threonine kinase signaling, response to cytokine stimulus, positive regulation of neuronal development, regulation of protein transport, regulation of cytokine production, protein translocation into nucleus, enzyme-linked protein signaling pathway, protein amino acid dephosphorylation, cell adhesion, and regulation of synaptic transmission.

As this very long list indicates, almost every aspect of neurobiology and interaction with the immune system has been identified from the large genetic epidemiology studies and recent expression studies. From a systems biology perspective, the identified pathways could potentially help design future therapeutic strategies for MS. However, more focused approaches that tease out pathways important in disease evolution in MS will be more helpful to the clinician in the future both for prediction and design of individualized medicine approaches.

A recently generated, weighted genetic risk score for MS utilizes 16 known susceptibility loci. This is a potentially useful concept to stratify patients for MS risk and develop a preventive strategy for the disease.[51] Could a primary care provider improve the odds for a child with a father or mother who has MS? Would it be possible to avert the onset of MS by identifying individuals with high genetic risk (i.e., a first-degree relative with MS), immunizing them for Epstein-Barr virus (EBV), optimizing their vitamin D intake early in life, and discouraging them from smoking? It is intriguing to think that genetic and environmental epidemiology studies are moving us closer to such primary prevention strategies for MS.

ENVIRONMENTAL RISK FACTORS IN MULTIPLE SCLEROSIS

Identification and quantification of environmental risks for MS have proven difficult because they rely on retrospective data from case-control studies in which all subjects are exposed to the same environment. Although highly impractical, the ideal study design would be to follow prospectively an entire population for 20 to 40 years to see if and how individuals will eventually develop MS and subsequently progressive MS. Therefore, we have to rely on replication of results and control for the potential biases associated with retrospective studies. A practical study design is a nested-cohort study that exploits for MS occurrence a population cohort already identified for exposure to given factor(s) for another disease. Many recent studies have taken this approach, albeit with the limitations associated with patients lost to follow-up due to the long time periods required to study MS.[52,53] Nevertheless, four environmental factors have emerged as strongly associated with MS: EBV, inadequate vitamin D, ultraviolet exposure, and smoking.[54,55] Many other environmental exposure factors, including infections (e.g., herpes simplex virus, cytomegalovirus and varicella zoster virus) and toxins (e.g., organic solvent and trace metals such as zinc), have been considered in the etiology of MS.[52,53,56–58] Although most of these results remained difficult to confirm at the time of this writing, we do discuss them in Chapter 6 as they relate to immunology.

Epstein–Barr Virus Infection and Multiple Sclerosis Risk

A lack of a relationship between MS risk and birth-order position makes it unlikely that early exposure to infections from siblings is solely important in MS.[52,53,59] Many viral infections have been considered in the etiology of MS, but the evidence remained unconvincing except in the case of EBV, which is further discussed below. In a small, nested case-control study of nurses, a positive serology for previous EBV exposure correlated with an increased risk of MS even after adjusting for smoking, ancestry, and latitude of residence at birth.[60] Another nested case-control study conducted among U.S. military personnel demonstrated elevated anti-EBV antibody titers 5 or more years before the onset of MS compared with controls.[61] Some of strongest evidence linking EBV with MS comes from pediatric MS studies. One would expect young children to have no exposure to EBV as opposed to young adults.[62–64] However, in children, elevated antibody titers to EBV nuclear antigen-1 increase the risk of MS prospectively.[65–67] It is unclear whether an EBV coinfection happens due to the same susceptibility factors that lead to MS or whether EBV exposure predisposes one to MS. It is also yet to be demonstrated that EBV infection acutely associates with MS.

Inadequate Vitamin D Intake and Lack of Sun Exposure and Multiple Sclerosis Risk

MS patients have lower serum 25-hydroxyvitamin D concentrations in the summer months compared to controls, a difference not seen in winter months.[68] Vitamin D supplementation, ~400 IU per day, decreases MS risk by twofold.[69] Since 25-hydroxyvitamin D levels in serum strongly correlate with ultraviolet B exposure, these studies clearly indicate vitamin D metabolism as a potential explanation for the increased risk of MS as a factor of distance from the Equator. Indeed, variants of *CYP27B1*, encoding the enzyme that converts 25-hydroxyvitamin D to its active form, have been associated with risk of MS.[70] This gene–environment interaction remains to be replicated but certainly is very plausible.

Three prospective trials of vitamin D in MS have been completed.[71–73] These studies found a clear correlation between increased serum 25-hydroxyvitamin D levels and decreased clinical and subclinical (MRI) relapsing activity in MS, an effect that seemed to work synergistically with IFNbeta treatment. There is no evidence that significantly higher doses are superior to 1,000 IU daily; however, a supplementation trial of 14,000 IU daily is under way.[74,75] Pending further studies, we usually prescribe 2,000 IU of vitamin D daily, seemingly a safe dose.[76] More importantly, a widespread application of vitamin D optimization in children, akin to fluoride supplementation for dental health, may be necessary for long-term primary prevention.

Smoking and Multiple Sclerosis Risk

Cigarette smoking increases the risk of MS by 1.8-fold compared with individuals who have never smoked.[77–79] Children exposed to second-hand, particularly parental, smoking appear to be at increased risk of developing MS.[80] Compared to their nonsmoking counterparts, patients who smoke cigarettes are more likely to convert from clinically isolated syndrome to definite MS, and smokers with relapsing-remitting MS are more likely to convert to secondary-progressive MS.[81] The risk of secondary progression is 3.6-fold higher among smokers compared with never-smokers, therefore increasing the chance that these patients will do worse in the long term.[82] Smoking seems to enhance the association between anti-EBNA antibodies but does not affect the HLA-DRB°1501-associated risk.[83] The exact mechanism of smoking's impact on MS is unknown. It is, however, likely that toxic tobacco byproducts damage axonal integrity, damage myelin, impair repair, or promote autoimmunity. One has to be careful, though, to tease out nicotine's effects, which have been associated both with increased functional efficiency in brain networks and a controversial slowing of neurodegenerative processes.[84,85] The association between tobacco use and MS is likely highly complex, with a need for further studies. Nevertheless, the existing studies underline that smoking cessation or, preferably, avoidance is a primary preventive approach in MS.

SUMMARY

The past two decades have seen highly focused, albeit expensive, efforts to create genetic and environmental epidemiology databases in MS. Today we are fortunate to have a better understanding of the etiology of MS. Efforts in the next decade will appropriately focus on surrogate markers of clinical heterogeneity in MS and the biological pathways involved in environment–gene interactions. Epigenetic modulation of MS risk will likely be a "hot target" for research efforts and potentially for therapeutics in MS.

REFERENCES

1. Mayr WT, Pittock SJ, McClelland RL, et al. Incidence and prevalence of multiple sclerosis in Olmsted County, Minnesota, 1985–2000. Neurology; 61(10):1373–1377, 2003.
2. Whetten-Goldstein K, Sloan FA, Goldstein LB, Kulas ED A comprehensive assessment of the cost of multiple sclerosis in the United States. Multiple Sclerosis; 4:419–425, 1998.
3. Group TIMSS Interferon beta-1b is effective in relapsing-remitting multiple sclerosis. I. Clinical results of a multicenter, randomized, double-blind, placebo-controlled trial. Neurology; 43:655–661, 1993.
4. Johnson KP, Brooks BR, Cohen JA, et al. Copolymer 1 reduces relapse rate and improves disability in relapsing-remitting multiple sclerosis: results of a phase III multicenter, double-blind placebo-controlled trial. The Copolymer 1 Multiple Sclerosis Study Group. Neurology; 45:1268–1276, 1995.
5. Rotstein Z, Hazan R, Barak Y, Achiron A Perspectives in multiple sclerosis health care: special focus on the costs of multiple sclerosis. Autoimmun Rev; 5:511–516, 2006.
6. Oksenberg JR, Barcellos LF The complex genetic aetiology of multiple sclerosis. J Neurovirol; 6(Suppl 2):S10–S14, 2000.
7. Ebers GC, Sadovnick AD, Risch NJ A genetic basis for familial aggregation in multiple sclerosis. Canadian Collaborative Study Group. Nature; 377:150–151, 1995.
8. Weinshenker BG, Epidemiology of multiple sclerosis. Neurol Clin; 14:291–308, 1996.
9. Ebers GC. A twin consensus in MS. Multiple Sclerosis; 11:497–499, 2005.
10. Orton SM, Herrera BM, Yee IM, et al. Sex ratio of multiple sclerosis in Canada: a longitudinal study. Lancet Neurology; 5:932–936, 2006.
11. Murray S, Bashir K, Penrice G, Womersley SJ. Epidemiology of multiple sclerosis in Glasgow. Scottish Med J; 49:100–104, 2004.
12. Kantarci OH, Weinshenker BG. Natural history of multiple sclerosis. Neurol Clin; 23:17–38, 2005.
13. Tutuncu M, Tang J, Zeid NA, et al. Onset of progressive phase is an age-dependent clinical milestone in multiple sclerosis. Multiple Sclerosis; 2012 Jun 26. [Epub ahead of print]
14. Kantarci OH, Spurkland A. Parent of origin in multiple sclerosis: understanding inheritance in complex neurologic diseases. Neurology; 71:786–787, 2008.
15. Herrera BM, Ramagopalan SV, Lincoln MR, et al. Parent-of-origin effects in MS: observations from avuncular pairs. Neurology; 71(11):799–803, 2008.
16. Ebers GC, Sadovnick AD, Dyment DA, et al. Parent-of-origin effect in multiple sclerosis observations in half-siblings. Lancet; 363(9423):1773–1774, 2004.
17. Kantarci OH, Barcellos LF, Atkinson EJ, et al. Men transmit MS more often to their children vs women: the Carter effect. Neurology; 67:305–310, 2006.
18. Herrera BM, Ramagopalan SV, Orton S, et al. Parental transmission of MS in a population-based Canadian cohort. Neurology; 69:1208–1212, 2007.
19. Hoppenbrouwers IA, Liu F, Aulchenko YS, et al. Maternal transmission of multiple sclerosis in a Dutch population. Arch Neurol; 65:345–348, 2008.
20. Pembrey ME, Bygren LO, Kaati G, et al. Sex-specific, male-line transgenerational responses in humans. Eur J Hum Genet; 14:159–166, 2006.
21. Kantarci OH, de Andrade M, Weinshenker BG. Identifying disease-modifying genes in multiple sclerosis. J Neuroimmunol; 123:144–159, 2002.
22. Hensiek AE, Seaman SR, Barcellos LF, et al. Familial effects on the clinical course of multiple sclerosis. Neurology; 68:376–383, 2007.
23. Games and Transatlantic Multiple Sclerosis Genetics Consortium. A meta-analysis of whole genome linkage screens in multiple sclerosis. J Neuroimmunol; 143:39–46, 2003.
24. Sawcer S, Compston A. The genetic analysis of multiple sclerosis in Europeans: concepts and design. J Neuroimmunol; 143:13–16, 2003.
25. Consortium IMSG. A high-density screen for linkage in multiple sclerosis. Am J Hum Genetics; 77:454–467, 2005.
26. Oksenberg JR, Barcellos LF, Cree BA, et al. Mapping multiple sclerosis susceptibility to the HLA-DR locus in African Americans. Am J Hum Genetics; 74:160–167, 2004.
27. Lincoln MR, Montpetit A, Cader MZ, et al. A predominant role for the HLA class II region in the association of the MHC region ith multiple sclerosis. Nature Genet; 37:1108–1112, 2005.
28. Barcellos LF, Sawcer S, Ramsay PP, et al. Heterogeneity at the HLA-DRB1 locus and risk for multiple sclerosis. Hum Mol Genet; 15:2813–2824, 2006.
29. Chao MJ, Ramagopalan SV, Herrera BM, et al. MHC transmission: insights into gender bias in MS susceptibility. Neurology; 76(3):242–6, 2011.
30. Chao MJ, Herrera BM, Ramagopalan SV, et al. Parent-of-origin effects at the major histocompatibility complex in multiple sclerosis. Hum Mol Genet; 19:3679–3689, 2010.
31. Kantarci OH. Sex-stratified inheritance of MS new horizons from studies in MHC region. Neurology; 76:210–212, 2010.
32. DeLuca GC, Ramagopalan SV, Herrera BM, et al. An extremes of outcome strategy provides evidence that

multiple sclerosis severity is determined by alleles at the HLA-DRB1 locus. Proc Natl Acad Sci USA; 104:20896–20901, 2007.

33. Patsopoulos NA, Esposito F, Reischl J, et al. Genome-wide meta-analysis identifies novel multiple sclerosis susceptibility loci. Ann Neurol; 70:897–912,

34. International Multiple Sclerosis Genetics C, Hafler DA, Compston A, et al. Risk alleles for multiple sclerosis identified by a genome-wide study. N Engl J Med; 357:851–862, 2007.

35. De Jager PL, Jia X, Wang J, et al. Meta-analysis of genome scans and replication identify CD6, IRF8 and TNFRSF1A as new multiple sclerosis susceptibility loci. Nat Genet; 41:776–782, 2009.

36. Genome-wide association study identifies new multiple sclerosis susceptibility loci on chromosomes 12 and 20. Nat Genet; 41:824–828, 2009.

37. Ebers GC, Kukay K, Bulman DE, et al. A full genome search in multiple sclerosis. Nature Genetics; 13:472–476, 1996.

38. Zhang Z, Duvefelt K, Svensson F, et al. Two genes encoding immune-regulatory molecules (LAG3 and IL7R) confer susceptibility to multiple sclerosis. Genes Immunity; 6:145–152, 2005.

39. Lundmark F, Salter H, Hillert J. An association study of two functional promotor polymorphisms in the myeloperoxidase (MPO) gene in multiple sclerosis. Multiple Sclerosis; 13:697–700, 2007.

40. O'Doherty C, Kantarci O, Vandenbroeck K. IL7RA polymorphisms and susceptibility to multiple sclerosis. N Engl J Med; 358:753–754, 2008.

41. Matiello M, Weinshenker BG, Atkinson EJ, Schaefer-Klein J, Kantarci OH. Association of IL2RA polymorphisms with susceptibility to multiple sclerosis is not explained by missense mutations in IL2RA. Mult Scler; 17:634–636, 2011.

42. Goris A, Heggarty S, Marrosu MG, Graham C, Billiau A, Vandenbroeck K. Linkage disequilibrium analysis of chromosome 12q14–15 in multiple sclerosis delineation of a 118-kb interval around interferon-gamma (IFNG) that is involved in male versus female differential susceptibility. Genes Immunity; 3:470–476, 2002.

43. Reboul J, Mertens C, Levillayer F, et al. Cytokines in genetic susceptibility to multiple sclerosis: a candidate gene approach. French Multiple Sclerosis Genetics Group. J Neuroimmunol; 102:107–112, 2000.

44. Vandenbroeck K, Cunningham S, Goris A, et al. Polymorphisms in the interferon-gamma/interleukin-26 gene region contribute to sex bias in susceptibility to rheumatoid arthritis. Arthritis Rheumatism; 48:2773–2778, 2003.

45. Kantarci OH, Goris A, Hebrink DD, et al. IFNG polymorphisms are associated with gender differences in susceptibility to multiple sclerosis. Genes Immunity; 6:153–161, 2005.

46. Dai Y, Masterman T, Huang WX, et al. Analysis of an interferon-gamma gene dinucleotide-repeat polymorphism in Nordic multiple sclerosis patients. Multiple Sclerosis; 7:157–163, 2001.

47. Goris A, Epplen C, Fiten P, et al. Analysis of an IFN-gamma gene (IFNG) polymorphism in multiple sclerosis in Europe: effect of population structure on association with disease. J Interferon Cytokine Res; 19:1037–1046, 1999.

48. Schrijver HM, Hooper-van Veen T, van Belzen MJ, et al. Polymorphisms in the genes encoding interferon-gamma and interferon-gamma receptors in multiple sclerosis. Eur J Immunogenetics; 31:133–140, 2004.

49. Bergkvist M, Olsson M, Sandberg-Wollheim M. No evidence for genetic linkage between development of multiple sclerosis and components of the IFN system and the JAK-STAT pathway. Multiple Sclerosis; 10:87–88, 2004.

50. Tuller T, Atar S, Ruppin E, Gurevich M, Achiron A. Global map of physical interactions among differentially expressed genes in multiple sclerosis relapses and remissions. Hum Mol Genet; 20:3606–3619,

51. De Jager PL, Chibnik LB, Cui J, et al. Integration of genetic risk factors into a clinical algorithm for multiple sclerosis susceptibility: a weighted genetic risk score. Lancet Neurol; 8:1111–1119, 2009.

52. Marrie RA. Environmental risk factors in multiple sclerosis aetiology. Lancet Neurology; 3:709–718, 2004.

53. Coo H, Aronson KJ. A systematic review of several potential non-genetic risk factors for multiple sclerosis. Neuroepidemiology; 23:1–12, 2004.

54. Ascherio A, Munger KL. Environmental risk factors for multiple sclerosis. Part II: Noninfectious factors. Ann Neurol; 61:504–513, 2007.

55. Ascherio A, Munger KL Environmental risk factors for multiple sclerosis. Part I: The role of infection. Ann Neurol; 61:288–299, 2007.

56. Marrie RA, Wolfson C, Sturkenboom MC, et al. Multiple sclerosis and antecedent infections: a case-control study. Neurology; 54:2307–2310, 2000.

57. Riise T, Moen BE, Kyvik KR. Organic solvents and the risk of multiple sclerosis. Epidemiology; 13:718–720, 2002.

58. Schiffer RB, McDermott MP, Copley C. A multiple sclerosis cluster associated with a small, north-central Illinois community. Arch Environmental Health; 56:389–395, 2001.

59. Sadovnick AD, Yee IM, Ebers GC, and Canadian Collaborative Study G. Multiple sclerosis and birth order: a longitudinal cohort study. Lancet Neurology; 4:611–617, 2005.

60. Wagner HJ, Munger KL, Ascherio A. Plasma viral load of Epstein-Barr virus and risk of multiple sclerosis. Eur J Neurol; 11:833–834, 2004.

61. Levin LI, Munger KL, Rubertone MV, et al. Temporal relationship between elevation of Epstein-Barr virus antibody titers and initial onset of neurological symptoms in multiple sclerosis. JAMA; 293:2496–2500, 2005.

62. Alotaibi S, Kennedy J, Tellier R, Stephens D, Banwell B. Epstein-Barr virus in pediatric multiple sclerosis. JAMA; 291:1875–1879, 2004.

63. Pohl D, Krone B, Rostasy K, et al. High seroprevalence of Epstein-Barr virus in children with multiple sclerosis. Neurology; 67:2063–2065, 2006.

64. Banwell B, Krupp L, Kennedy J, et al. Clinical features and viral serologies in children with multiple sclerosis: a multinational observational study. Lancet Neurol; 6:773–781, 2007.

65. Ascherio A, Munger KL, Lennette ET, et al. Epstein-Barr virus antibodies and risk of multiple sclerosis a prospective study. JAMA; 286:3083–3088, 2001.

66. DeLorenze GN, Munger KL, Lennette ET, Orentreich N, Vogelman JH, Ascherio A. Epstein-Barr virus and multiple sclerosis: evidence of association from a prospective study with long-term follow-up. Arch Neurol; 63:839–844, 2006.

67. Sundstrom P, Juto P, Wadell G, et al. An altered immune response to Epstein-Barr virus in multiple sclerosis: a prospective study. Neurology; 62:2277–2282, 2004.

68. Soilu-Hanninen M, Airas L, Mononen I, Heikkila A, Viljanen M, Hanninen A. 25-Hydroxyvitamin D levels in serum at the onset of multiple sclerosis. Multiple Sclerosis; 11:266–271, 2005.

69. Munger KL, Zhang SM, O'Reilly E, et al. Vitamin D intake and incidence of multiple sclerosis. Neurology; 62:60–65, 2004.

70. Ramagopalan SV, Dyment DA, Cader MZ, et al. Rare variants in the CYP27B1 gene are associated with multiple sclerosis. Ann Neurol; 70:881–886, 2011.

71. Runia TF, Hop WC, de Rijke YB, Buljevac D, Hintzen RQ. Lower serum vitamin D levels are associated with a higher relapse risk in multiple sclerosis. Neurology; 79:261–266,

72. Loken-Amsrud KI, Holmoy T, Bakke SJ, et al. Vitamin D and disease activity in multiple sclerosis before and during interferon-beta treatment. Neurology; 79:267–273, 2012.

73. Stewart N, Simpson S, Jr., van der Mei I, et al. Interferon-beta and serum 25-hydroxyvitamin D interact to modulate relapse risk in MS. Neurology; 79:254–260, 2012.

74. Ascherio A, Marrie RA. Vitamin D in MS: A vitamin for 4 seasons. Neurology; 79:208–210, 2012.

75. Smolders J, Hupperts R, Barkhof F, et al. Efficacy of vitamin D(3) as add-on therapy in patients with relapsing-remitting multiple sclerosis receiving subcutaneous interferon beta-1a: a Phase II, multicenter, double-blind, randomized, placebo-controlled trial. J Neurol Sci; 311:44–49, 2011.

76. Wingerchuk DM, Lesaux J, Rice GP, Kremenchutzky M, Ebers GC. A pilot study of oral calcitriol (1,25-dihydroxyvitamin D3) for relapsing-remitting multiple sclerosis. J Neurol Neurosurg Psychiatry; 76:1294–1296, 2005.

77. Handel AE, Williamson AJ, Disanto G, Dobson R, Giovannoni G, Ramagopalan SV. Smoking and multiple sclerosis: an updated meta-analysis. PLoS One; 6:e16149, 2011.

78. Hernan MA, Olek MJ, Ascherio A. Cigarette smoking and incidence of multiple sclerosis. Am J Epidemiol; 154:69–74, 2001.

79. Riise T, Nortvedt MW, Ascherio A. Smoking is a risk factor for multiple sclerosis. Neurology; 61:1122–1124, 2003.

80. Mikaeloff Y, Caridade G, Tardieu M, Suissa S. Parental smoking at home and the risk of childhood-onset multiple sclerosis in children. Brain; 130:2589–2595, 2007.

81. Healy BC, Ali EN, Guttmann CR, et al. Smoking and disease progression in multiple sclerosis. Arch Neurol; 66:858–864, 2009.

82. Hernan MA, Jick SS, Logroscino G, Olek MJ, Ascherio A, Jick H. Cigarette smoking and the progression of multiple sclerosis. Brain; 128:1461–1465, 2005.

83. Simon KC, van der Mei IA, Munger KL, et al. Combined effects of smoking, anti-EBNA antibodies, and HLA-DRB1°1501 on multiple sclerosis risk. Neurology; 74:1365–1371

84. Wylie KP, Rojas DC, Tanabe J, Martin LF, Tregellas JR. Nicotine increases brain functional network efficiency. Neuroimage; 63:73–80, 2012.

85. Thiriez C, Villafane G, Grapin F, Fenelon G, Remy P, Cesaro P. Can nicotine be used medicinally in Parkinson's disease? Exp Rev Clin Pharmacol; 4:429–436, 2011.

Chapter 4

The Role of Magnetic Resonance Imaging in Multiple Sclerosis

Abstract

MRI is an extremely effective tool to diagnose and manage several neurological conditions. It offers high-resolution, noninvasive, *in vivo* imaging without radiation exposure. In addition, it provides structural and functional information superior to other currently available imaging modalities. It has relatively few contraindications. Its greater sensitivity to disease activity compared with clinical outcome measures favors its use as a metric in clinical trials, often as a primary outcome measure or as surrogate marker, especially when testing new drugs. This chapter discusses the role of MRI sequences in the diagnosis and management of MS and reviews advanced MRI methods used in research studies. It also briefly discusses the role of MRI in diagnosing other white matter diseases.

INTRODUCTION

MRI is a critically important, state-of-the-art tool to diagnose and manage several neurological conditions. It offers high-resolution, noninvasive, *in vivo* imaging without exposure to ionizing radiation or isotopes. In addition, with several available pulse sequences scrutinizing different physicochemical, physiological, and pathological aspects of CNS diseases, it provides structural and functional information superior to other currently available imaging modalities. It has relatively few contraindications, the most serious being the use of certain implantable medical devices and prostheses containing ferromagnetic metals. Over the past three decades, MRI has revolutionized the diagnosis and management of leukoencephalopathies and MS.[1] The incorporation of specific MRI findings represents the most significant change to determining the diagnosis of MS since the introduction and subsequent modifications of the 2001 McDonald criteria.[2-4] As discussed in Chapters 1 and 2, MRI-derived measures are also among the strongest predictors for conversion to MS following a clinically isolated demyelinating syndrome (clinically isolated syndrome [CIS]).[5-7] MRI plays an important role in the diagnostic criteria of other CNS neuroinflammatory diseases such as neuromyelitis optica (NMO),[8,9] pediatric MS,[10] and acute

disseminated encephalomyelitis (ADEM),[11] in addition to MS (see Chapter 2). Because it is more sensitive to disease activity than clinical outcome measures, MRI-derived metrics are frequently used in clinical trials, often as primary outcome measures or as surrogate markers, especially in trials of new therapeutics. However, the rationale behind its "exclusive" use in clinical trials is controversial.[12]

In this chapter, we discuss the role of routinely available MRI sequences in the diagnosis and management of MS, briefly review some advanced MRI methods used in research studies, and discuss the overall role of MRI in disease management. We also briefly discuss two commonly encountered white matter diseases, ADEM and NMO, that are unrelated to MS. This chapter expands on many concepts introduced in Chapters 1 and 2. The reader is encouraged to refer to these chapters as needed.

CONVENTIONAL MRI IN THE CLINIC: COMMONLY USED SEQUENCES AND APPLICATIONS

T2-Weighted MRI: Classic Determinant of Overall White Matter Lesion Load

T2-weighted MRI sequences are the classic method used to visualize MS plaques *in vivo* (Fig. 4.1). T2-weighted images are very sensitive to classic white matter lesions, regardless of their chronicity.[13] However, they show poor specificity to the disease process at the tissue level because many conditions in addition to demyelination appear hyperintense on these scans. These include inflammation, edema, cell infiltration, remyelination, Wallerian degeneration, axonal loss, ischemic changes, neoplasms, and infections. Often T2-weighted images use fast spin echo-based techniques. Of note, the commonly used FLAIR images are also T2-weighted (see discussion later in this chapter).

The location of T2-weighted, hyperintense lesions is of great importance from the standpoint of MS diagnosis because it differentiates MS from its numerous mimickers. For this reason, lesion location features prominently in the current diagnostic criteria for MS.[2,3,14]

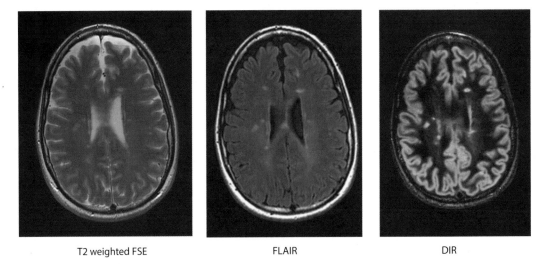

T2 weighted FSE   FLAIR   DIR

Figure 4–1. Fast spin echo (FSE) T2-weighted, FLAIR, and double inversion recovery (DIR) image of typical MS lesions. Note the easier identification of juxtacortical lesion on FLAIR compared to T2-weighted image (left frontal midsagittal area); note that the same lesion is even easier to identify on DIR. DIR also reveals a number of other cortical and juxtacortical lesions. In addition, standard white matter lesions are very sensitively identified on DIR.

In advanced MS, the originally multifocal T2 lesions present as a confluent signal change. At the same time, brain atrophy also progresses. As a result of these two processes, the lesion load may actually *decrease* in advanced cases. This is one of the reasons for the "MRI paradox": the correlation between standard T2-lesion load and disability is relatively weak, with the potential exception of early relapsing–remitting MS (RRMS) cases, where the correlation is modest.[7,15–17] There are several reasons for this paradox, including (1) the overall nonspecificity of T2-weighted sequences; (2) the fact that "lesion load" does not consider lesion location, and some locations in the brain, such as the brainstem, corticospinal tract, and cerebellum, correlate more closely with disability when damaged; and (3) while T2-weighted sequences are sensitive to classic demyelinated white-matter lesions, they are insensitive to cortical and deep gray matter pathology and to nonlesional changes in normal-appearing gray and white matter. The strongest correlation between functional outcome measures and MRI metrics occurs with advanced and volumetric MRI modalities that concentrate on gray matter features or features in normal-appearing white and gray matter (NAWM and NAGM).[15,18]

FLAIR IMAGES

FLAIR (fluid attenuated inversion recovery) images are also T2-weighted, but they are acquired through an additional inversion-recovery pulse designed to minimize signal arising from unbound water (i.e., the CSF). FLAIR has greater sensitivity to cerebral hemispheric lesions, especially juxtacortical ones.[19] FLAIR, in general, has a slightly greater sensitivity to cortical lesions, especially to ones also involving the underlying white matter (leukocortical or juxtacortical lesions). However, the vast majority of intracortical and especially subpial cortical lesions remain undetected with FLAIR. Double inversion recovery (DIR) imaging is a newer technique used for cortical lesion detection and is discussed among the advanced imaging sequences in this chapter. The main advantage of FLAIR is increased visualization of lesions adjacent to CSF-filled spaces. While practicing neurologists prefer FLAIR images over standard T2-weighted sequences, FLAIR images do have a major, often forgotten shortcoming: their relative insensitivity to posterior fossa lesions. Of note, posterior fossa structures are very commonly involved in MS; therefore, the above needs to be taken into consideration when reviewing especially newly diagnosed (or to-be-diagnosed) cases (Fig. 4.2).[20,21]

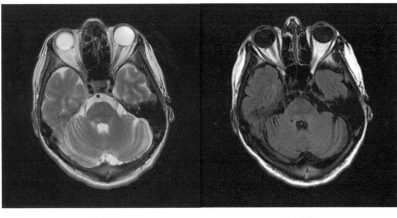

FSE T2   FLAIR

Figure 4–2. The insensitivity of FLAIR to infratentorial lesions. Note that while numerous hyperintense lesions are clearly visualized in the pons and middle cerebellar peduncle on the T2-weighted image, they are barely visible and easily could be missed on FLAIR.

Special Notes on Spinal Cord Imaging

Practicing neurologists often seem to overlook cord lesions, although they are common in MS (Fig. 4.3). The significance of cord involvement is also underlined in the new diagnostic criteria for MS.[2,3] T2-weighted scans are optimal for visualizing cord lesions. On sagittal scans, MS lesions rarely extend beyond one spinal cord segment longitudinally. This contrasts markedly with the cord lesions of NMO (Devic's disease), which often extend longitudinally over three or more cord segments, as discussed in Chapter 2 and later in this chapter. Axial cord images commonly show involvement of less than half (usually a quarter to a third) of the cord area on axial cut with white and often gray matter involvement. STIR (short tau inversion recovery) imaging is also often used to detect cord lesions and may have better sensitivity.[22] STIR sequences also provide fat suppression, which results in increased sensitivity, not only in cord imaging but also in the imaging of optic nerves.[23,24] Some advanced MRI sequences are also particularly useful in spinal cord imaging,

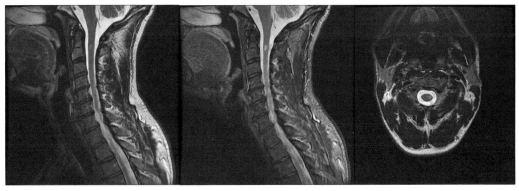

Sagittal FSE T2   STIR   Axial T2

Figure 4–3. Typical MS-related spinal cord lesions in the upper cervical cord. Note that the hyperintense lesion is less than 1 spinal cord segment long and is more sensitively detected on the short-tau inversion recovery image (STIR) compared to standard T2-weighted sagittal scan. On the axial cut, the lesion occupies ~25% of the cord surface area, which is also typical for MS lesions.

most notably magnetization-transfer MRI, as discussed later in this chapter.

COMMONLY UTILIZED PULSE

Deep Gray Matter T2 Hypointensity and its Correlations with Disability

One group of investigators has extensively reported hypointensity in the thalamus, deep gray nuclei, and cortical gray matter on standard T2-weighted images (Fig. 4.4).[25–29] This is a newer finding in MS. The presence of these lesions appears to correlate with an increased incidence of cognitive problems, fatigue, brain atrophy, and overall disability. This MRI finding, along with that of T1 hypointensities (or T1 black holes, as discussed later), may alert the clinician to a potentially more disabling disease course in individual cases. Although not yet proven, the finding likely represents pathological iron deposition. Other processes resulting in susceptibility artifacts, including the presence of free radicals, may also explain these changes. Newer imaging techniques, including susceptibility-weighted imaging (SWI),[30] allow for easier quantification and advanced visualization of this finding.

PROTON DENSITY-WEIGHTED IMAGING

Proton density-weighted imaging has slowly passed out of favor for the past several years, and many institutions stopped acquiring these scans altogether. While they are less helpful than FLAIR in delineating periventricular lesions, proton density scans are sensitive to infratentorial lesions and, overall, represent a good compromise between conventional T2-weighted and FLAIR images.

T1-Weighted MRI

T1-weighted scans may look unimpressive compared to their T2-weighted counterparts; in many cases, especially on passing observation, T1-weighted scans appear completely normal in MS, without any obvious pathology. There are currently three main uses for T1-weighted images: (1) the standard T1 "precontrast" scans facilitate identification of "T1 black holes" or T1 hypointense lesions; (2) 3D (volume acquisition) T1-weighted studies like MPRAGE or MDEFT allow accurate gray–white matter segmentation for volumetric studies and also serve as a "registration template" for other MRI studies; and (3) after the injection of chelated gadolinium-based contrast dye, T1-weighted scans permit the

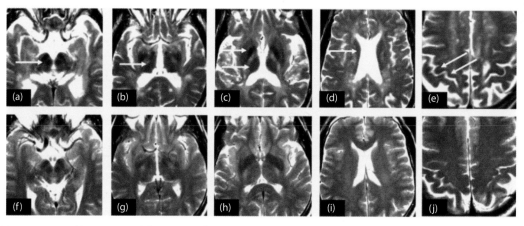

Figure 4–4. T2 hypointensity of deep gray nuclei in MS. Standard T2-weighted images of a 43-year-old man with relapsing–remitting MS with mild to moderate disability (**A–E**) compared to an age-matched healthy subject (**F–J**). Note bilateral hypointensity of various deep gray matter areas (*arrows*), including the red nucleus (**A**), thalamus (**B, C**), lentiform nucleus (**B, C**), caudate (**D**), and rolandic cortex (**E**) compared with the healthy subject. The patient also has brain atrophy (note enlarged CSF spaces). (Reproduced with permission from Pirko I, Lucchinetti CF, Sriram S, Bakshi R. Gray matter involvement in multiple sclerosis. Neurology; 68:634–642, 2007.)[18]

identification of blood–brain barrier (BBB) leakage, a common phenomenon accompanying new lesion formation in MS. BBB leakage distinguishes "active scans" from inactive ones, and currently available therapeutic modalities best treat this phenomenon. In patients treated with disease-modifying agents (DMAs), the reduction in new lesion formation should result in a corresponding decrease in visualization of new gadolinium-enhancing lesions.

Hypointense lesions on T1-weighted images form a subset of the classic T2-weighted hyperintense lesions.[31] This phenomenon can be seen with two largely independent mechanisms. First, acute T1 black holes represent an early transient stage in lesion formation,[32,33] thought to be caused by lesional infiltrates in emerging lesions and associated "focal edema." This is expected to resolve.[34,35] However, approximately 30% of MS patients also develop persistent T1 "black holes" that do not resolve (Fig. 4.1).[36] These areas may represent more severe tissue loss and, specifically, areas of axonal damage.[37,38] In contrast to T2 hyperintense lesion load, T1 black hole load correlates well with chronic disability.[15,39–41] Therefore, T1 black holes, especially when seen early in MS onset, are worrisome and should prompt appropriate treatment decisions as discussed later.

T1 black holes are most commonly located in the cerebral white matter; however, abnormalities, likely of the same etiology and significance, have also been reported in the spinal cord.[42] When correlated with histology findings,[37] the degree of hypointensity correlated best with axonal density.[38] On advanced MRI, T1 black holes are associated with low magnetization-transfer ratios (MTR). These are even lower than in T1 isointense lesions and are another indicator of more profound tissue damage.[43] The most hypointense, "darkest" black holes are CSF-filled spaces in the parenchyma, but in most cases, the MRI intensity is higher than that of CSF in these areas, indicating that these "holes" still contain CNS tissue. On magnetic resonance spectroscopy (MRS), the hallmark of chronic black holes is severely decreased NAA, a marker of axonal *or* neuronal integrity and density.[44] Investigators recently established a murine model of T1 black holes, which may permit the identification of immune mechanisms responsible

for this more severe form of tissue damage in MS.[45]

Spontaneous T1 Hyperintensities on Noncontrast Scans

Another interesting, newly reported finding—so far, by one group only—is the presence of spontaneous T1 hyperintensity on conventional spin echo-based T1-weighted studies (Fig. 4.5.).[46] This is more common in secondary progressive MS (SPMS) and may appear as hyperintense perilesional rims (two thirds of lesions) or as a homogeneous hyperintensity (one third of lesions). Like T1 black holes, these areas reportedly have good correlation with disability and brain atrophy measures but not with disease duration. If confirmed, this finding may provide a readily available biomarker for a more disabling, progressive disease course.

Gadolinium-Enhancing Lesions: The Significance of "Active Scans"

Gadolinium enhancement is the hallmark of newly forming "active lesions," with BBB leakage and the presence of inflammatory infiltrates. Chelated gadolinium is the most commonly used positive contrast material, detected as hyperintensity on T1-weighted images (Fig. 4.6). Of note, negative contrast materials do exist. These include iron-based and particulate materials containing SPION-s or USPIO-s ([ultra]small super-paramagnetic iron oxide [nano] particle). These contrast materials are useful for labeling and enable cell—or macromolecule-specific imaging. These are best detected as hypointensity on T2*-weighted images, where they cause susceptibility effects; some may also have mild-to-moderate T1 effects. Given that negative contrast materials currently only have research applications and are unlikely to gain FDA approval in the near future, we will not discuss them in this chapter. However, the reader may wish to consult the numerous available studies in the literature, in animal models as well as smaller-scale human studies.[47–50]

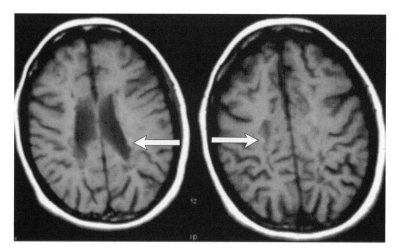

Figure 4–5. Spontaneous T1 hyperintensity on noncontrast T1-weighted images of a SPMS case. Note that hyperintense areas can be seen at lesion edges, or in a uniformly hyperintense fashion. The scans also demonstrate substantial central and cortical atrophy. (Reproduced with permission from Bakshi R, Dmochowski J, Shaikh ZA, Jacobs L. Gray matter T2 hypointensity is related to plaques and atrophy in the brains of multiple sclerosis patients. J Neurol Sci; 185:19–26, 2001.[148])

In routine clinical imaging with gadolinium, the dose and the delay between administration and scanning are equally important determinants of the outcome. The recommended standard dose is 0.1 mmol/kg, and a delay of 5 minutes after administration is advisable; this most commonly is accomplished by administering gadolinium and running a "gadolinium-insensitive" sequence, such as a multislice T2-weighted scan, to "use the scanning delay wisely." Thinner slices or 3D acquisition is important for the sensitive detection of enhancement. Higher field strength is also helpful—the relaxation-enhancement properties of this rare earth metal are even more pronounced in that setting.

A "sensitizing" magnetization transfer pulse[51] incorporated into the T1-weighted sequence can also be of help, which, in this setting, can be considered "background noise reduction" to render the areas of enhancement more visible. (Classic MT-MRI uses proton-density or T2-weighted sequences, as discussed later.) Whereas gadolinium-enhancing lesions signal newly emerging lesions, in most cases their presence will not result in new clinically obvious relapses. These scans are 5 to 10 times more sensitive to inflammatory activity than clinical observation alone.[52] This increased sensitivity to "new pathology" compared to clinical observation alone is the main reason for using gadolinium-enhancing lesion-based quantitative

metrics as outcome measures in clinical trials of emerging MS therapies. While they efficiently capture inflammatory disease activity, gadolinium-enhancing lesions do not correlate well with disability on longitudinal studies: the mean number of enhancing lesions in the first 6 months after the diagnosis of MS showed a weak correlation with disability 1 and 2 years later.[53] Of note, gadolinium enhancement does not always accompany the formation of new lesions, and preexisting lesions often enlarge without evidence for enhancement. Gadolinium-enhancing lesions are strong predictors of subsequent relapses. This observation is critically important for the practicing neurologist; this active stage is exactly what the currently approved DMAs best address. As a result, clinicians often base treatment initiation and "upgrade" decisions on this biomarker of MS in routine practice. In terms of lesion development, gadolinium enhancement is typically observable in the first 4 to 6 weeks of lesion formation.[54,55] It is very rarely detectable beyond 2 to 3 months. When enhancement lasts longer, the treating neurologist should consider alternative diagnoses, including neurosarcoidosis and neoplasm. In SPMS, especially in patients no longer having superimposed relapses, gadolinium enhancement is infrequent and may not be observable at all.[56,57] In primary progressive MS (PPMS), only as few as 5% of patients will have detectable gadolinium enhancement.[58] However, in the first 5 years of PPMS, up to

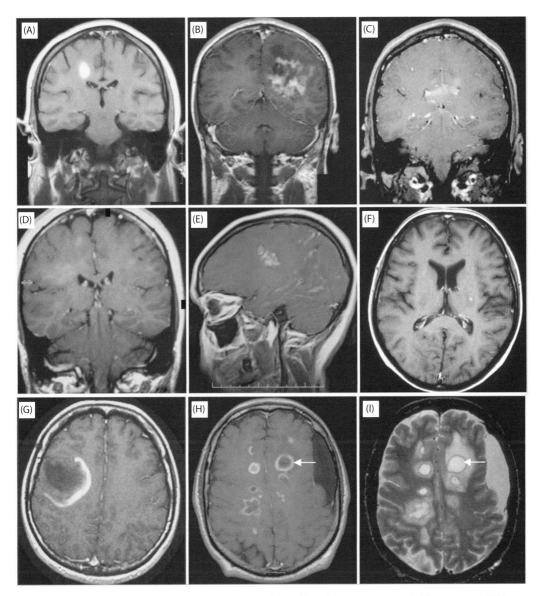

Figure 4–6. Examples of different enhancement patterns observable in biopsy-proven MS: (**A**) homogenous; (**B**) heterogeneous; (**C**) patchy and diffuse; (**D**) cotton-ball; (**E**) nodular; (**F**) punctate; (**G**) open ring; (**H**) multiple closed rings; (**I**) T2 hypointense rims colocalize with ring enhancement (*arrow*; T2-weighted MRI). These T2 hypointense rims colocalize with the location of macrophages. (Adapted from Lucchinetti CF, Gavrilova RH, Metz I, et al. Clinical and radiographic spectrum of pathologically confirmed tumefactive multiple sclerosis. Brain; 131:1759–1775, 2008.[149])

40% may be associated with enhancing lesions,[59] supporting the notion as discussed in Chapter 1 of PPMS representing the onset of progressive MS after a period of radiologically isolated syndrome.

Gadolinium-enhancing lesions may differ in appearance. They may appear homogenously enhancing, heterogeneous/nodular enhancing, or ring or open ring enhancing[52,54,60–62] (in which case the opening is typically "upward" toward the cortex).[63,64] Open ring-enhancing lesions may be more specific for demyelinating lesions in general. Ring-enhancing lesions are typically larger, may exhibit a shorter duration of enhancement,[65] and have a lower apparent diffusion-coefficient (ADC)[66] and MTR.[67] In some cases, they may predict the evolution of lesions to T1 black holes and correlate with a higher likelihood of brain atrophy.[33] However, in the largest biopsy-proven cohort of demyelinating diseases, no association existed between ring-enhancing lesions and increased risk for disability. Of note, ring-enhancing lesions are often seen with other etiologies, including gliomas, metastases, and abscesses. Larger ring-enhancing lesions often demonstrate a T2 hypointense border ("T2 dark rim or ring") when caused by inflammatory demyelination (Fig. 4.6).[68]

Is Gadolinium Dangerous?

Gadolinium in its native, nonchelated form is highly toxic, like most rare earth metals; however, in chelated form, as in MRI contrast material, it is very safe. However, cases of nephrogenic systemic fibrosis have recently emerged as a result of gadolinium administration. Perhaps the most important fact about nephrogenic systemic fibrosis is that to date, *no such case has been reported in patients with normal renal function.* The most common predisposing factors are severely compromised renal function, especially in the context of transplantation and accompanying liver failure. It is important to monitor the estimated glomerular filtration rate in patients at risk; if that is normal, it is highly unlikely that gadolinium would cause any problems. The incidence is also higher with double- or triple-dose administration, which should be avoided. There is a difference between various gadolinium-based contrast agents in the incidence of this potentially serious adverse effect. The website of the International Society for Magnetic Resonance in Medicine provides regular updates regarding this topic (www.ismrm.org). Another important point is related to contrast dye allergy: while allergy to standard iodine-based x-ray, including CT scan, contrast dye, is not uncommon, allergy to chelated gadolinium is exceptionally rare and seldom encountered in routine clinical settings.

MRI IN THE DIAGNOSTIC CRITERIA OF MULTIPLE SCLEROSIS

The most important addition to the McDonald criteria over its predecessors is the incorporation of MRI-based paraclinical markers.[2] Since the original inception of the McDonald criteria in 2001, expert panels have developed two revisions through a review process, most recently in 2010.[14,69] They established specific "dissemination in space" and "dissemination in time" criteria to include more MRI-based, clinically silent activity, as discussed in Chapter 1. MS-related changes can literally appear anywhere in the white matter (and also in the gray matter, as discussed later). However, the most common location is the periventricular white matter, where ovoid lesions often occur. The large axis of the oval is nearly perpendicular to the large axis of the lateral ventricles. These lesions, similar to most but not all MS lesions, seem to surround veins. Lesions in the corpus callosum result in the typical Dawson's fingers configuration on sagittal T2-weighted images.[70,71] In addition to periventricular lesions (1), the 2010 dissemination in space criteria also include juxtacortical (2), infratentorial (3), and spinal cord lesions (4). Of note, gadolinium enhancement is not necessary to fulfill dissemination in space criteria (i.e., the chronicity of the lesions doesn't matter). Lesions must be present in two of the above four locations to meet dissemination in space criteria.

In contrast to MS lesions, T2 lesions in nonspecific small-vessel ischemic changes tend to spare the U-fibers, and lesions are typically not detected in the periventricular areas. Such nonspecific lesions are virtually never seen infratentorially except in the pons, where they can be observed in a low proportion of cases. Small-vessel ischemic changes do not cause signal abnormalities in the spinal cord, whereas cord lesions very often accompany MS. Therefore, cord imaging increases the diagnostic certainty for a true demyelinating disease.[72] In progressive forms of MS, especially in PPMS, where myelopathy-related symptoms dominate the clinical picture, cord atrophy and increasing cord lesion load may be the only MRI manifestations of the disease.

The 2010 revision of the McDonald criteria greatly simplified the criteria for dissemination in time. Initially, either new enhancing or new non-enhancing lesions needed to develop between defined time points, but now a single scan is sufficient to establish dissemination-in-time criteria, as long as the scan includes different stages of lesion formation. This includes the presence of both enhancing ("new") and nonenhancing ("old") lesions on the same scan, as proposed earlier by the Magnetic Resonance Network in Multiple Sclerosis (MAGNIMS) group in Europe (Fig. 4.7).[73,74] While this seems a logical extension to the McDonald criteria and certainly allows for earlier diagnosis of MS, one must be especially careful in interpreting scans of a single time point. If different pathologies, such as the coexistence of persistently enhancing venous angiomas and MS-related T2 hyperintense lesions, contribute to "lesion formation," one could erroneously conclude that there is evidence for dissemination in time. In other words, the specificity of the diagnosis may be compromised by the introduction of the "single scan" modification for dissemination in time, where clinicians' experience and attention to detail are essential.

PPMS typically presents as a slowly progressive myelopathy. MRI in most patients with PPMS demonstrates a cord-predominant lesion formation pattern and a paucity of enhancing lesions compared to RRMS cases, although a pattern indistinguishable from SPMS cases can also be observed. The 2010 MRI criteria for PPMS have further simplified the diagnosis of progression-onset MS. It requires 1 year of slow progression and two of the following three findings: (1) limited evidence of dissemination in space in the brain, with one or more periventricular, juxtacortical, and infratentorial locations demonstrating lesions; (2) evidence of dissemination in space in the cord with two or more characteristic T2-weighted lesions; and (3) positive CSF OCB (oligoclonal band) elevation and/or IgG index elevation).

Despite the considerable attention given to the development of these MRI criteria, one must note that CNS diseases other than MS may also meet these criteria. In other words, the criteria are not 100% specific to MS. MS therefore remains a clinical diagnosis with contributing data derived from history, clinical examination, laboratory findings, and MRI findings. Any one of these components alone is insufficient.

Misdiagnosing Multiple Sclerosis by MRI: A Word of Caution

Many patients visit tertiary care centers after receiving a diagnosis of "MS" based solely on a suggestive MRI appearance. If the overall clinical picture (especially the symptoms and temporal characteristics of the presentation) is inconsistent with MS, the mere presence of T2 hyperintense lesions in the brain may not indicate MS. While MRI has very high sensitivity in detecting CNS pathology, its actual specificity is very low. As a result, several CNS diseases have MRI features that are easily mistaken for MS. In some diseases, even the clinical features may

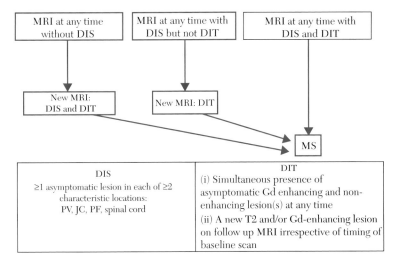

Figure 4–7. MRI criteria of MS in 2010: dissemination in space (DIS) and dissemination in time (DIT). Note that the new criteria allow DIT to be fulfilled on one single scan if the scan shows the simultaneous presence of enhancing and nonenhancing lesions suggestive of different time points of lesion formation. (Reproduced with permission from Montalban X, Tintore M, Swanton J, et al. MRI criteria for MS in patients with clinically isolated syndromes. Neurology; 74:427–434, 2010.[74])

suggest an inflammatory demyelinating disease when the actual diagnosis is different. A workshop of the European Magnetic Resonance Network in Multiple Sclerosis (MAGNIMS) group was held in 2005 with a goal to define "MRI red flags" derived from evidence-based findings and "educated guesses" to avoid erroneous diagnoses of MS.[75] For example, T1 hypo-intense and T2 hyper-intense lesions in the spinal cord of more than three vertebral segments in length should prompt a thorough evaluation for NMO. The preferential involvement of temporal poles and external capsule should suggest cerebral autosomal dominant arteriopathy with subcortical infarcts and leukoencephalopathy (CADASIL). Alternatively, nonspecific white matter lesions and dilated Virchow-Robin spaces with hippocampal and amygdala atrophy may suggest hyperhomocysteinemia. Table 4.1 summarizes the identified sets of MRI features suggestive of specific etiologies. The presence of these specific features in the proper clinical setting should trigger a targeted workup of the affected patients.

THE ROLE OF MRI IN PROGNOSIS OF CLINICALLY ISOLATED SYNDROME

The first presentation of MS commonly includes well-characterized subacute-onset demyelinating syndromes including optic neuritis, transverse myelitis, or isolated brainstem/cerebellar syndromes. The best-established predictor of conversion from these CIS events to MS is the number of lesions on the initial scan. As established through the National Hospital series in London (Fig. 4.8)[5–7,76,77] and confirmed in other, usually smaller studies, the 1-year conversion rate to MS in those with abnormal scans was 30%.

None from the normal scan group converted to MS at this early time point. At 5 years, 65% of those with an abnormal MRI converted to MS versus 3% with a normal MRI. Corresponding figures were 83% and 11% at 10 years; 88% and 19% at 14 years; and 82% and 21% at 20 years. The reason for the somewhat fluctuating percentages is that the availability of patients and follow-up scans differed at the various study time points.[77] As evident from these data, the majority of conversions to MS occurred in the first few years after the initial demyelinating event. Those who converted with an ambiguous MRI at presentation typically also had milder disease.

A study in 2008 addressed the association of these findings with disability risk using the 20-year data.[77] In those converting to MS, a correlation of T2 lesion volume with change in Expanded Disability Status Scale (EDSS) score was most evident in the first 5 years. The estimated lesion growth rate over the duration of the study was 0.80 cm^3/year in patients with RRMS and 2.89 cm^3/year in those who developed SPMS; the difference was statistically significant. The study established that lesion volume and change at earlier time points correlate with disability after 20 years. Lesion volume increases for at least 20 years in relapse-onset MS, and the rate of lesion growth is over three times higher in those who develop SPMS than in those who remain with RRMS.

RADIOLOGICALLY ISOLATED SYNDROME

An interesting scenario arises when MRI findings strongly suggestive of MS are seen in the context of a workup for an unrelated complaint; for example, in the context of headache or

Conversion to MS following CIS

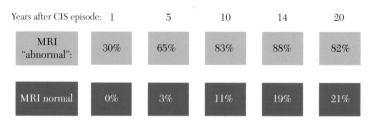

Figure 4–8. Conversion risk to clinically definite MS from CIS, using the National Hospital ("Queen Square") series data.

Table 4–1 MRI Red Flags Suggestive of a Diagnosis Other than MS

Brain white matter	Disease
Normal	NMO (absent or few lesions), ATM
Large lesions	AMS (sometimes confluent or perilesional edema), BCS (concentric whorls of alternating rings of enhancement), PACNS (with mass effect)
Symmetrically distributed lesions	ADEM, AFL
Poorly defined lesion margins	ADEM, pattern III MS
Absent or rare Dawson's fingers, corpus callosum and periventricular lesions	ADEM
Absent MRI activity at follow-up	ADEM (with exceptions)
T2 hyperintensity of the temporal pole, U-fibers at the vertex, external capsule, and insular regions	CADASIL
Multiple bilateral microhemorrhagic foci	CADASIL, SVD
Frequent sparing of corpus callosum and cerebellum	CADASIL, SVD
Lesions in the center of corpus callosum, sparing periphery	Susac's syndrome
Hemorrhages	PACNS
Simultaneous enhancement of all lesions	ADEM, PACNS, sarcoidosis
Infarcts	SID, PACNS, SVD
Punctiform parenchymal enhancement	PACNS, sarcoidosis, NBD
Predominance of lesions at cortical/subcortical junction	SID
Diffuse white matter involvement	NBD, encephalitis (HIVE), SVD, CADASIL
Cerebral venous sinus thrombosis	NBD
Large, infiltrating brainstem lesions	NBD
Anterior temporal and inferior frontal lobe involvement, associated with enhancement or mass effect	Encephalitis (HSE)
Isolated lesions with ring enhancement	Abscesses
Mass effect	Abscesses
Multifocal, asymmetrical lesions starting in a juxtacortical location and progressively enlarging	PML
Large lesions with absent or rare mass effect	PML
Extensive, bilateral periventricular abnormalities in isolation	B12D, ACD
Cortical gray matter	
Cortical/subcortical lesions crossing vascular territories	MELAS
Prevalent involvement versus white matter	Encephalitis
Infiltrating lesions that do not remain in gray or white matter abnormalities	Abscesses
Deep gray matter	
Bilateral lesions	ADEM (at the gray/white matter junction), CADASIL
Lacunar infarcts	CADASIL, SVD
T1 hyperintensity of the pulvinar	FD
Multiple discrete lesions in the basal ganglia and thalamus	Susac's syndrome
Large, infiltrating basal ganglia lesions	NBD
Infiltrating lesions w/o respect to gray or white matter boundaries	Abscesses
T2 hyperintense lesions in the dentate nuclei	AFL (CTX)
Spinal cord	
Large, swelling lesions	NMO (with corresponding T1 hypointensity), ADEM, ATM, Sjögren's syndrome
Diffuse abnormalities in the posterior columns	B12D, ACD
Other	
No "occult" changes in the NAWM	NMO, Lyme disease, SID (except in NSLE)
Pontine lacunar infarcts	CADASIL, SVD

(Continued)

Table 4–1 Continued

Brain white matter	Disease
Dilation of Virchow-Robin spaces	HHC, PACNS
Diffuse lactate increase on brain MRS	MELAS
Meningeal enhancement	Susac's syndrome, PACNS, NBD, meningitis, Lyme disease, sarcoidosis
Hydrocephalus	Sarcoidosis
Absence of optic nerve lesions	PML
Regional atrophy	HHC (hippocampus and amygdala), NBD (brainstem)

ACD, acquired copper deficiency; ADEM, acute disseminated encephalomyelitis; AFL, adult forms of leukoencephalopathies; AMS, acute multiple sclerosis (Marburg type); B12D, vitamin B12 deficiency; BCS, Balo's concentric sclerosis; FD, Fabry's disease; HHC, hyperhomocysteinemia; HIVE, HIV encephalitis; HSE, herpes simplex encephalitis; MELAS, mitochondrial encephalopathy with lactic acidosis and stroke-like episodes; MRS, magnetic resonance spectroscopy; NAWM, normal-appearing white matter; NBD, Behçet's disease with CNS involvement; NMO, neuromyelitis optica; NSLE, neuropsychiatric systemic lupus erythematosus; PACNS, primary angiitis of the CNS; PML, progressive multifocal leukoencephalopathy; SID, systemic immune-mediated disease; SSP, subacute sclerosing panencephalitis; SVD, small vessel disease.

Adapted from Charil A, Yousry TA, Rovaris M, et al. MRI and the diagnosis of multiple sclerosis: expanding the concept of "no better explanation." Lancet Neurol; 5:841–852, 2006.[147]

head-injury workup. This scenario is commonly labeled "radiologically isolated syndrome" (RIS) to maintain some resemblance to the wording of CIS. However, RIS is a somewhat of a misnomer because these patients by definition do not have symptoms attributable to a demyelinating disease. Therefore, the term "syndrome" (symptom complex) is not really applicable. As with CIS, it is imperative to screen for MS mimickers in this population. In a preclinical MS study of 22 patients, 8 converted to clinically definite MS over an observation period of up 10 years.[78] In a similar cohort of 44 patients, radiological progression was identified in 59% of cases, but only 10 (22.8%) converted to either CIS or definite MS. The presence of contrast-enhancing lesions on the initial MRI was predictive of dissemination in time on repeat MRI.[79] One of the largest studies to date included 70 patients, with a clinical conversion rate of 33% during a mean follow-up period of 5.2 years.[80] Asymptomatic spinal cord lesions are especially strong predictors of conversion to MS: in 25 RIS cases with cervical cord lesions, 21 (84%) progressed clinically to CIS (n = 19) or PPMS (n = 2) over a median time of 1.6 years.[81] Although most RIS cases do not have any obvious neurological symptoms at presentation, some of the studies did uncover subtle but detectable findings on neurological examination[79] or via extensive cognitive testing, which clearly demonstrated cognitive abnormalities in RIS similar to MS.[82] RIS cases definitely need radiological and clinical follow-up, and treatment decisions should be considered if radiological or clinical conversion is confirmed and associated with a high-disability risk profile.

THE ROLE OF MRI IN TREATMENT DECISIONS

MRI has three main roles in the clinical management of MS: (1) it helps establish the diagnosis itself and exclude other diagnoses; (2) it clarifies risk of conversion to MS in CIS and RIS; and (3) it provides a glimpse at the inflammatory activity via gadolinium-enhanced scans, and at overall disease activity by comparing lesion-load changes at multiple time points, which aids in treatment initiation and upgrade decisions. CIS patients at high risk for conversion may be treated early, especially if the overall disability-risk profile also appears high (e.g., in the presence of many cord lesions, T1 black holes, brain atrophy, and/or T2 hypointense, deep gray nuclei). If the risk for conversion and the potential disability profile are low, a "wait-and-see" approach is preferable. In general, treatment decisions should always be individualized and customized to the given case. It is imperative to give patients sufficient information and seek their input. Educating patients can be time-consuming, but agreement and trust between patients and physicians are key components of patient care in complex chronic diseases like MS. It is important to remember that not all MS cases are universally disabling; benign MS is a well-recognized entity.[53] The pros and cons of early treatment versus watchful waiting and as-needed intervention[54–86] are discussed elsewhere in this book.

MRI also plays an important part in treatment monitoring and can help to determine treatment failure. In general, the currently available DMAs best address the active inflammatory stage of MS, evidenced by gadolinium-enhancing new lesion formation by MRI. If an untreated patient develops lesions, especially multiple lesions, treatment should begin. Increased inflammatory activity in an already-treated patient may indicate a need to upgrade to a stronger form of immunomodulation (e.g., from low-dose interferons or glatiramer acetate to high-dose interferons). Mitoxantrone and natalizumab are best for patients whose disease fails to stabilize on conventional injectable DMAs from the standpoint of MRI-detectable inflammatory profile. In progressive forms of MS, the currently available immunomodulatory therapies are largely ineffective. In the low proportion of SPMS cases with evidence of inflammatory activity on MRI, standard DMAs may provide some help. Advanced MRI can also clarify progression by demonstrating gradually decreased NAA levels, increased atrophy by MRI volumetry, and changes in normal-appearing white matter. Sadly, despite our ability to identify these changes, the currently available DMAs cannot meaningfully address the progressive "neurodegenerative" component of MS.

SPECIAL DIAGNOSTIC CONSIDERATIONS: MRI IN TUMEFACTIVE DEMYELINATION

As discussed in Chapter 2, a small but well-defined subset of CIS patients present with unusually large or tumefactive lesions. These lesions often present as neoplasms, metastatic lesions, or even abscesses. They are atypical lesions, often requiring biopsy for correct diagnosis. Obviously, it is very important to get the diagnosis right to administer appropriate treatment. Irradiation typically causes MS to become highly active and results in the formation of new lesions and severely damaged tissue. A few subtle features distinguish these lesions from neoplasms even on conventional MRI scans. T2 hypointense rims or arcs and open-ring enhancement are, in general, more suggestive of demyelination than competing etiologies (Fig. 4.6). However, similar hypointense rims and arcs also appear in neoplasms and in abscesses. In a larger study of ring-enhancing lesions, 54% of tumefactive MS lesions had T2 hypointense borders, 57% showing rims and 43% arcs. The hypointense borders may correspond with the location of macrophages in these lesions.[68,87]

One of the most sensitive methods available using conventional techniques is to examine lesion characteristics on diffusion-weighted images and ADC maps. These are part of the standard MS workup at several institutions, but even when not routinely performed, these sequences are certainly available and used daily in stroke workup. The behavior of peripheral ADC patterns at the lesion edge is the most informative. Peripheral restriction is more common in demyelination than in abscesses or tumors ($p = .006$), whereas central restriction is seen only in abscesses. In demyelination, restricted diffusion (low ADC, 33%), increased diffusion (high ADC, 60%), and normal diffusion (homogenously isointense, 7%) were seen in a recent study that included biopsy-proven demyelinating lesions.[87] On serial imaging, four of seven (57%) patients demonstrated changes in ADC patterns, and changes to ADC patterns were extremely uncommon in comparative abscess and neoplasm cohorts.

MRS of tumefactive MS lesions may show elevated choline, lactate, and lipid peaks and a decreased NAA peak. However, low-grade neoplasms also may demonstrate exactly the same spectrum. A changing MRS pattern over time may be more suggestive of demyelination than neoplasm, similar to the changing behavior on ADC maps.[88] An algorithm (Fig. 4.9) was also recently proposed for the evaluation of these masses using perfusion MRI, diffusion MRI, and MRS characteristics.[89]

ADVANCED MRI TECHNIQUES

It is beyond the scope of this chapter to provide a comprehensive review of all research

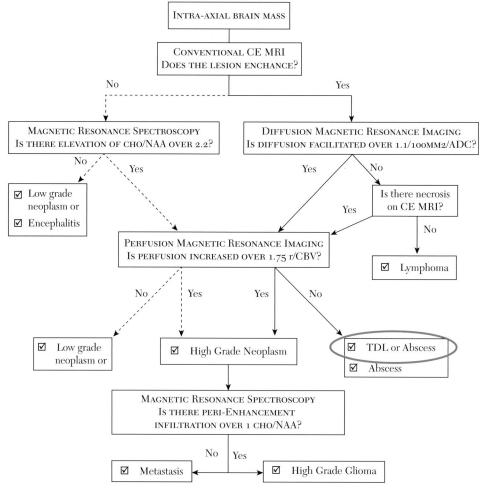

Figure 4–9. Proposed diagnostic algorithm of idiopathic intra-axial brain masses, including tumefactive demyelination (TDL). By a rational combination of postcontrast scans, MRS, and perfusion MRI, TDL and abscesses can be differentiated from masses of other etiology. Of note, ADC maps may be particularly useful for further differentiating TDL from abscesses. (Figure from Al-Okaili RN, Krejza J, Woo JH, et al. Intraaxial brain masses: MR imaging-based diagnostic strategy—initial experience. Radiology; 243:539–550, 2007.[89])

MRI sequences that are not yet available for routine clinical care. Many of these advanced MRI methods unfortunately may not find their way into clinical practice for a variety of reasons. These include lack of the required pulse sequences and postprocessing programs in the standard software package of scanners. These methods also require time- and labor-intensive postprocessing, as do most quantitative MRI methods such as volumetric scans to determine atrophy or volumetric lesion load, MTR histogram and map analysis, and DTI-based studies. Below we summarize the main applications of currently utilized research MRI methods in MS research, which may become available to practicing clinicians via clinical trials and research protocols.

Magnetization-Transfer Imaging

Magnetization-transfer imaging (MTI) was first performed in MS patients in the 1990s.[90] The physical principle behind MTI, the use of a saturation pulse directed at macromolecules such as myelin and subsequent transfer of magnetization to the mobile proton pool, has been known and used in nuclear magnetic resonance for decades. MTI is especially suited to study the influence of large macromolecules, including myelin, on their microenvironment. MT imaging is overall very sensitive to tissue integrity. The MT ratio decreases in lesional areas with the decrease proportionate to the magnitude of tissue abnormalities. MTR may normalize as part of normal lesion evolution[91,92] or may remain decreased.[92–94] The partial recovery of MTR may accompany tissue repair and remyelination, and as such, this pulse sequence is the focus of upcoming and current clinical trials trying to address neuroregeneration and remyelination.[95–98] MT-MRI is also a sensitive measure of nonlesional pathology observed in the NAWM and NAGM.[99–103] Changes in NAWM and NAGM are often detectable very early in MS and correlate, at least moderately, with future disability according to most[102–104] but not all[105] studies.

In addition to its use in brain imaging, MT imaging can also occur in the spinal cord.[106] MT-derived measures of cord pathology are especially important as biomarkers for progressive forms of MS, most of which present clinically as progressive myelopathies; however, cord lesion load, in general, shows only limited correlation with disability in these cases, whereas MT-MRI may be able to capture the progressive pathology and provide a quantitative measure of disease burden.

In contrast to MS and CIS, NAWM shows no abnormalities on MT-MRI in ADEM and NMO. Thus, MTI may be useful in distinguishing between MS and ADEM cases, although this observation requires further validation.[107]

Double-Inversion Recovery Imaging

DIR imaging is a relatively recent innovation in MS research. DIR is similar to FLAIR; it is a T2- or proton density-weighted sequence with two independent inversion recovery pulses, one in addition to the CSF-suppression pulse as in FLAIR. There is an additional pulse calibrated to suppress signal arising from normal white matter. This sequence has an inherently low signal-to-noise ratio but an excellent contrast-to-noise ratio to identify lesions. Although this aspect of DIR is rarely discussed, it is probably the most sensitive sequence to visualize "standard" white-matter lesions. In addition, it improves the detection of cortical lesions, especially leukocortical lesions. As per recent histology–MRI comparative studies, it captures only a fraction of cortical plaques when compared to histology, with an overall sensitivity of only 18% (Fig. 4.1).[108,109]

Diffusion-Weighted and Diffusion-Tensor Imaging

Diffusion-weighted MRI (DWI) and diffusion-tensor imaging (DTI) enable insight into the "degrees of freedom" of molecular water movement and provide information on tissue integrity and "diffusion directionality." DWI of the brain takes advantage of the tendency of water to diffuse more easily in directions parallel to fibers than perpendicular to them. Monitoring changes in free and restricted diffusion of water can identify various pathological processes, including stroke, ischemia, brain tumors, and white matter diseases. Several parameters have been used to describe numerically the tissue processes captured by DWI. One of the most important measures is the ADC, a measure of random displacement of water in a particular direction of interest. In general, the ADC of brain structures always tends to be lower than that of free water due to diffusion-limiting membranes, myelinated axons, and, overall, the directional organization of CNS tissue, especially in the white matter. A direction-independent measure of diffusion is the mean diffusivity index or D, also known as directionally averaged ADC. D is the average of the ADC measured in three orthogonal directions. Mean diffusivity is lower in coherently organized and higher in "disorganized" tissue. In normal-appearing brain tissue, increases in D and ADC have been observed in MS patients, consistent with subtle tissue damage.[110,111] The D and ADC tend to be higher in lesions than in NAWM and especially high in acute lesions. Subtle increases in D values often precede the appearance of gadolinium-enhancing lesions by a few weeks and may represent the earliest sign of the focal tissue abnormalities leading to lesion formation.[112]

DTI studies investigate the directional predominance of water movements and can be used for detailed tractography. A common DTI-derived measure is fractional anisotropy

(FA). FA can be considered a measure of directional restriction of tissue architecture from the standpoint of water diffusion. Higher FA represents more coherent tissue organization. Therefore, white-matter areas always have a higher FA than gray matter areas, especially in areas of neatly organized parallel fiber bundles. Fractional anisotropy in MS is often decreased in lesions, NAWM, and enhancing lesions.[113–117] Importantly, it can be lower in white matter not only as a result of white-matter lesions or NAWM pathology but also where fiber bundles cross. D and FA may change in opposite directions as a result of MS pathology, such that higher mean diffusivity and lower FA can be seen in lesions compared to NAWM; this is most prominent in lesions with extensive tissue damage, such as T1 black holes.[117–120]

Magnetic Resonance Spectroscopy

MRS allows insight into the biochemical ingredients of a studied voxel or voxels of interest *in vivo*. Studied nuclei most commonly include protons (^1H); studies of phosphorus and sodium also take place occasionally but require special hardware, including separate coils tuned to the appropriate frequencies at the given field strength. It is commonly done on single voxels as well as entire slices (chemical shift imaging) of MRS measures describing the entire brain. The spatial resolution of MRS is usually orders of magnitude lower than that of standard MR imaging, with voxel sizes rarely lower than 1 mL in human imaging.

MRS may be helpful in two critical ways from the standpoint of clinical patient care. First, it may help in the diagnosis of masslike lesions, including tumefactive demyelinating lesions, and second, it may serve as a useful surrogate marker in upcoming neuroprotective treatment trials. MRS markers provide partial insight into both demyelinating and axonal/neuronal pathologies and can also detect inflammation, gliosis, inflammatory infiltration, and changes related to ischemia. However, none of the changes detectable by MRS can be attributed to just one single, straightforward etiology.[92,121,122] In areas of active inflammation, the choline, lactate, and lipid peaks are often increased. Choline peak increase is considered a cell membrane turnover marker,

and its elevation may accompany immune cell infiltration, demyelination and remyelination, and gliosis. Myo-inositol is frequently viewed as a marker of gliosis. Creatinine is classically considered as the "standard peak" that is not changed in most CNS pathological conditions; however, several studies have demonstrated that creatinine can and does change even in MS in certain disease stages and location. With the universal availability of quantitative "absolute spectroscopy" that provides actual numerical concentration values as opposed to metabolite ratios to characterize metabolic alterations, the use of creatinine as the "standard peak" may no longer be needed, depending on the application.

Areas of axonal and neuronal damage or dysfunction may reveal a relative decrease of NAA. NAA decrease may indicate a metabolic abnormality and not necessarily irreversible axonal loss or neuronal damage. Selective serotonin reuptake inhibitors may result in increased NAA concentration in MS patients' CNS; similar observations have been made in neurodegenerative diseases and animal models.[123] NAA may become an especially intriguing marker with the recent interest in progressive forms of MS and in upcoming restorative therapies. Its changes may reflect axonal and neuronal dysfunction; however, controversy remains about the overall role of this metabolite. The classic dogma is that NAA is an osmotic regulator of neurons and axons. A novel hypothesis suggests that NAA serves as a glutamate reservoir and may be converted into glutamate in an energetically favorable set of reactions that also produce NADH. Glutamate is needed for neuronal function and survival and is also utilized by astrocytes and oligodendrocytes, while NADH may serve as an additional energy reservoir for these metabolically active cells.[124]

Volumetric Studies of the Brain and Spinal Cord in Multiple Sclerosis

MRI readily detects brain and spinal cord atrophy, some of the strongest measures that correlate with disability.[125–129] While it is easy to recognize atrophy on a scan by observation alone, currently there are no fully reliable automated methods to generate atrophy information that could be readily reported to practicing clinicians. However, this is routinely done in the context of research studies and clinical trials. Atrophy is most prominent in the progressive stage of advanced MS, but it is also detectable in the initial stage, both in the cortex as well as in the deep gray nuclei, most notably the thalamus. In addition, atrophy continues even when new lesion formation and gadolinium enhancement are no longer detectable in progressive MS and is, overall, at least partially independent of lesion load in most studies.[130–134] MS-related atrophy includes both gray and white matter loss, with the potential predominance of gray-matter atrophy emerging in more recent studies.[18,135] The disease stage may also determine where atrophy is most prominent. Cortical atrophy predominates early on, whereas in advanced cases, especially in SPMS, white-matter atrophy may be significant. Several publications report progressive gray-matter atrophy in the early years of MS.[136–138]

Field Strength and MRI

Over the past 5 to 10 years, higher-field-strength systems have become available at a growing number of centers, including 3 Tesla and, at many institutions, up to 7 Tesla for human imaging. It is important to note that the current FDA approval of imaging systems goes up to 4 Tesla; therefore, higher-Tesla scanners can be used only for research and not for current patient care. In general, higher field strength results in a higher signal-to-noise ratio, which enables higher resolution acquisition in less time by reducing the need for oversampling, and allows for a better contrast-to-noise ratio in some studies. However, the relaxation properties are different at higher field strength, and several artifacts appear that are of no relevance in lower-field-strength studies, most notoriously pronounced susceptibility-based artifacts. Higher-field-strength MRI systems may also induce undesired changes to physiology such as myoclonic activity due to eddy currents, excessive energy (heat) absorption in the tissue, and others. It becomes critically important to monitor the specific absorption rate at these higher field strengths and to use pulse sequences that allow for the acquisition of the desired "weightedness" without overstepping specific absorption rate boundaries.

MRI IN NON-MS DEMYELINATING DISEASES

Acute Disseminated Encephalomyelitis

The hallmark of ADEM is perivenous demyelination. Overall, ADEM remains relatively poorly defined compared to MS or NMO. Although discussed extensively in a clinical context in Chapter 2, we discuss the relevant MRI features further here. It usually presents in children as a one-time postinfectious demyelinating condition following the trigger event by 2 to 4 weeks. It almost always correlates with encephalopathy, pyramidal signs, hemiplegia, spinal cord involvement, seizures, and aphasia. Less commonly, optic neuritis or other cranial neuropathies may be present.[11] While relapsing forms have been described in specific cases, especially in children, they tend to be in the same stage of lesion formation from the standpoint of time. They often include not only white but also gray matter structures, and unlike MS, they often do not show gadolinium enhancement upon initial presentation.

A recent classification suggestion of ADEM[11] proposed four patterns of cerebral involvement to describe the MRI findings: (1) ADEM with small lesions (<5 mm); (2) ADEM with large, confluent, or tumefactive lesions, with frequent extensive perilesional edema and mass effect; (3) ADEM with additional symmetric bithalamic involvement; and (4) acute hemorrhagic encephalomyelitis (AHEM) or acute hemorrhagic leukoencephalitis (AHLE), where T2 hypointensities are detected within the T2 hyperintense areas, suggestive of the presence of blood or blood degradation products (Fig. 4.10). Of note, it is unclear if all the above patterns truly represent ADEM, other leukoencephalopathies, or simply pediatric MS, which presents with a different MRI appearance than is typical in adults, especially in children before puberty. In contrast to MS, advanced MRI markers of normal-appearing white and gray matter tend not to show abnormalities in ADEM. An international study of ADEM proposed the following three ADEM diagnostic criteria: atypical clinical symptoms for MS, absence of oligoclonal bands, and gray matter involvement[139] (see detailed discussion in Chapter 2). These criteria must be

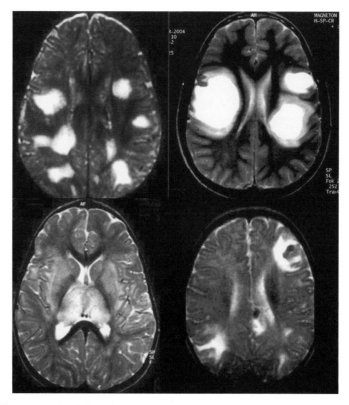

Figure 4–10. The four proposed radiological presentations of ADEM, clockwise from top left: (1) multiple white matter lesions; (2) tumefactive presentation; (3) acute hemorrhagic encephalomyelitis (AHEM); (4) bilateral thalamic involvement.

evaluated in a prospective cohort of ADEM cases and may be modified in the future. More recently, an important study related to pediatric MS and ADEM attempted to differentiate the two often very confusing entities. They suggest that any two of the following criteria must be present to distinguish MS from ADEM: (1) absence of a diffuse bilateral lesion pattern; (2) presence of T1 black holes; and (3) presence of two or more periventricular lesions. As per the authors, MS patients at first attack could be distinguished from monophasic ADEM patients with 81% sensitivity and 95% specificity using these criteria.[140] Another group reviewed the above criteria and called it the best compromise for ADEM/MS differentiation with its sensitivity of 75% and specificity of 95% in their cohort, compared to the KIDMUS criteria of 11% sensitivity with 100% specificity, versus 61% sensitivity and 91% specificity of the Barkhof-Fazekas criteria.

Neuro-myelitis Optica

Although NMO was considered for decades as a "variant of MS," recent research has completely redefined this disease and concluded that it has different epidemiology, pathology, radiological findings, and response to therapy than classic MS. A group recently identified the serum marker NMO IgG seen in up to 80% of all cases; when seen, it is virtually pathognomonic for NMO (specificity close to 100%).[141,142] It is likely that NMO IgG is actually pathogenic in the right environment and not just a biomarker.[143] It is both surprising and significant that NMO's marker antibody is unrelated to myelin or oligodendrocytes but is about a water channel on astrocytic end-feet. This is a new direction in demyelinating disease research. NMO is now considered a disease primarily targeting astrocytes. The presence of demyelination is the only remaining commonality between MS and NMO spectrum disorders.

However, NMO lesions usually account for more tissue destruction than MS lesions. NMO pathology involves very characteristic elements never seen in MS such as eosinophilic infiltration, loss of aquaporin-4 staining in lesions (vs. upregulation of aquaporin-4 immunoreactivity in MS lesions), and nonlesional pathology in normally aquaporin-4-rich areas characterized by aquaporin-4 loss without severe inflammation. Hence, we use the term "aquaporinopathy" in Chapter 2 to describe NMO spectrum disorders.

It is critically important to differentiate NMO from MS. NMO not only responds poorly to standard MS DMAs but may even worsen on interferon therapy. However, it shows a reasonable response to immunosuppressive medications and to agents that selectively suppress or modify B-cell function and/or antibody production. Investigators proposed carefully considered diagnostic criteria in 1999, which were subsequently modified and simplified.[5,9] MRI findings, including the presence of a longitudinally extensive cord lesion over three or more spinal cord segments, are integral to the criteria (Fig. 4.11). Of note, while not part of the criteria, optic nerve lesions also tend to be "longitudinally extensive" and often cross the optic chiasm, a feature that would be unusual in MS-related optic neuritis. Active NMO spinal cord lesions often appear to have a mass effect ("swollen cord" appearance) and can be mistaken for cord infarcts or tumors. Unlike MS, NMO cord lesions on axial scans may involve more than half of the cord cross-cut surface area, including gray and white matter areas, and they most often involve central cord areas. In up to 10% of cases at initial presentation, an unusual pattern may be seen in the diencephalon and brainstem lesions, which may include the hypothalamus and areas adjacent to the fourth ventricle. Interestingly, the above-mentioned brain areas have a high density of aquaporin-4, the antigen recognized by NMO IgG,[144,145] as illustrated in Chapter 2. NAWM and NAGM abnormalities are less common in NMO[68,146] and appear to involve only areas directly hit by active disease, such as the corticospinal tract as well as the optic radiation. The reader is encouraged to review Chapter 2 for more clinical detail on aquaporinopathies or NMO spectrum disorders.

SUMMARY

MRI of the brain and spinal cord is the single most important paraclinical marker of demyelinating diseases. MRI-based markers are routinely used in the diagnosis, differential diagnosis, prognosis, and monitoring of common white-matter diseases. MRI also provides a very useful aid to treatment monitoring and planning. In MRI research, a growing number of advanced techniques have revolutionized our understanding of MS and other inflammatory demyelinating diseases. However, despite the very obvious advances that neuroimaging

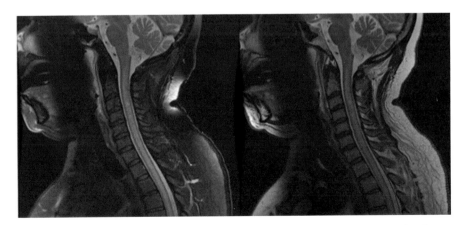

Figure 4–11. Longitudinally extensive transverse myelitis (LETM) in the context of NMO. Note that the entire visualized cord demonstrates T2 hyperintense signal change, which is mainly centrally located and gives rise to a "swollen cord" appearance. All these are very typical for NMO.

has brought to the field of clinical neuroimmu-nology, one must remember the relative lack of specificity of standard MRI techniques. No paraclinical diagnostic modality can replace solid clinical judgment, but MRI represents an important supplement to the decision-making process.

REFERENCES

1. Noseworthy JH, Lucchinetti C, Rodriguez M, Weinshenker BG. Multiple sclerosis. N Engl J Med; 343:938–952, 2000.
2. McDonald WI, Compston A, Edan G, et al. Recommended diagnostic criteria for multiple sclerosis: guidelines from the International Panel on the diagnosis of multiple sclerosis. Ann Neurol; 50:121–127, 2001.
3. Polman CH, Reingold SC, Edan G, et al. Diagnostic criteria for multiple sclerosis: 2005 revisions to the "McDonald Criteria." Ann Neurol; 58:840–846, 2005.
4. Polman CH, Reingold SC, Banwell B, et al. Diagnostic criteria for multiple sclerosis: 2010 revisions to the McDonald criteria. Ann Neurol; 69:292–302, 2011.
5. Morrissey SP, Miller DH, Kendall BE, et al. The significance of brain magnetic resonance imaging abnormalities at presentation with clinically isolated syndromes suggestive of multiple sclerosis. A 5-year follow-up study. Brain; 116 (Pt 1):135–146, 1993.
6. Brex PA, Ciccarelli O, O'Riordan JI, Sailer M, Thompson AJ, Miller DH. A longitudinal study of abnormalities on MRI and disability from multiple sclerosis. N Engl J Med; 346:158–164, 2002.
7. O'Riordan JI, Thompson AJ, Kingsley DP, et al. The prognostic value of brain MRI in clinically isolated syndromes of the CNS. A 10-year follow-up. Brain; 121 (Pt 3):495–503, 1998.
8. Wingerchuk DM, Hogancamp WF, O'Brien PC, Weinshenker BG. The clinical course of neuromyelitis optica (Devic's syndrome). Neurology; 53:1107–1114, 1999.
9. Wingerchuk DM, Lennon VA, Pittock SJ, Lucchinetti CF, Weinshenker BG. Revised diagnostic criteria for neuromyelitis optica. Neurology; 66:1485–1489, 2006.
10. Callen DJ, Shroff MM, Branson HM, et al. MRI in the diagnosis of pediatric multiple sclerosis. Neurology; 72:961–967, 2009.
11. Tenembaum S, Chitnis T, Ness J, Hahn JS. Acute disseminated encephalomyelitis. Neurology; 68:S23–S36, 2007.
12. Daumer M, Neuhaus A, Morrissey S, Hintzen R, Ebers GC. MRI as an outcome in multiple sclerosis clinical trials. Neurology; 72:705–711, 2009.
13. Paty DW, Li DK. Interferon beta-1b is effective in relapsing-remitting multiple sclerosis. II. MRI analysis results of a multicenter, randomized, double-blind, placebo-controlled trial. UBC MS/MRI Study Group and the IFNB Multiple Sclerosis Study Group. Neurology; 43:662–667, 1993.
14. Polman CH, Reingold SC, Banwell B, et al. Diagnostic criteria for multiple sclerosis: 2010 revisions to the McDonald criteria. Ann Neurol; 69:292–302, 2011.
15. Zivadinov R, Leist TP. Clinical-magnetic resonance imaging correlations in multiple sclerosis. J Neuroimaging; 15:10S–21S, 2005.
16. Molyneux PD, Filippi M, Barkhof F, et al. Correlations between monthly enhanced MRI lesion rate and changes in T2 lesion volume in multiple sclerosis. Ann Neurol; 43:332–339, 1998.
17. Sailer M, O'Riordan JI, Thompson AJ, et al. Quantitative MRI in patients with clinically isolated syndromes suggestive of demyelination. Neurology; 52:599–606, 1999.
18. Pirko I, Lucchinetti CF, Sriram S, Bakshi R. Gray matter involvement in multiple sclerosis. Neurology; 68:634–642, 2007.
19. Filippi M, Yousry T, Baratti C, et al. Quantitative assessment of MRI lesion load in multiple sclerosis. A comparison of conventional spin-echo with fast fluid-attenuated inversion recovery. Brain; 119 (Pt 4):1349–1355, 1996.
20. Stevenson VL, Gawne-Cain ML, Barker GJ, Thompson AJ, Miller DH. Imaging of the spinal cord and brain in multiple sclerosis: a comparative study between fast FLAIR and fast spin echo. J Neurol; 244:119–124, 1997.
21. Moseley IF, Miller DH, Gass A. The contribution of magnetic resonance imaging to the assessment of optic nerve and spinal cord involvement in multiple sclerosis. J Neurol Neurosurg Psychiatry; 64 Suppl 1:S15–S20, 1998.
22. Bot JC, Barkhof F, Lycklama a Nijeholt GJ, et al. Comparison of a conventional cardiac-triggered dual spin-echo and a fast STIR sequence in detection of spinal cord lesions in multiple sclerosis. Eur Radiol; 10:753–758, 2000.
23. Moseley IF, Miller DH, Gass A. The contribution of magnetic resonance imaging to the assessment of optic nerve and spinal cord involvement in multiple sclerosis. J Neurol Neurosurg Psychiatry; 64 Suppl 1:S15–S20, 1998.
24. Campi A, Pontesilli S, Gerevini S, Scotti G. Comparison of MRI pulse sequences for investigation of lesions of the cervical spinal cord. Neuroradiology; 42:669–675, 2000.
25. Grimaud J, Millar J, Thorpe JW, Moseley IF, McDonald WI, Miller DH. Signal intensity on MRI of basal ganglia in multiple sclerosis. J Neurol Neurosurg Psychiatry; 59:306–308, 1995.
26. Bakshi R, Dmochowski J, Shaikh ZA, Jacobs L. Gray matter T2 hypointensity is related to plaques and atrophy in the brains of multiple sclerosis patients. J Neurol Sci; 185:19–26, 2001.
27. Tjoa CW, Benedict RH, Weinstock-Guttman B, Fabiano AJ, Bakshi R. MRI T2 hypointensity of the dentate nucleus is related to ambulatory impairment in multiple sclerosis. J Neurol Sci; 234:17–24, 2005.
28. Bakshi R, Benedict RH, Bermel RA, et al. T2 hypointensity in the deep gray matter of patients with multiple sclerosis: a quantitative magnetic resonance imaging study. Arch Neurol; 59:62–68, 2002.
29. Bermel RA, Puli SR, Rudick RA, et al. Prediction of longitudinal brain atrophy in multiple sclerosis by gray matter magnetic resonance imaging T2 hypointensity. Arch Neurol; 62:1371–1376, 2005.
30. Haacke EM, Ayaz M, Khan A, et al. Establishing a baseline phase behavior in magnetic resonance imaging to determine normal vs. abnormal iron content in the brain. J Magn Reson Imaging; 26:256–264, 2007.

31. Uhlenbrock D, Sehlen S. The value of T1-weighted images in the differentiation between MS, white matter lesions, and subcortical arteriosclerotic encephalopathy (SAE). Neuroradiology; 31:203–212, 1989.

32. Levesque I, Sled JG, Narayanan S, et al. The role of edema and demyelination in chronic T1 black holes: a quantitative magnetization transfer study. J Magn Reson Imaging; 21:103–110, 2005.

33. Bagnato F, Jeffries N, Richert ND, et al. Evolution of T1 black holes in patients with multiple sclerosis imaged monthly for 4 years. Brain; 126:1782–1789, 2003.

34. Brex PA, Molyneux PD, Smiddy P, et al. The effect of IFNbeta-1b on the evolution of enhancing lesions in secondary progressive MS. Neurology; 57:2185–2190, 2001.

35. Losseff NA, Miller DH, Kidd D, Thompson AJ. The predictive value of gadolinium enhancement for long-term disability in relapsing-remitting multiple sclerosis—preliminary results. Mult Scler; 7:23–25, 2001.

36. van Waesberghe JH, Kamphorst W, De Groot CJ, et al. Axonal loss in multiple sclerosis lesions: magnetic resonance imaging insights into substrates of disability. Ann Neurol; 46:747–754, 1999.

37. van Walderveen MA, Kamphorst W, Scheltens P, et al. Histopathologic correlate of hypointense lesions on T1-weighted spin-echo MRI in multiple sclerosis. Neurology; 50:1282–1288, 1998.

38. Bitsch A, Kuhlmann T, Stadelmann C, Lassmann H, Lucchinetti C, Bruck W. A longitudinal MRI study of histopathologically defined hypointense multiple sclerosis lesions. Ann Neurol; 49:793–796, 2001.

39. van Walderveen MA, Lycklama ANGJ, Ader HJ, et al. Hypointense lesions on T1-weighted spin-echo magnetic resonance imaging: relation to clinical characteristics in subgroups of patients with multiple sclerosis. Arch Neurol; 58:76–81, 2001.

40. van Walderveen MA, Barkhof F, Hommes OR, et al. Correlating MRI and clinical disease activity in multiple sclerosis: relevance of hypointense lesions on short-TR/short-TE (T1-weighted) spin-echo images. Neurology; 45:1684–1690, 1995.

41. Truyen L, van Waesberghe JH, van Walderveen MA, et al. Accumulation of hypointense lesions ("black holes") on T1 spin-echo MRI correlates with disease progression in multiple sclerosis. Neurology; 47:1469–1476, 1996.

42. Losseff NA, Wang L, Miller DH, Thompson AJ. T1 hypointensity of the spinal cord in multiple sclerosis. J Neurol; 248:517–521, 2001.

43. Hiehle JF, Jr., Grossman RI, Ramer KN, Gonzalez-Scarano F, Cohen JA. Magnetization transfer effects in MR-detected multiple sclerosis lesions: comparison with gadolinium-enhanced spin-echo images and nonenhanced T1-weighted images. AJNR Am J Neuroradiol; 16:69–77, 1995.

44. Brex PA, Parker GJ, Leary SM, et al. Lesion heterogeneity in multiple sclerosis: a study of the relations between appearances on T1 weighted images, T1 relaxation times, and metabolite concentrations. J Neurol Neurosurg Psychiatry; 68:627–632, 2000.

45. Pirko I, Nolan TK, Holland SK, Johnson AJ. Multiple sclerosis: pathogenesis and MR imaging features of T1 hypointensities in murine model. Radiology; 246:790–795, 2008.

46. Janardhan V, Suri S, Bakshi R. Multiple sclerosis: hyperintense lesions in the brain on nonenhanced T1-weighted MR images evidenced as areas of T1 shortening. Radiology; 244:823–831, 2007.

47. Pirko I, Johnson A, Ciric B, et al. In vivo magnetic resonance imaging of immune cells in the central nervous system with superparamagnetic antibodies. Faseb J; 18:179–182, 2004.

48. Pirko I, Fricke ST, Johnson AJ, Rodriguez M, Macura SI. Magnetic resonance imaging, microscopy, and spectroscopy of the central nervous system in experimental animals. NeuroRx; 2:250–264, 2005.

49. Dousset V, Brochet B, Deloire MS, et al. MR imaging of relapsing multiple sclerosis patients using ultra-small-particle iron oxide and compared with gadolinium. AJNR Am J Neuroradiol; 27:1000–1005, 2006.

50. Vellinga MM, Oude Engberink RD, Seewann A, et al. Pluriformity of inflammation in multiple sclerosis shown by ultra-small iron oxide particle enhancement. Brain; 131:800–807, 2008.

51. Silver N, Lai M, Symms M, Barker G, McDonald I, Miller D. Serial gadolinium-enhanced and magnetization transfer imaging to investigate the relationship between the duration of blood–brain barrier disruption and extent of demyelination in new multiple sclerosis lesions. J Neurol; 246:728–730, 1999.

52. Thompson AJ, Miller D, Youl B, et al. Serial gadolinium-enhanced MRI in relapsing/remitting multiple sclerosis of varying disease duration. Neurology; 42:60–63, 1992.

53. Kappos L, Moeri D, Radue EW, et al. Predictive value of gadolinium-enhanced magnetic resonance imaging for relapse rate and changes in disability or impairment in multiple sclerosis: a meta-analysis. Gadolinium MRI Meta-analysis Group. Lancet; 353:964–969, 1999.

54. Miller DH, Rudge P, Johnson G, et al. Serial gadolinium enhanced magnetic resonance imaging in multiple sclerosis. Brain; 111 (Pt 4):927–939, 1988.

55. Cotton F, Weiner HL, Jolesz FA, Guttmann CR. MRI contrast uptake in new lesions in relapsing-remitting MS followed at weekly intervals. Neurology; 60:640–646, 2003.

56. Kidd D, Thorpe JW, Kendall BE, et al. MRI dynamics of brain and spinal cord in progressive multiple sclerosis. J Neurol Neurosurg Psychiatry; 60:15–19, 1996.

57. Tubridy N, Coles AJ, Molyneux P, et al. Secondary progressive multiple sclerosis: the relationship between short-term MRI activity and clinical features. Brain; 121 (Pt 2):225–231, 1998.

58. Thompson AJ, Kermode AG, Wicks D, et al. Major differences in the dynamics of primary and secondary progressive multiple sclerosis. Ann Neurol; 29:53–62, 1991.

59. Ingle GT, Sastre-Garriga J, Miller DH, Thompson AJ. Is inflammation important in early PPMS? A longitudinal MRI study. J Neurol Neurosurg Psychiatry; 76:1255–1258, 2005.

60. Thorpe JW, Kidd D, Moseley IF, et al. Serial gadolinium-enhanced MRI of the brain and spinal cord in early relapsing-remitting multiple sclerosis. Neurology; 46:373–378, 1996.

61. Grossman RI, Braffman BH, Brorson JR, Goldberg HI, Silberberg DH, Gonzalez-Scarano F. Multiple sclerosis: serial study of gadolinium-enhanced MR imaging. Radiology; 169:117–122, 1988.

62. Grossman RI, Gonzalez-Scarano F, Atlas SW, Galetta S, Silberberg DH. Multiple sclerosis: gadolinium enhancement in MR imaging. Radiology; 161:721–725, 1986.

63. Masdeu JC, Moreira J, Trasi S, Visintainer P, Cavaliere R, Grundman M. The open ring. A new imaging sign in demyelinating disease. J Neuroimaging; 6:104–107, 1996.

64. Masdeu JC, Quinto C, Olivera C, Tenner M, Leslie D, Visintainer P. Open-ring imaging sign: highly specific for atypical brain demyelination. Neurology; 54:1427–1433, 2000.

65. Minneboo A, Uitdehaag BM, Ader HJ, Barkhof F, Polman CH, Castelijns JA. Patterns of enhancing lesion evolution in multiple sclerosis are uniform within patients. Neurology; 65:56–61, 2005.

66. Leist TP, Gobbini MI, Frank JA, McFarland HF. Enhancing magnetic resonance imaging lesions and cerebral atrophy in patients with relapsing multiple sclerosis. Arch Neurol; 58:57–60, 2001.

67. Morgen K, Jeffries NO, Stone R, et al. Ring-enhancement in multiple sclerosis: marker of disease severity. Mult Scler; 7:167–171, 2001.

68. Schwartz KM, Erickson BJ, Lucchinetti C. Pattern of T2 hypointensity associated with ring-enhancing brain lesions can help to differentiate pathology. Neuroradiology; 48:143–149, 2006.

69. Polman CH, Reingold SC, Edan G, et al. Diagnostic criteria for multiple sclerosis: 2005 revisions to the "McDonald Criteria." Ann Neurol; 58:840–846, 2005.

70. Gean-Marton AD, Vezina LG, Marton KI, et al. Abnormal corpus callosum: a sensitive and specific indicator of multiple sclerosis. Radiology; 180:215–221, 1991.

71. Offenbacher H, Fazekas F, Schmidt R, et al. Assessment of MRI criteria for a diagnosis of MS. Neurology; 43:905–909, 1993.

72. Bot JC, Barkhof F, Lycklama a Nijeholt G, et al. Differentiation of multiple sclerosis from other inflammatory disorders and cerebrovascular disease: value of spinal MR imaging. Radiology; 223:46–56, 2002.

73. Rovira A, Swanton J, Tintore M, et al. A single, early magnetic resonance imaging study in the diagnosis of multiple sclerosis. Arch Neurol; 66:587–592, 2009.

74. Montalban X, Tintore M, Swanton J, et al. MRI criteria for MS in patients with clinically isolated syndromes. Neurology; 74:427–434, 2010.

75. Charil A, Yousry TA, Rovaris M, et al. MRI and the diagnosis of multiple sclerosis: expanding the concept of "no better explanation." Lancet Neurol; 5:841–852, 2006.

76. Chard DT, Brex PA, Ciccarelli O, et al. The longitudinal relation between brain lesion load and atrophy in multiple sclerosis: a 14-year follow-up study. J Neurol Neurosurg Psychiatry; 74:1551–1554, 2003.

77. Fisniku LK, Brex PA, Altmann DR, et al. Disability and T2 MRI lesions: a 20-year follow-up of patients with relapse onset of multiple sclerosis. Brain; 131:808–817, 2008.

78. Siva A, Saip S, Altintas A, Jacob A, Keegan BM, Kantarci OH. Multiple sclerosis risk in radiologically uncovered asymptomatic possible inflammatory-demyelinating disease. Mult Scler; 15:918–927, 2009.

79. Okuda DT, Mowry EM, Beheshtian A, et al. Incidental MRI anomalies suggestive of multiple sclerosis: the radiologically isolated syndrome. Neurology; 72:800–805, 2009.

80. Lebrun C, Bensa C, Debouverie M, et al. Association between clinical conversion to multiple sclerosis in radiologically isolated syndrome and magnetic resonance imaging, cerebrospinal fluid, and visual evoked potential: follow-up of 70 patients. Arch Neurol; 66:841–846, 2009.

81. Okuda DT, Mowry EM, Cree BA, et al. Asymptomatic spinal cord lesions predict disease progression in radiologically isolated syndrome. Neurology; 76:686–692, 2011.

82. Lebrun C, Blanc F, Brassat D, Zephir H, de Seze J; CFSEP. Cognitive function in radiologically isolated syndrome. Mult Scler; 16:919–925, 2010.

83. Pittock SJ, McClelland RL, Mayr WT, et al. Clinical implications of benign multiple sclerosis: a 20-year population-based follow-up study. Ann Neurol; 56:303–306, 2004.

84. Pittock SJ, Weinshenker BG, Noseworthy JH, et al. Not every patient with multiple sclerosis should be treated at time of diagnosis. Arch Neurol; 63:611–614, 2006.

85. Wingerchuk DM. Current evidence and therapeutic strategies for multiple sclerosis. Semin Neurol; 28:56–68, 2008.

86. Frohman EM, Havrdova E, Lublin F, et al. Most patients with multiple sclerosis or a clinically isolated demyelinating syndrome should be treated at the time of diagnosis. Arch Neurol; 63:614–619, 2006.

87. Abou Zeid N, Pirko I, Erickson B, et al. Diffusion-weighted imaging characteristics of biopsy-proven demyelinating brain lesions. Neurology; 78:1655–1662, 2012.

88. Butteriss DJ, Ismail A, Ellison DW, Birchall D. Use of serial proton magnetic resonance spectroscopy to differentiate low-grade glioma from tumefactive plaque in a patient with multiple sclerosis. Br J Radiol; 76:662–665, 2003.

89. Al-Okaili RN, Krejza J, Woo JH, et al. Intraaxial brain masses: MR imaging-based diagnostic strategy—initial experience. Radiology; 243:539–550, 2007.

90. Dousset V, Grossman RI, Ramer KN, et al. Experimental allergic encephalomyelitis and multiple sclerosis: lesion characterization with magnetization transfer imaging. Radiology; 182:483–491, 1992.

91. Filippi M, Rocca MA. Magnetization transfer magnetic resonance imaging in the assessment of neurological diseases. J Neuroimaging; 14:303–313, 2004.

92. Inglese M, Grossman RI, Filippi M. Magnetic resonance imaging monitoring of multiple sclerosis lesion evolution. J Neuroimaging; 15:22S–29S, 2005.

93. Dousset V, Gayou A, Brochet B, Caille JM. Early structural changes in acute MS lesions assessed by serial magnetization transfer studies. Neurology; 51:1150–1155, 1998.

94. Oreja-Guevara C, Charil A, Caputo D, Cavarretta R, Sormani MP, Filippi M. Magnetization transfer magnetic resonance imaging and clinical changes in patients with relapsing-remitting multiple sclerosis. Arch Neurol; 63:736–740, 2006.

95. Barkhof F, Bruck W, De Groot CJ, et al. Remyelinated lesions in multiple sclerosis: magnetic resonance image appearance. Arch Neurol; 60:1073–1081, 2003.

96. Schmierer K, Scaravilli F, Altmann DR, Barker GJ, Miller DH. Magnetization transfer ratio and myelin

in postmortem multiple sclerosis brain. Ann Neurol; 56:407–415, 2004.

97. Gass A, Barker GJ, Kidd D, et al. Correlation of magnetization transfer ratio with clinical disability in multiple sclerosis. Ann Neurol; 36:62–67, 1994.

98. Rovaris M, Viti B, Ciboddo G, et al. Brain involvement in systemic immune mediated diseases: magnetic resonance and magnetisation transfer imaging study. J Neurol Neurosurg Psychiatry; 68:170–177, 2000.

99. Filippi M, Iannucci G, Tortorella C, et al. Comparison of MS clinical phenotypes using conventional and magnetization transfer MRI. Neurology; 52:588–594, 1999.

100. Chen JT, Collins DL, Freedman MS, Atkins HL, Arnold DL. Local magnetization transfer ratio signal inhomogeneity is related to subsequent change in MTR in lesions and normal-appearing white-matter of multiple sclerosis patients. Neuroimage; 25:1272–1278, 2005.

101. Laule C, Vavasour IM, Whittall KP, et al. Evolution of focal and diffuse magnetisation transfer abnormalities in multiple sclerosis. J Neurol; 250:924–931, 2003.

102. Rovaris M, Agosta F, Sormani MP, et al. Conventional and magnetization transfer MRI predictors of clinical multiple sclerosis evolution: a medium-term follow-up study. Brain; 126:2323–2332, 2003.

103. Santos AC, Narayanan S, de Stefano N, et al. Magnetization transfer can predict clinical evolution in patients with multiple sclerosis. J Neurol; 249:662–668, 2002.

104. Traboulsee A, Dehmeshki J, Brex PA, et al. Normal-appearing brain tissue MTR histograms in clinically isolated syndromes suggestive of MS. Neurology; 59:126–128, 2002.

105. Rocca MA, Agosta F, Sormani MP, et al. A three-year, multi-parametric MRI study in patients at presentation with CIS. J Neurol, 2008.

106. Bot JC, Blezer EL, Kamphorst W, et al. The spinal cord in multiple sclerosis: relationship of high-spatial-resolution quantitative MR imaging findings to histopathologic results. Radiology; 233:531–540, 2004.

107. Inglese M, Salvi F, Iannucci G, Mancardi GL, Mascalchi M, Filippi M. Magnetization transfer and diffusion tensor MR imaging of acute disseminated encephalomyelitis. AJNR Am J Neuroradiol; 23:267–272, 2002.

108. Geurts JJ, Pouwels PJ, Uitdehaag BM, Polman CH, Barkhof F, Castelijns JA. Intracortical lesions in multiple sclerosis: improved detection with 3D double inversion-recovery MR imaging. Radiology; 236:254–260, 2005.

109. Seewann A, Kooi EJ, Roosendaal SD, et al. Postmortem verification of MS cortical lesion detection with 3D DIR. Neurology; 78:302–308, 2012.

110. Cercignani M, Bozzali M, Iannucci G, Comi G, Filippi M. Magnetisation transfer ratio and mean diffusivity of normal appearing white and grey matter from patients with multiple sclerosis. J Neurol Neurosurg Psychiatry; 70:311–317, 2001.

111. Cercignani M, Inglese M, Pagani E, Comi G, Filippi M. Mean diffusivity and fractional anisotropy histograms of patients with multiple sclerosis. AJNR Am J Neuroradiol; 22:952–958, 2001.

112. Rocca MA, Cercignani M, Iannucci G, Comi G, Filippi M. Weekly diffusion-weighted imaging of normal-appearing white matter in MS. Neurology; 55:882–884, 2000.

113. Griffin CM, Chard DT, Ciccarelli O, et al. Diffusion tensor imaging in early relapsing-remitting multiple sclerosis. Mult Scler; 7:290–297, 2001.

114. Ciccarelli O, Werring DJ, Wheeler-Kingshott CA, et al. Investigation of MS normal-appearing brain using diffusion tensor MRI with clinical correlations. Neurology; 56:926–933, 2001.

115. Ciccarelli O, Parker GJ, Toosy AT, et al. From diffusion tractography to quantitative white matter tract measures: a reproducibility study. Neuroimage; 18:348–359, 2003.

116. Ciccarelli O, Toosy AT, Hickman SJ, et al. Optic radiation changes after optic neuritis detected by tractography-based group mapping. Hum Brain Mapp; 25:308–316, 2005.

117. Werring DJ, Clark CA, Barker GJ, Thompson AJ, Miller DH. Diffusion tensor imaging of lesions and normal-appearing white matter in multiple sclerosis. Neurology; 52:1626–1632, 1999.

118. Filippi M, Cercignani M, Inglese M, Horsfield MA, Comi G. Diffusion tensor magnetic resonance imaging in multiple sclerosis. Neurology; 56:304–311, 2001.

119. Rovaris M, Gass A, Bammer R, et al. Diffusion MRI in multiple sclerosis. Neurology; 65:1526–1532, 2005.

120. Rovaris M, Filippi M. Diffusion tensor MRI in multiple sclerosis. J Neuroimaging; 17 Suppl 1:27S–30S, 2007.

121. Narayana PA. Magnetic resonance spectroscopy in the monitoring of multiple sclerosis. J Neuroimaging; 15:46S–57S, 2005.

122. Tartaglia MC, Arnold DL. The role of MRS and fMRI in multiple sclerosis. Adv Neurol; 98:185–202, 2006.

123. Mostert JP, Sijens PE, Oudkerk M, De Keyser J. Fluoxetine increases cerebral white matter NAA/Cr ratio in patients with multiple sclerosis. Neurosci Lett; 402:22–24, 2006.

124. Clark JF, Doepke A, Filosa JA, et al. N-acetylaspartate as a reservoir for glutamate. Med Hypotheses; 67:506–512, 2006.

125. Zivadinov R, Bakshi R. Role of MRI in multiple sclerosis II: brain and spinal cord atrophy. Front Biosci; 9:647–664, 2004.

126. Kutzelnigg A, Lassmann H. Cortical lesions and brain atrophy in MS. J Neurol Sci; 233:55–59, 2005.

127. Bermel RA, Bakshi R. The measurement and clinical relevance of brain atrophy in multiple sclerosis. Lancet Neurol; 5:158–170, 2006.

128. De Stefano N, Battaglini M, Smith SM. Measuring brain atrophy in multiple sclerosis. J Neuroimaging; 17 Suppl 1:10S–15S, 2007.

129. Simon JH. Brain atrophy in multiple sclerosis: what we know and would like to know. Mult Scler; 12:679–687, 2006.

130. Miller DH, Barkhof F, Frank JA, Parker GJ, Thompson AJ. Measurement of atrophy in multiple sclerosis: pathological basis, methodological aspects and clinical relevance. Brain; 125:1676–1695, 2002.

131. Losseff NA, Wang L, Lai HM, et al. Progressive cerebral atrophy in multiple sclerosis. A serial MRI study. Brain; 119 (Pt 6):2009–2019, 1996.

132. Fox NC, Jenkins R, Leary SM, et al. Progressive cerebral atrophy in MS: a serial study using registered, volumetric MRI. Neurology; 54:807–812, 2000.

133. Jasperse B, Valsasina P, Neacsu V, et al. Intercenter agreement of brain atrophy measurement in multiple sclerosis patients using manually-edited SIENA and SIENAX. J Magn Reson Imaging; 26:881–885, 2007.

134. Anderson VM, Fernando KT, Davies GR, et al. Cerebral atrophy measurement in clinically isolated syndromes and relapsing remitting multiple sclerosis: a comparison of registration-based methods. J Neuroimaging; 17:61–68, 2007.

135. Zivadinov R, Cox JL. Neuroimaging in multiple sclerosis. Int Rev Neurobiol; 79:449–474, 2007.

136. Tiberio M, Chard DT, Altmann DR, et al. Gray and white matter volume changes in early RRMS: a 2-year longitudinal study. Neurology; 64:1001–1007, 2005.

137. Sastre-Garriga J, Ingle GT, Chard DT, Ramio-Torrenta L, Miller DH, Thompson AJ. Grey and white matter atrophy in early clinical stages of primary progressive multiple sclerosis. Neuroimage; 22:353–359, 2004.

138. Sastre-Garriga J, Ingle GT, Chard DT, et al. Grey and white matter volume changes in early primary progressive multiple sclerosis: a longitudinal study. Brain; 128:1454–1460, 2005.

139. de Seze J, Debouverie M, Zephir H, et al. Acute fulminant demyelinating disease: a descriptive study of 60 patients. Arch Neurol; 64:1426–1432, 2007.

140. Callen DJ, Shroff MM, Branson HM, et al. Role of MRI in the differentiation of ADEM from MS in children. Neurology; 72:968–973, 2009.

141. Lennon VA, Wingerchuk DM, Kryzer TJ, et al. A serum autoantibody marker of neuromyelitis optica: distinction from multiple sclerosis. Lancet; 364:2106–2112, 2004.

142. Lennon VA, Kryzer TJ, Pittock SJ, Verkman AS, Hinson SR. IgG marker of optic-spinal multiple sclerosis binds to the aquaporin-4 water channel. J Exp Med; 202:473–477, 2005.

143. Hinson SR, Pittock SJ, Lucchinetti CF, et al. Pathogenic potential of IgG binding to water channel extracellular domain in neuromyelitis optica. Neurology; 69:2221–2231, 2007.

144. Pittock SJ, Weinshenker BG, Lucchinetti CF, Wingerchuk DM, Corboy JR, Lennon VA. Neuromyelitis optica brain lesions localized at sites of high aquaporin 4 expression. Arch Neurol; 63:964–968, 2006.

145. Pittock SJ, Lennon VA, Krecke K, Wingerchuk DM, Lucchinetti CF, Weinshenker BG. Brain abnormalities in neuromyelitis optica. Arch Neurol; 63:390–396, 2006.

146. Yu CS, Zhu CZ, Li KC, et al. Relapsing neuromyelitis optica and relapsing-remitting multiple sclerosis: differentiation at diffusion-tensor MR imaging of corpus callosum. Radiology; 244:249–256, 2007.

147. Charil A, Yousry TA, Rovaris M, et al. MRI and the diagnosis of multiple sclerosis: expanding the concept of "no better explanation." Lancet Neurol; 5:841–852, 2006.

148. Bakshi R, Dmochowski J, Shaikh ZA, Jacobs L. Gray matter T2 hypointensity is related to plaques and atrophy in the brains of multiple sclerosis patients. J Neurol Sci; 185:19–26, 2001.

149. Lucchinetti CF, Gavrilova RH, Metz I, et al. Clinical and radiographic spectrum of pathologically confirmed tumefactive multiple sclerosis. Brain; 131:1759–1775, 2008.

Chapter 5

Neuropathology: Clues to Pathogenesis

Abstract

Understanding the pathology of MS is critical to develop working models of the basic pathogenesis of the disease. Classical analyses of MS focused on staging the lesion based on the character of its inflammatory response and the presence of myelin debris detected as sudanophilic material in macrophages. More recent classification of acute lesions has emphasized four basic patterns of pathology with clear implications for therapy. Demonstrated immunoglobulin and complement in ~40% of acute pathological specimens correlate perfectly with plasma-exchange response in patients with devastating acute attacks unresponsive to steroids. CD8+ T cells predominate over CD4+ T cells in all acute pathological patterns along with the constitutive expression of class I MHC and neural elements; this rationale allows a possible role for cytotoxic T cells in the pathogenesis of all forms of acute MS. This chapter will focus primarily on the pathology of MS but will also discuss how it differs from associated disorders. We will describe both the classical nomenclature and theoretical implications of the disease as well as a new classification system based on the findings of autopsied cases of acute MS as well as cerebral biopsies obtained during the earliest phases of the disease course. We will attempt to compare and contrast the classical approach to the neuropathology of MS to the newer findings and provide insights into new therapeutic strategies and, most importantly, etiology.

TRADITIONAL CLASSIFICATION OF INFLAMMATORY DEMYELINATING PATHOLOGY

Pathological classification of demyelinating diseases traditionally divides these disorders into three basic groups: (1) perivenous encephalomyelitis, as observed with classic peri-infectious or postimmunization idiopathic acute disseminated encephalomyelitis (ADEM); (2) demyelinating disorders associated with a systemic disease, such as central pontine myelinolysis (with a rapid, upward shift in sodium in the serum), Marchiafava-Bignami disease associated with alcohol intoxication, and progressive multifocal leukoencephalopathy (PML) associated with JCV, a polyoma virus infection (formerly known as papova virus), usually in an immunocompromised host; and (3) classic MS, which subdivides into classic Charcot type, acute Marburg type, concentric sclerosis (Balo's type), and neuromyelitis optica (NMO, Devic's type). This traditional classification evolved over years. It is presented here to provide the reader with a historical perspective from which to interpret future studies.

Acute Disseminated Encephalomyelitis

This disorder occurs primarily in children after acute infections or after vaccination, although some rare adult forms have been recorded. It occurs after exposure to a number of different viruses or bacteria, including measles, mumps, chicken pox, rubella, and whooping cough, or after vaccination targeting one of these conditions. The relationship between vaccination and disease onset remains controversial, but the association seems most likely when the onset of the neurological finding occurs within 2 weeks after the vaccination or systemic illness. Studies showed a relatively high incidence of the disease after Semple rabies vaccine, and the affected children demonstrated reactivity to myelin antigens approximately 2 weeks after the initial exposure.[1] The pattern and pathology of disease closely resemble experimental autoimmune encephalomyelitis (EAE), a disease induced in a number of experimental animals. In EAE, after receiving the antigens or peptides via immunization, the animals develop meningitis and perivenous inflammation with scant demyelination approximately 12 days after immunization. The majority return to normal; however, depending on the inoculation and types of adjuvants used, the disease persists (but does not progress) in some animals, resulting in permanent demyelination and axonal injury. Similar patterns occur in ADEM.

At necropsy in ADEM, the brain and spinal cord appear normal; however, sectioned areas reveal a slight gray discoloration of the white matter located around small blood vessels. These areas are visible even with the naked eye and become increasingly apparent by histology,

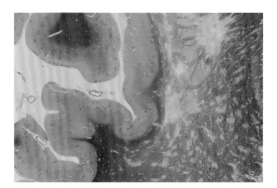

Figure 5–1. A large mounted section showing demyelination in the cerebral white matter from a patient with ADEM. The distribution of the lesions is characteristics of ADEM. Most of the very patchy demyelination surrounds individual veins. None of these coalesce into large lesions, as would be seen in MS. This is a Luxol fast blue preparation. Note the absence of lesions within the cortex. Demyelinating lesions have a stringy appearance as a result of following the venules.

which allows observation of the characteristic perivenous inflammatory process surrounding each specific small venule. Scant demyelination occurs, but in a perivascular distribution that differs greatly from classic MS (Fig. 5.1), which

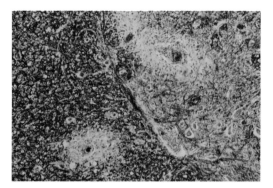

Figure 5–2. Paraffin-embedded section stained with Luxol fast blue of ADEM. This is a classic example of the pathology from a patient with ADEM. This comes from a young boy who presented with a viral illness, which was followed by a devastating inflammatory demyelinating disease and eventual death. The section shows the classical perivenular inflammatory cells, and there is also demyelination, which again just surrounds the venules. This is very characteristic of this type of demyelination, which differs greatly from acute MS, in which lesions are large and well demarcated. All of the myelin sheaths stained blue are normal, and there are no inflammatory cells infiltrating within this normal-appearing white matter. On the right side of the figure are some neurons, indicating that this is a lesion of the deep gray matter. There is no inflammation around the neurons, even though many of them appear to have swollen cytoplasm.

exhibits scattered sharply demarcated, larger demyelinated lesions throughout the brain and spinal cord. Lesions rarely occur in the spinal cord in ADEM, even though there is evidence of inflammatory CNS injury, mostly in the realm of microglial cell proliferation and astrogliosis. Most brain lesions show astrocytic hypertrophy and hyperplasia and, in later stages, intense gliosis. This is usually the norm; however, rare cases end in early death, usually as a result of respiratory insufficiency. Some patients experience persistent neurological deficits such as subacute dementia, blindness, or tetraplegia. While some investigators believe that the disease recurs, many cases of presumed recurrence later prove to be classic MS. It is unclear whether recurrent forms of ADEM truly exist in adults. Inflammatory cells apparently mediate the pathogenesis of the disorder with scant demyelination. An autoimmune process results in myelin antigen presentation that recruits inflammatory cells to the lesion. These cells then secrete various myelin-destroying factors as "collateral damage" (Fig. 5.2). That is, the process is not primarily a disease of myelin but rather a disease of inflammation of the brain and spinal cord, where myelin is destroyed as an "innocent bystander."

Occasionally, the disease can result in hemorrhagic lesions, in which case it is called acute hemorrhagic leukoencephalitis (AHLE). The majority of these cases result in pyrexia, coma, and, ultimately, death. All attempts to isolate infectious agents have been negative. Hemorrhagic lesions also correlate frequently with neutrophil migration into the perivascular spaces with evidence of thrombosed capillaries surrounding necrotic tissue. Rare acute cases may only show neutrophil leukocyte infiltration without many mononuclear infiltrates. (See Chapter 2 for a detailed clinical discussion of ADEM and AHLE.)

Demyelinating Disorders Associated with Systemic Disease

The best-known of these include central pontine myelinolysis (associated with a rapid shift in sodium in the serum), Marchiafava-Bignami disease (associated with alcohol intoxication), and PML (associated with polyoma virus infection, usually in an immunocompromised host).

CENTRAL PONTINE MYELINOLYSIS

Chronic alcoholism and malnutrition are frequent underlying factors of this disorder. More recently, studies have linked central pontine myelinolysis to systemic disorders, including viral hepatitis, chronic pulmonary disease, and chronic neoplasia. Signs of the underlying disease localize to symptoms associated with the pontine lesion. Necropsy is notable for a gray softening in the central part of the upper and middle pons impinging on the tegmentum. Physiologically, myelin breakdown occurs in a sharply defined area but with relative preservation of nerve cell bodies and axons. The condition is linked in most cases with biochemical shifts in sodium, particularly a rapid rise in plasma sodium in patients who present with hyponatremia as a result of a systemic illness.[2] Experiments supporting this hypothesis induced hyponatremia in adult animals subsequently given rapid infusions of sodium, after which they developed central pontine myelinolyis indistinguishable from the human disease.[3]

MARCHIAFAVA-BIGNAMI SYNDROME

This disorder, first described in the early 1900s, is characterized by specific demyelination in the corpus callosum and commonly follows consumption of crude red wine.[4] A high incidence of cases before the 1950s, which has decreased remarkably since then, implied that a toxic factor in the production of local red wine induced the process. On necropsy, sharply demarcated lesions appear exclusively in the corpus callosum along with symmetrical lesions in the anterior commissures and the cerebellar peduncles. Unlike most other demyelinating diseases, this disorder is remarkable for loss of axon cylinders. Oligodendrocytes are completely lost in the lesion, and the astrocytic response is only slight. Many patients also have other evidence of chronic alcohol intoxication, including Wernicke's encephalopathy. This disorder is not associated with all forms of alcoholism. Some have suggested that chronic forms of intoxication might produce similar lesions or that possibly methyl alcohol in locally made wine is a contributing factor.

PML

PML, first described in the late 1950s, presents with an insidious onset of dementia, weakness, visual loss, and, sometimes, ataxia. The disease usually progresses to death within 6 months; however, a few patients experience a more benign course and may survive for several years. Patients are middle-aged at onset with underlying immune-compromised conditions such as Hodgkin's disease, leukemia, lymphoma, sarcoidosis, tuberculosis, cancer, and HIV. Most recently, this disorder has also been associated with immunosuppressive drugs; one of these, natalizumab (Tysabri) is now an FDA-approved drug for MS. The disease does not present with abnormalities in the CSF, and only biopsy or necropsy can confirm a diagnosis. Polymerase chain reaction of the CSF for the JC DNA virus can aid the diagnosis. The cardinal pathological feature is the presence of ~30-nanometer viral particles, which appear as inclusion bodies in the oligodendrocytes. Studies have demonstrated that PML occurs almost exclusively as the result of the JC strain of polyoma virus. Most of the population have antibodies against these viruses in their serum. Normally, the virus persists in the kidney or in B cells. Pathogenesis occurs when an immune-compromised system allows the virus to enter the CNS, where it can infect oligodendrocytes and eventually give rise to an oligodendrogliopathy. Neurological findings localize almost exclusively to the brain; in contrast with MS, there are no known cases of pathology localized exclusively to the spinal cord or optic nerves. Lesions are usually large and confluent and may appear as softening or necrotic areas with even, cystic changes by imaging. Microscopic examination shows evidence of confluent foci of demyelination.

Pathologists describe the cytological features around the lesion as enlarged astrocytes, many of which may appear to be in a precancerous state. There are relatively few inflammatory cells and rare lymphocytes as a result of the patient's compromised immune system. The most important histological feature is the presence of intranuclear inclusions found exclusively within swollen oligodendrocytes. These may be either basophilic or eosinophilic in nature. PML lesions are characteristically destructive of myelin; the sparing of axons is only relative, and the lesion may be necrotic at its center. It is sometimes difficult to distinguish from an infarct. There is widespread hypertrophy of microglial cells. Electron microscopy and immunofluorescence techniques can detect the virus. The large swelling in oligodendrocytes is diagnostic for the disorder.

The occasional appearance of this disorder in MS patients given natalizumab (Tysabri) is unfortunate and frequently creates confusion regarding whether the lesion can be ascribed to MS or PML. The distinction may be difficult to make by standard imaging techniques and may require a biopsy for definitive diagnosis.

Classic Multiple Sclerosis

The pathology of MS is completely limited to the CNS; that is, the brain and spinal cord. Even though occasional MS patients report symptoms associated with inflammatory demyelinating polyradiculoneuropathy, most suffer no alteration of the peripheral nervous system. Upon examination, the pathology of MS demonstrates a sharp demarcation at the root entry zone with frequent demyelination at the CNS but with preserved myelin in the peripheral root (Fig. 5.3). In addition, MS patients rarely demonstrate pathological abnormalities outside the nervous system. In contrast to other established autoimmune disorders or suspected autoimmune disorders, MS carries with it only a minimally increased incidence or risk of other autoimmune disorders such as diabetes mellitus, thyroid disease, scleroderma, systemic lupus erythematosus, or myasthenia gravis. Neither pathological nor epidemiological studies have linked MS with any of these diseases.[5,6] If MS is ultimately proven to be an autoimmune disorder, it will be unique in its specificity to one organ system and lack of a significant association in family members with other autoimmune processes. The pathological process begins in the CNS and, as a result, includes inflammatory cells, which may either induce damage or help to repair lesions.

In contrast to ADEM, classic MS is clearly differentiated pathologically by the well-circumscribed, sharply demarcated primary demyelinating lesions. Pathological disease found outside the CNS is often secondary to nonneurological illness such as infection of the renal or respiratory tracts, atelectasis, or pressure sores. In most cases, especially chronic ones, the brain appears slightly atrophic with widened cerebral sulci and slight ventricular dilatation. Sectioning of the brain, pons, and spinal cord clearly demonstrates circumscribed, irregular gray, firm lesions (Fig. 5.4). Lesions often affect the optic nerve, particularly in the intraorbital portions. Sectioning of the brain reveals numerous large plaques in the deep white matter and the cerebral hemispheres, some extending into the subcortical myelin (Fig. 5.5). Other plaques are scattered haphazardly in the cerebral cortex, although they typically follow white matter tracts.

Lesion distribution preferentially involves the cerebral hemispheres and, in particular, the periventricular white matter. In addition, more

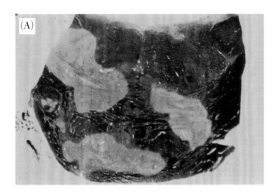
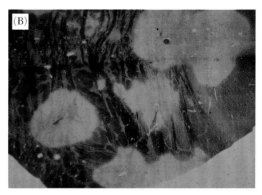

Figure 5–3. (**A**) Block section of the brainstem showing demyelinated plaques. This patient died of MS. Note the very chronic lesions of MS that show an absence of myelin (brown) staining. These lesions are extremely well demarcated from each other. Many of the lesions cross the midline, as can be seen in the bottom lesion. These brainstem lesions are extremely common in MS patients and are found in most patients who die of the disease. (**B**) Demyelination in the brainstem with myelin stained dark brown. This shows areas of multiple white matter plaques, many of which surround blood vessels, but the lesions are extremely well demarcated from each other. Some are beginning to become confluent with each other. This is extremely common in chronic MS and results in many of the stereotypic diagnostic lesions observed, such as medial longitudinal fasciculus lesions.

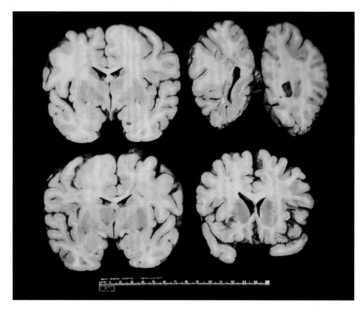

Figure 5–4. Cross-section of the brain from a patient who died of MS. Note multiple areas of abnormality throughout the subcortical white matter. In addition, there are lesions in the gray matter, particularly in the putamen and the thalamus. There is some evidence of cerebral atrophy, as manifested by thin sulci surrounding the surface of the brain.

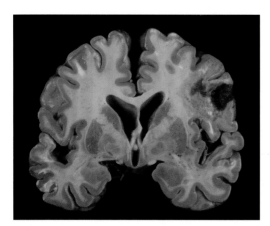

Figure 5–5. Freshly cut pathological specimen from a patient who died of acute MS. Note the large hemorrhagic lesion in the left subcortical white matter. This lesion shows evidence of necrosis and significant acute blood products and hemosiderin deposit.

lesions cluster near the cortex (so-called *cortical demyelination*). The lesions may involve the inferior and anterior quadrants of the lateral ventricles and frequently occur at the junctions of gray and white matter. Recent studies[7] have demonstrated pathology in the gray matter as well as the white matter. Cortical (i.e., gray matter) pathology has emerged as a critical

aspect of the pathogenesis of MS, associated with disease progression and cognitive impairment. Recently, investigators have demonstrated that, in select cases, gray-matter lesions can spread to white matter.[8]

HISTOLOGY OF THE LESIONS

Considerable disagreement exists over the earliest pathological change in MS. In the 1960s, a group of investigators characterized early lesions by degeneration of oligodendrocytes and myelin, relative axonal preservation, and microglial proliferation.[9] In many lesions, these features are recognizable. Early investigation focused almost exclusively on autopsy material, in which the patient may have had the disease for more than 30 years. More recent attempts to classify acute lesions offer better understanding of the heterogeneity of the pathology.

OLD PLAQUES

Elements of axons and astrocytic processes predominate in very old plaques, and the plaques are usually more hypocellular than the surrounding tissue (Fig. 5.6). In the chronic stages, inflammatory cells are usually not present;

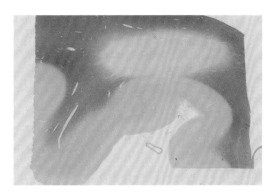

Figure 5–6. Whole mount from autopsy material from a patient with chronic MS. Note the well-demarcated lesion. This lesion has been stained with Luxol fast blue. The lesion is immediately subcortical and shows an absence of inflammatory cells. Many would call this a burnt-out plaque. Normal-appearing white matter also appears without evidence of abnormality. There are no lesions extending into the area of the cortex. This is an old established plaque using the traditional classification.

however, there is significant axonal loss (as will be discussed later in this chapter). Astrogliosis (Fig. 5.7), inflammation, perivascular lipofuscin deposition, and vascular hyalinization have been observed even in the normal-appearing white matter of patients with disease duration of 40 years or more. The edges of the plaques demonstrate hyaline deposition in blood vessels, although the deposition is relatively scattered and, at the present time, of unknown significance. Investigators now focus on this area via MRI. Most old plaques have been confirmed as demyelinating or else classified as "shadow plaques."

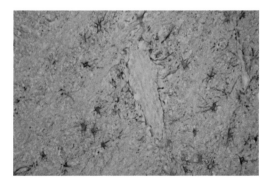

Figure 5–7. Example of a paraffin-embedded tissue stained for glial fibrillary acidic protein (GFAP). This specimen is taken from a patient with acute MS. This lesion surrounds a blood vessel. The tissue has been stained with immunoperoxidase technique for GFAP, and thus astrocytes stain pink or red. These are the same fibrils that are seen by electron microscopy in the previous electron micrograph.

SHADOW PLAQUES

Shadow plaques are lesions in which myelin loss is only partial and lacks a clear-cut outline. The etiology of these plaques of only partial myelin loss has spawned a number of explanations. Currently, many scientists believe that shadow plaques represent areas of remyelination. In these lesions, the myelin is thinner than observed normally in reference to the axon diameter. The lesions show inflammation, but the inflammatory process may be necessary for remyelination.

Acute Multiple Sclerosis, Marburg Type

This relatively acute form of MS is associated with multiple large demyelinated lesions in the CNS but rarely involves the spinal cord[10] (Fig. 5.8). It often follows an illness characterized by fever with rapid deterioration, and death ensues within a few months. Common features include extensive myelin destruction and severe axonal loss (Fig. 5.9). Widespread edema appears especially in the early stages of the disease with significant early axonal degeneration. Many lesions are large with ventricular shift mimicking a brain tumor. Often a

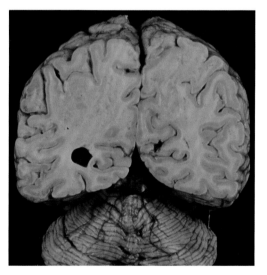

Figure 5–8. Cross-section of the brain from a patient dying of acute fulminant MS. This patient died of a very large lesion in the right cerebral white matter. One can detect abnormalities in both the right and left posterior white matter. The right subcortical lesion shows evidence of edema. This is typical of the Marburg type of MS. The cerebellum appears normal.

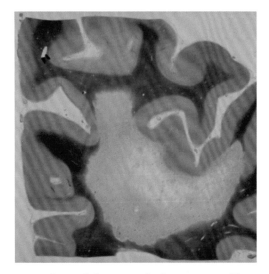

Figure 5–9. Whole mount of a large section of brain from a patient with a large demyelinating plaque with evidence of necrosis in the center. This section is typical of a Marburg-type lesion. The lesion has been stained with Luxol fast blue. Note that the lesion extends up to the area of the cortex but does involve the subcortical fibers. The lesion takes up the majority of the subcortical white matter in this section of the brain. The normal myelin is shown as dark blue; the pink cortex shows no active lesions. As is typical, the demyelinating plaque is sharply demarcated from the area of normal myelin. However, in the center of the plaque, there is absence of neuritic tissue, evidence of a cavitation consistent with an area of necrosis. The lesion has relatively few inflammatory cells. There is an absence of mononuclear cells within the lesion. Therefore, this is a chronic plaque.

cerebral biopsy is necessary to distinguish the two possibilities. Advances in MRI have shown that large lesions are fairly common and do not usually lead to a poor prognosis or death.[11] Therefore, a diagnosis of fulminant MS of the Marburg type should be reserved for cases with a severe clinical presentation rather than MRI (see Chapter 2).

Balo's Concentric Sclerosis

This very rare form of MS was first recognized in 1928.[12] Characterized by a random, relatively fulminant course, this condition reveals alternating zones of myelinated and demyelinated tissue at necropsy. These zones occur in a concentric pattern or in more irregular arrangements (Fig. 5.10). Spongy, partially remyelinated axons typically appear in areas of preserved myelin. A 1994 study

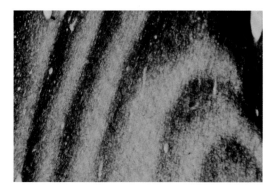

Figure 5–10. This is a highly magnified image of the pathology from a patient with Balo's concentric sclerosis. The lesion has been stained with Luxol fast blue to detect the myelin. The areas of dark myelin are clearly visible with the dark blue stain, and these are separated by bands of light-staining material in which there is a relative absence of myelin. This is very typical of the concentric lesions seen in this disorder. All of these lesions present on MRI as large edematous lesions. The prognosis of this condition is variable. Some patients do quite well despite the presence of these very large lesions, whereas others have persistent neurological deficits. The different distribution of myelin staining in the lesion is thought to be a result of decreased amounts of messenger RNA for myelin gene products in the areas that are poorly stained with the Luxol fast blue.

found the highest oligodendroglial densities in areas of normal-appearing white matter or partially remyelinated areas and lowest in demyelinated areas.[13] Messenger-RNA levels of myelinating genes follow the same pattern and were lowest in the demyelinated areas. The findings support the hypothesis that oligodendroglial loss is the primary event in this pathogenic demyelinating process. These authors felt that the partially myelinated areas represent places of ongoing myelin breakdown rather than remyelination of previously demyelinated areas. However, as discussed in Chapter 2, demyelination can alternate with remyelination.

Neuro-myelitis Optica

NMO (Devic's disease), as originally defined, is a relatively rare disorder usually classified under the heading of MS. However, it has become more prevalent after more recent classification and updated terminology have broadened the inclusion criteria.[14] As discussed in Chapters 2 and 4, its major characteristics include optic nerve involvement and extensive longitudinal lesions (at least three consecutive spinal cord segments). Involvement of the optic nerve and spinal cord can occur simultaneously or within weeks of each other. Investigators recently identified the antigen against aquaporin-4 that is responsible for this process;[15,16] hence, the *aquaporinopathy* has become the preferred term to describe any type of NMO spectrum disorder. Derived from screened blood samples on fixed tissue of cerebellum, muscle, and gut, the findings show immunofluorescent staining surrounding blood vessels. Of interest, aquaporin-4 is primarily present and associated with astrocytes.[16] This water channel is critical at the node of Ranvier and may facilitate axon propagation.

NMO has many pathological features distinct from MS. Consistent with the immunofluorescence pattern observed by the pathogenic antibody, the disease preferentially destroys small and medium-sized blood vessels, primarily arteries rather than veins. In addition, along with high numbers of macrophages, microglial cells, and lymphocytes, there is also a preponderance of eosinophils, which often proves helpful with the pathological diagnosis.[17] The pathogenesis of NMO may be more of an ischemic process rather than a classical demyelinating process, a hypothesis supported by the antibody binding to blood vessels and the intense destruction of blood vessel elements. In contrast to MS, there is a relative lack of direct oligodendrocyte or myelin involvement.

NEUROPATHOLOGY OF MS: ESTABLISHED CLASSIFICATION SYSTEM

Key to the pathogenesis of MS is determining whether the myelin sheath or oligodendrocytes are the primary target of attack. Based on pathological results, classical neuropathologists have argued either hypothesis. The majority of classical neuropathologists characterize the pathology based on various subclassifications.

Acute Active Plaques

Most classical neuropathologists characterize an active plaque by hypercellularity at the edge of the lesion (Fig. 5.11), increased vascularization, and evidence of lipid products resulting from myelin breakdown (Fig. 5.12). Sudanophilic lipids may be present in microglial cells, presumably at the active edge of myelin destruction. However, active lesions with retained histochemical lipid reaction can also contain myelin debris.[9] The nature of the cells at the edge of the active plaque has provoked controversy (Fig. 5.13A and 5.13B). Some have argued that these cells are activated astrocytes, while others favor activated microglial cells or macrophages (Fig. 5.13C). Some have claimed that oligodendrocyte damage is an initial event

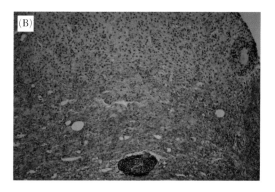

Figure 5–11. (**A**) Paraffin-embedded tissues stained with hematoxylin–eosin from an acute MS lesion. There is an intense inflammatory response surrounding the blood vessel in the lower right-hand corner. Using the classical nomenclature, this is an acute active lesion. All of the cells with pale nuclei are likely astrocytes or macrophages. Many of the inflammatory (darkly staining) cells would be revealed as of the CD8 T-cell phenotype. (**B**) Paraffin-embedded section stained with Luxol fast blue shows a well-demarcated lesion of MS. The top of the lesion, which does not stain with the blue reaction product, shows almost complete demyelination. The lesion is extremely hypercellular. In addition, there are two blood vessels with intense inflammatory response surrounding them. One of these vessels is outside the area of the plaque in the bottom of the figure, and the other is at the edge of the plaque in the top right-hand portion of the figure. In the classical nomenclature, this is an active plaque.

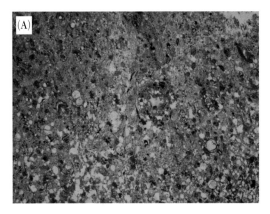 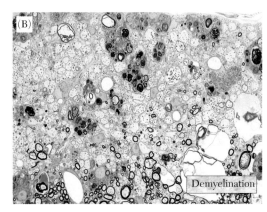

Figure 5–12. (**A**) Evidence of acute, fulminant demyelination in a biopsy from a patient with MS. In the center of this araldite-embedded section, there is evidence of necrosis with destruction of the CNS structures. In addition, there are multiple inflammatory cells, a majority of which are macrophages, which have evidence of intracytoplasmic myelin debris. Many of the myelin sheaths have been completely disrupted. There are a few remaining myelin sheaths at the very edge of the lesion. Even in the area outside of the lesion, there is an intense amount of macrophage infiltration, characteristic of acute MS. This is a 1-μ-thick section stained with toluidine blue. (**B**) Araldite-embedded section stained with paraphenylene-diamine. This relatively high-magnification light-microscopy image shows evidence of primary demyelination. One can see multiple axons that are completely demyelinated. Inside the axons are small mitochondria. In addition, there are cells consuming myelin debris with myelin ovoids. In the bottom of the panel is an area of relatively normal myelination. The figure also represents evidence of myelinolysis, which results in the large vesicular pattern of myelin destruction (lower right).

in MS lesions, while others have denied this and actually emphasized the hyperplasia of these cells at the edge of the lesion. The experimental models have demonstrated immune attack by microglial cells or monocytes. Neuronal degeneration appears to be a major part of the destruction, even in the early plaque. The early inflammation in plaques may be a reparative process. Most acute plaques are not particularly edematous (Fig. 5.14). However, electron microscopy has demonstrated interstitial edema and cellular edema in the astrocytic cytoplasm associated with intense peri-cuffing by lymphocytes and mononuclear cells (Fig. 5.15).

Inactive Plaque

In contrast to the active plaque, classical neuropathologists classify lesions without intense mononuclear inflammatory cells as inactive (Fig. 5.16A and 5.16B). These plaques are characterized primarily by astrocytic proliferation and hyperplasia (Fig. 5.16C). There can be significant axonal loss (Fig. 5.17). The timing of how an active plaque becomes inactive is completely unknown. However, experimental animal models (albeit imperfect models of MS) suggest that the process occurs within 2 to 3 weeks.

Chronic Active Plaque

Some investigators use the term "chronic active plaque" to describe lesions with chronic demyelination that have received a second "hit" of demyelination within the original demyelinated area. These lesions are characterized by intense inflammation and destruction of the myelin sheath (Fig. 5.18). Sudanophilic material is present in these lesions, primarily in microglial cells or macrophages, which contain myelin proteins when stained for myelin-basic protein or myelin oligodendrocyte glycoprotein (MOG).

Chronic Burnt-out Plaque

Most investigators agree on the final late consequences of MS lesions. This lesion is characterized by the relative absence of cells. There are few inflammatory cells or oligodendrocytes but more axonal injury than described in active plaques. Occasionally, individual cells appear in the center of the lesion. Many of these older lesions are in the cortex (Fig. 5.19). After staining these lesions for specific cell surface markers, some investigators have suggested that these cells are progenitor oligodendrocytes

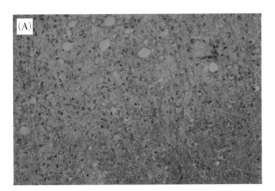

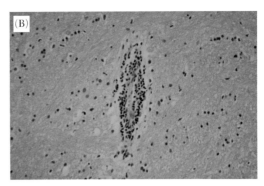

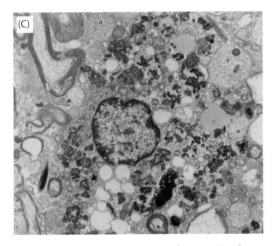

Figure 5–13. (**A**) Demyelinated lesion from a biopsy of a patient with acute MS. This section shows a hypercellular area within a lesion. Many of these cells with small nuclei are oligodendrocytes that appear to proliferate in the area of demyelination, rather typical of a pattern I lesion in which oligodendrocytes are preserved or may actually proliferate within the lesion. (**B**) This paraffin-embedded section from an acute MS lesion shows evidence of inflammatory cells surrounding a venule. Most of these inflammatory cells are also expanding outside of the area surrounding the blood vessel. There is decreased staining immediately around the blood vessel for eosin. However, the eosin staining appears relatively normal outside of the blood vessel, suggesting that this plaque is in the early stages of evolution. In the classical nomenclature of MS, this is an acute active plaque. (**C**) Electron micrograph from a patient biopsy for acute MS. Multiple demyelinated axons are shown in the field; however, a few myelinated axons are present. In addition, there is evidence of myelin degradation that is seen surrounding some of the processes, and there is a macrophage in the upper left-hand corner of the field showing typical large vesicles, likely representing lipid myelin debris, which dissolves as a result of the fixation process. Many times the lipids are disrupted and are not visible by electron microscopy, which then results in empty vacuoles. However, other aspects of the myelin debris are seen in this figure, represented by a dark osmophilic material.

with remyelination-inducing potential under the right stimuli.[18]

The general paradigm of the pathology of MS and the temporal evaluation derives, in part, from the data in EAE. This model, which has been studied by most experimental neuropathologists in MS, has significantly shaped opinion about the evolution of the MS lesion. However, other experimental models, especially those induced by virus, show a primary oligodendrogliopathy in association with the infiltration of inflammatory cells into the lesion. This heterogeneity has led to a new classification system that incorporates many of these findings and provides some clues as to pathogenesis.

NEW CLASSIFICATION SYSTEM

Clearly, the different theories of MS etiology and pathology raised the need for a more

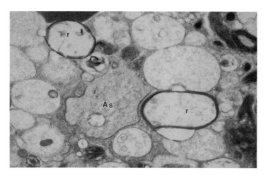

Figure 5–14. Electron micrograph from a patient with acute MS. In the center of the field is an astrocyte (As) with glial fibrillary material. In addition, there are two thinly myelinated axons, which represent remyelination (r). In addition, there are multiple other axons with no myelin surrounding them. At the edge of the field, there are normally myelinated axons as well as myelin debris, which is darkly stained osmophilic material. Most of the osmophilic materials in the figure are astrocytic processes.

unifying hypothesis; namely, that demyelination and neurological injury differ in subgroups of MS patients, and this explains the heterogeneous pathology in lesions from large numbers of patients. This heterogeneity supports the hypothesis of distinct etiologies or, preferably, distinct genetic responses of the host to the pathological event. However, the pattern of pathology appears to remain the same for all the lesions from an individual patient. The major therapeutic implication of this new classification is to target treatment to aspects of pathogenesis rather

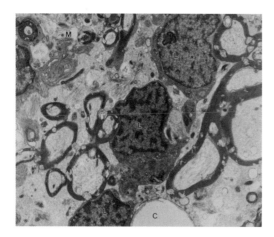

Figure 5–15. Electron micrograph from biopsy of acute MS. These are inflammatory cells, likely lymphocytes (L), which are in intimate contact with myelin sheaths. A capillary (C) appears at the bottom of the figure.

than to the traditional clinical MS subtypes (relapsing–remitting, secondary progressive, and primary progressive MS). There are clear indicators of heterogeneity in MS: variable clinical course, complex genetics, and the partial response to established treatments such as interferon beta, glatiramer acetate, and even immunosuppressive approaches by powerful therapeutic antibodies that delete immune subsets. There is also a conflicting therapeutic response to acute aggressive immunosuppression.

Groundbreaking, ongoing international collaboration in the context of the MS Lesion Project established a new paradigm to classify actively demyelinating MS lesions into four immunopathological subtypes. These distinct patterns were homogenous within a given patient, suggesting that the targets and mechanisms of tissue injury in active MS lesions differ between patient subsets.[19–25] Using experimental models such as EAE to discern early events in the disease course, these studies demonstrated the superiority of immune detection of myelin-degrading products within macrophages for determining the activity level of a lesion. Even simple approaches, such as staining with Luxol fast blue and demonstrating blue-labeling reaction product within macrophages, correlate well with recent activity. More precise approaches, such as immunostaining against myelin-basic protein or MOG, demonstrated positive immunocytochemical reaction processes inside macrophages.

In contrast, the presence of inflammatory cells, including T lymphocytes and B cells, did not correlate strongly with disease activity or patterns of acute pathology. This contradicts the classical hypothesis described previously, where the presence or absence of inflammatory cells was central to the classification. Therefore, in the new classification, the level of inflammatory infiltration was independent of the type of acute pathology.

Bases of New Classification System

Based on the level of oligodendrocyte survival, we can divide the acute pathology of MS into two major subtypes, lesions that preserve oligodendrocytes and lesions that allow oligodendrocytes to die[24] (Table 5.1).

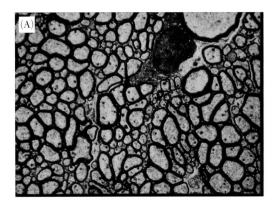

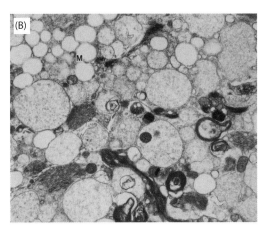

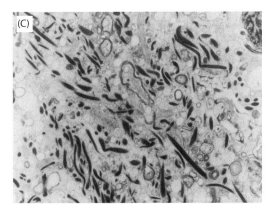

Figure 5–16. (**A**) Electron micrograph from a normal area of the CNS. The axons are surrounded by normal myelin sheaths, which stain dark brown or black due to dark osmophilic material. The cell in the top panel shows a relatively round nucleus. The cell has very dense, dark cytoplasm with the characteristic features of an oligodendrocyte. An oligodendrocyte such as this is known to myelinate 50 to 100 axons. In the center of many axons are small round structures, which are mitochondria. (**B**) Multiple demyelinated axons without active inflammation are seen by electron microscopy. Macrophage (**M**)-engulfing myelin debris is seen at the top of the figure. (**C**) Electron micrographs showing dark osmophilic fibrils. These fibrils are from astrocytes. They represent the fibrils that usually stain with antibodies to glial fibrillary acidic protein. These are very common in activated astrocytes and in both acute and chronic MS lesions.

OLIGODENDROCYTE PRESERVATION

These lesions demonstrate oligodendrocyte survival or recruitment; that is, stains for specific oligodendrocyte markers, in particular *in situ* hybridization for proteolipid protein (PLP) expression, reveal a relatively normal number of oligodendrocytes within the center of the lesion. In these studies, a 30% reduction of oligodendrocytes still constitutes evidence of oligodendrocyte survival.

Lesions characterized by oligodendrocyte survival and recruitment separate into two main categories (Fig. 5.20). Pattern I lesions have evidence of T cells and macrophages as

presumed effectors of damage in the absence of B cells and immunoglobulin deposition (Fig. 5.21). In contrast, pattern II lesions contain abundant antibody (Fig. 5.22) and deposition of the terminal components (Fig. 5.23) of the complement system, which are the mediators of injury.

OLIGODENDROCYTE DEATH

These lesions yield minimal or no reactivity after staining for oligodendrocytes. This, again, occurs in acute plaques rather than in established, burnt-out plaques, where the absence of oligodendrocytes would be the expected

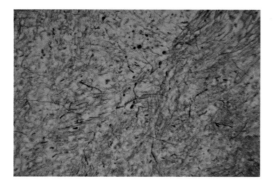

Figure 5–17. This paraffin-embedded section from an acute MS lesion shows axonal loss within 2 weeks of neurological deficits. The edge of the lesion is well demarcated, and one can see the relatively normal expression of the Bielschowsky silver staining of axons. Some of the axons show a dark, round, bulbous appearance. These are axons that have been transected, and the Bielschowsky stain has accumulated at the edge of the transection. Axonal transection is common in many acute MS lesions. Many of the axons also show aberrant morphology with accumulation of the silver reaction product. (Adapted from Rodriguez M, Scheithauer BW, Forbes G, Kelly PJ. Oligodendrocyte injury is an early event in lesions of multiple sclerosis. Mayo Clinic Proc; 68:627–636, 1993.[50])

finding in the classical classification system. In contrast, in acute cases with macrophages demonstrating degradation of myelin proteins, the absence of oligodendrocytes suggested a primary oligodendrogliopathy as the primary inciting event for pathogenesis.

Lesions with oligodendrocyte loss also group into two patterns, patterns III and IV. Pattern III lesions, characterized by oligodendrocyte loss, show evidence of apoptosis within the lesion itself and preferential loss of myelin-associated glycoprotein as compared to myelin-basic protein or PLP (Fig. 5.24). Pattern IV lesions display oligodendrocyte degeneration (Fig. 5.25) within the periplaque white matter as well as within the plaque itself. This is a pattern observed exclusively in patients with primary progressive MS.

PATTERN I LESIONS (OLIGODENDROCYTE PRESERVATION)

In this pattern, a minor reduction in oligodendrocytes (≤30%) occurs in the areas of myelin breakdown (Fig. 5.26). In addition, all of these cases correlate with rapid remyelination. There is no evidence of acute oligodendrocyte death, either because it may have occurred earlier or because the techniques for detecting cell death

may lack sufficient sensitivity to detect oligodendrocyte death within the lesion. Staining with MOG markers demonstrates numerous oligodendrocytes in these lesions, and similarly *in situ* hybridization for PLP demonstrates intense RNA expression of PLP message (Fig. 5.27) within oligodendrocytes, showing that these cells are not destroyed in these very acute cases (Fig. 5.28). Electron microscopy demonstrates the presence of perivascular infiltrates intimately associated with myelin sheaths, not oligodendrocytes. Oligodendrocytes look normal by electron microscopy (Fig. 5.29). There is absence of immunoglobulin-mediated injury.

Among the possible mechanisms of pattern I lesions is T-cell–mediated disease with primary macrophage activation, characterized by primary demyelination with variable oligodendrocyte death. Many findings in pattern I lesions share characteristics of EAE, indicating that the process may be a "collateral damage" reaction by immunotoxins secreted primarily by either lymphocytes or macrophages.

PATTERN II LESIONS (OLIGODENDROCYTE PRESERVATION)

Characterized by the abundant expression of immunoglobulin and complement, pattern II lesions also show oligodendrocyte survival and recruitment. In this situation, plasma cells and immunoglobulins are intimately associated with complement activation, as demonstrated by staining for the terminal components of the complement cascade. In addition, there is concomitant loss of myelin proteins, such as myelin-associated glycoprotein, myelin-basic protein, PLP, and MOG, which supports a process directed against myelin rather than against oligodendrocytes. Pattern II lesions appear to be a T-cell–dependent, antibody-mediated process. Antibody deposition may be the primary mechanism of lesion formation. There is variable oligodendrocyte necrosis rather than apoptosis and selective areas of oligodendrocyte recruitment. Thus, experimental models of EAE appear to support this model, which is associated with anti-MOG antibodies.[26] In EAE, animals immunized with myelin-basic proteins recruit T cells into the CNS lesions without initiating demyelination. However, if these animals then receive a dose of an antibody directed against MOG, intense demyelination occurs.[27] When the antibody is withheld,

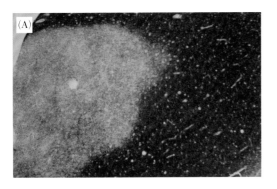
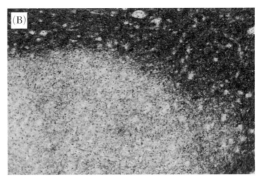
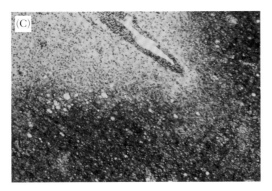

Figure 5–18. (**A**) Paraffin-embedded section stained with Luxol fast blue. This figure shows a well-demarcated lesion surrounding a blood vessel in the center of the plaque. The lesion is hypercellular, but many of these cells are astrocytes or macrophages, which remain in the lesion. There are few T or B cells in the lesion. This is from autopsy material showing a chronic active lesion using the traditional nomenclature system. (**B**) Evidence of oligodendrocyte proliferation in a chronic acute demyelinated lesion. This is a paraffin-embedded section stained with a combination of Luxol fast blue and hematoxylin. At the edge of the lesion, there is normal blue staining (bottom right of the panel), characteristic of normal myelin. Within the lesion itself, there are large numbers of cells. The majority of these have the morphologic features of oligodendrocytes, which are proliferating within the area of demyelination. Many inflammatory cells are seen, consistent with this being a chronic active plaque. (**C**) Paraffin-embedded section stained with Luxol fast blue. This is a relatively sharply demarcated lesion. There is also an intense inflammatory response surrounding the venule. There is already evidence of ongoing demyelination by the absence of blue reaction product. Many of the cells inside the lesions are macrophages, which have taken up the Luxol fast reaction product, indicating that this lesion continues to be active. The lesion does not yet have a very clear, sharply demarcated border, indicating that the lesion is probably still evolving. Using the classical nomenclature system, this is a chronic active plaque.

demyelination does not occur. This provides direct evidence that immunoglobulin induces demyelination, at least in the experimental model and possibly in the human disease. Of interest, there has been a precise correlation between the presence of this pattern of acute demyelination and patient response to plasma exchange.[28]

PATTERN III LESIONS (OLIGODENDROCYTE LOSS)

Pattern III lesions are notable for oligodendrocyte destruction, primarily apoptosis (Fig. 5.30). This oligodendrocyte destruction occurs

primarily at the borders of the active lesions (Fig. 5.31). The dying oligodendrocytes localize to areas of active myelin destruction. This pattern is characteristic of all the lesions or lesion areas of an individual patient. Routine histological stains demonstrate more evidence of oligodendrocyte apoptosis rather than necrosis. In addition, staining with MOG to identify oligodendrocytes demonstrates the apoptotic nuclei within the oligodendrocytes stained with this specific surface antigen. This pattern is consistent with the concept of dying-back oligodendrogliopathy,[29,30] in which there is degeneration of the inner glial loop of the myelin sheath as visualized by electron

Table 5–1 Patterns of Acute MS Pathology

Pattern	Oligodendrocytes	Immune	Oligodendrogliopathy	% cases
I	Preserved	T cells, macrophages	No	12
II	Preserved	T cells, macrophages, B cells, Ig, complement	No	53
III	Diminished	T cells, microglia	Yes	30
IV	Diminished	T cells, microglia	Yes	5

microscopy images of MS lesions.[30] The cell body of the oligodendrocyte appears unable to maintain the myelin. This was originally described in mice treated with cuprizone, an oligodendrocyte-damaging toxin resulting in demyelination exclusively in specific areas of the nervous system.[31] As a result of oligodendrocyte injury, the most distal extension of myelin, the inner glial loop, degenerates first (Fig. 5.32), which is consistent with the dying-back oligodendrogliopathy. Similar observations occur in animal infections with mouse hepatitis virus (MHV) or Theiler's murine encephalomyelitis virus (TMEV), which induces demyelination. Thus far, there is no evidence of virus in MS lesions, even though electron microscopy has revealed a number of unusual paracrystalline arrays (fingerprint bodies)((Fig. 5.33), and elemental structures suggestive of infectious material. However, these "rod-like bodies" (Fig. 5.34)

most likely represent precipitation of proteinaceous material as a result of the fixation process necessary for electron microscopy.

PATTERN IV LESIONS (OLIGODENDROCYTE LOSS)

These lesions are characterized by demyelination of groups of axons by electron microscopy (Fig. 5.35). Lesions in this pattern are characterized by oligodendrocyte destruction localized to the borders of active lesions. There is also evidence of oligodendrocyte death in areas of myelin destruction. However, pattern IV is notable for primary damage to oligodendrocytes in the apparently normal peri-white matter with secondary demyelination. Oligodendrocyte degeneration occurs not only within the plaque itself but also within the so-called normal-appearing white matter. Again, persistent virus infections or toxins provide experimental support for this pathological pattern.

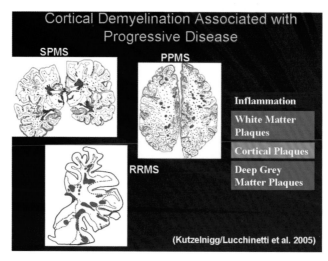

Figure 5–19. This shows the distribution of white matter plaques, cortical plaques, and deep gray matter plaques in typical MS. SPMS, secondary progressive MS; PPMS, primary progressive MS; RRMS, relapsing–remitting MS. Note the varied distribution of lesions in the various clinical forms of MS. (Reproduced with permission from Kutzelnigg A, Lucchinetti CF, Stadelmann C, et al. Cortical demyelination and diffuse white matter injury in multiple sclerosis. Brain; 128:2705–2712, 2005.[46])

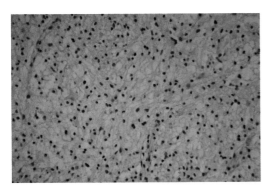

Figure 5–20. Acute demyelination with oligodendrocyte preservation. Survival of oligodendrocytes as detected by *in situ* hybridization for PLP RNA, which marks oligodendrocytes. The lesion is completely demyelinated due to the absence of Luxol fast blue. Despite complete demyelination, the oligodendrocytes persist. (Adapted from Lucchinetti CF, Brueck W, Rodriguez M, Lassmann H. Multiple sclerosis: lessons from neuropathology. Seminars in neurology; 18:337–349, 1998.[22])

Inflammation: CD4 and CD8 T Cells

Controversy exists over the nature of the inflammatory response present in the MS plaques. Some investigators suggest that CD4 T cells are present in the lesions and propose, as in EAE, that these Th1[+] and, more recently,

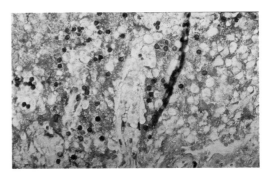

Figure 5–22. Immunoglobulin deposition. This is a paraffin-embedded section stained with the immunoperoxidase technique for immunoglobulin. The brown deposit shows the immunoglobulin deposited throughout the white matter plaque. In addition, there are some very dark brown cells that are either plasma cells or B cells, which express immunoglobulin on their surface and in their cytoplasm. This immunoglobulin deposit is found exclusively in pattern II lesions, in which the pathogenic mechanism of myelin destruction appears to be a combination of immunoglobulin plus terminal components of a complement cascade. (Adapted from Lucchinetti C, Bruck W, Parisi J, Scheithauer B, Rodriguez M, Lassmann H. Heterogeneity of multiple sclerosis lesions: implications for the pathogenesis of demyelination. Ann Neurol; 47:707–717, 2000.[25])

Th17[+] cells mediate myelin destruction. However, after examining a large number of MS lesions, some investigators have come to a different conclusion, clearly demonstrating that the CD8[+] T cell is the dominant T cell in

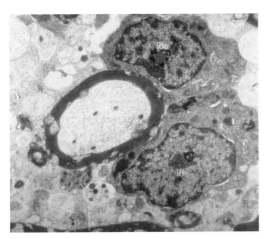

Figure 5–21. Electron micrograph from a patient undergoing biopsy for acute MS. Two mononuclear cells are in intimate contact with the exterior membrane of the myelin sheaths. This represents classical pattern I-type demyelination, and in this situation, these mononuclear cells, which are likely either T cells or macrophages, come in contact with the outer membrane of the myelin sheath. This is in contrast to the pattern III lesions with dying-back oligodendrogliopathy, where the degeneration begins in the inner glial loops. Nu = nucleus. (Adapted from Rodriguez M, Scheithauer B. Ultrastructure of multiple sclerosis. Ultrastructural Pathol; 18:3–13, 1994.[30])

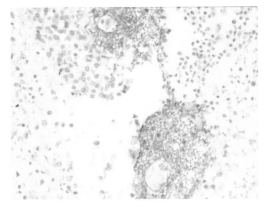

Figure 5–23. Paraffin-embedded tissue stained for C9neo, the final component of the complement cascade. The staining is shown with the red reaction product by immunoperoxidase technique. The blue stain shows nuclei of inflammatory cells in this lesion. This pattern of staining is characteristic of pattern II lesions in which the mechanism of injury is thought to be the combination of immunoglobulins and complement that attacks the myelin sheath. (Adapted from Lucchinetti C, Bruck W, Parisi J, Scheithauer B, Rodriguez M, Lassmann H. Heterogeneity of multiple sclerosis lesions: implications for the pathogenesis of demyelination. Ann Neurol; 47:707–717, 2000.[25])

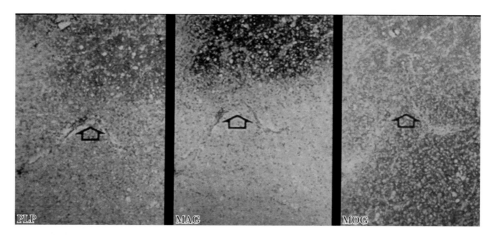

Figure 5–24. Autopsy material from a patient with MS. This shows evidence of pattern III oligodendrocyte pathology in an acute MS. This lesion has been stained for PLP, myelin-associated glycoprotein (MAG), and MOG. There is normal staining for PLP and MOG but an absence of staining for MAG. This is characteristic of pattern III lesions. MAG is a protein expressed on the inner surface of the myelin sheath and is in direct contact with the axons. This is precisely where the degeneration begins in the process of oligodendrocyte pathology or oligodendrodystrophy that is common in pattern III lesions. The process begins in the inner glial loop, where MAG is localized. As a result, MAG is lost from these lesions, whereas other proteins of myelin, such as PLP and MOG, are preserved. Arrow points to the edge of the lesion. (Adapted from Lucchinetti C, Bruck W, Parisi J, Scheithauer B, Rodriguez M, Lassmann H. Heterogeneity of multiple sclerosis lesions: implications for the pathogenesis of demyelination. Ann Neurol; 47:707–717, 2000.[25])

the lesion.[32] This is particularly noteworthy in view of the fact that the CD4 T cell permeates the lesions in most autoimmune processes. In contrast, CD8-mediated pathology is usually associated with infection or toxic etiologies. In a paper published in 1986, investigators analyzed 16 postmortem brains from patients with progressive MS and two biopsy specimens. They stained for T-cell subsets, B cells, and HLA-DR antigens. The perivascular cuffs consisted primarily of T cells, primarily of the CD8 phenotype with a very

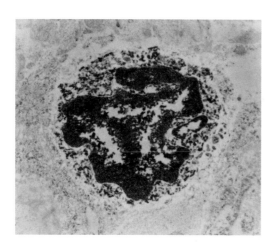

Figure 5–25. Electron micrograph showing apoptosis in a patient undergoing biopsy for acute MS. The cell shown in the center is undergoing apoptosis. The nucleus is beginning to condense with a dark osmophilic material. There also appears to be degeneration in the cytoplasm. This is likely a dying oligodendrocyte; apoptosis of oligodendrocytes is a characteristic of pattern III lesions.

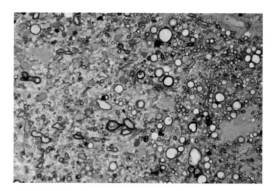

Figure 5–26. Araldite-embedded section, 1 micron thick, stained with toluidine blue (pattern I lesion). This is from an acute lesion from a patient undergoing a biopsy for MS. A number of myelinating axons appear normal; however, in the left part of the figure there is clear degeneration of the myelin sheath with infiltration of a large number of rather large cells that are macrophages engulfing myelin debris. The axons appear swollen, indicative of interstitial edema, which is typical of some of these very large edematous lesions characterized as Marburg-type lesions. Oligodendrocytes are preserved in the lesion.

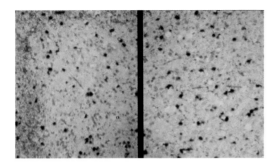

Figure 5–27. Pattern I-type pathology with preserved oligodendrocytes. This is an example of a lesion that has been stained for PLP. *In situ* hybridization has been performed looking for PLP messenger RNA, which directly marks the oligodendrocyte. The dark reaction product shows oligodendrocytes present in this acutely demyelinated plaque. This section has also been counterstained for MOG by immunoperoxidase, which shows the red reaction product at the edge of the plaque. The figure on the left-hand side shows the edge of the plaque with an essentially normal number of oligodendrocytes both within the plaque and outside of it. The figure on the right-hand side is within the center of the plaque and, again, shows the presence of the oligodendrocytes with the black reaction products in the center of the plaque. These are characteristics of pattern I lesions, in which there is oligodendrocyte preservation despite the presence of demyelination. This occurs even though this is an acute lesion. These oligodendrocytes have either been preserved or, as the result of a stimulus, have actually undergone proliferation so that their numbers are normal or even elevated. (Adapted from Lucchinetti CF, Brueck W, Rodriguez M, Lassmann H. Multiple sclerosis: lessons from neuropathology. Semin Neurol; 18:337–349, 1998.[22])

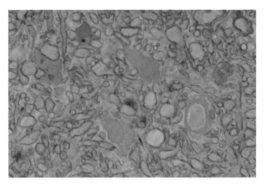

Figure 5–28. Example of an araldite-embedded section stained with toluidine blue. This 1-μ section shows four oligodendrocytes, all within the vicinity of thinly myelinated axons. All of the axons in this figure show the thin myelin characteristic of remyelination. The four oligodendrocytes in such close proximity imply that these cells have recently divided or proliferated. Most of the axons are normal; however, rare axons are beginning to degenerate, with the accumulation of blue reaction product inside the axon. This is typical for pattern I lesions.

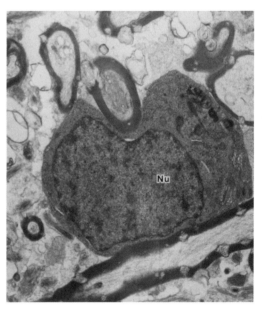

Figure 5–29. Electron micrograph from a biopsy of a patient with acute MS (pattern I lesion). This is from a relatively normal area near the edge of the lesion that shows a normal oligodendrocyte. Nu indicates the nucleus of the cell. This cell is in intimate contact with myelin sheaths. There is a longitudinal axon in the bottom of the figure with normal myelin as well as number of axons cut at cross-sections with relatively normal myelin. Normal oligodendrocytes such as this surrounding the normal-appearing white matter are characteristic of lesions with pattern I-type pathology, where oligodendrocytes are preserved.

low number of CD4 T cells. The CD8:CD4 ratio was as high as 50:1, and CD8⁺ T cells were predominant in the normal-appearing white matter. In presumably active lesions, the majority of T cells were CD8⁺; however, in many of these histological samples, macrophages were the predominant phenotype. Of interest, no brain had more CD4 than CD8 T cells, demonstrating that the overrepresentation of CD8⁺ T cells was a consistent factor of lesions in all MS patients. Of interest, CD8⁺ T cells predominate irrespective of the pattern of active demyelination based on the new classification system. In all active lesions, irrespective of the manner of tissue destruction, the CD8⁺ T cells predominate. Another study demonstrated increased high-affinity beta-adrenergic receptor densities in CD8⁺ T cells in MS patients.[33] The authors suggest that peripheral sympathetic dysregulation plays a role in immune pathogenesis of the disease process in MS.

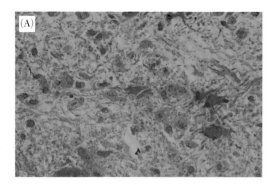

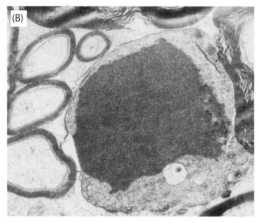

Figure 5–30. (**A**) Araldite-embedded section from a pattern III lesion. There is active demyelination with proliferation of astrocytes. No oligodendrocytes are seen in the lesion. (Adapted from Rodriguez M, Scheithauer B. Ultrastructure of multiple sclerosis. Ultrastructural Pathol; 18:3–13, 1994.[30]) (**B**) Electron micrograph from the same patient in (**A**) shows an oligodendrocyte undergoing apoptosis. This oligodendrocyte is not as far advanced as the cell shown in Figure 5.25. However, there is very dense condensation of the nucleus. The cytoplasm in this cell, however, has not yet begun to degenerate. The image demonstrates the presence of the oligodendrocyte, since there is a double plasma membrane surrounding this cell, which goes on to make contact with the myelinated sheath at the bottom left of the figure. The width of the myelin sheath in reference to the axon diameter appears relatively normal. This is characteristic of a pattern III lesion in which there is primary injury to the oligodendrocytes, which then results in degeneration of myelin.

Members of the ICAM and LFA Superfamily

Other investigators have examined distribution of the immunoglobulin superfamily members, ICAM-1, ICAM-2, and ICAM-3, and the beta 2 integrin LFA-1 in MS.[34] These authors demonstrated the presence of ICAM-1 and ICAM-2 in endothelial cells, with ICAM-3 restricted to infiltrating leukocytes. They

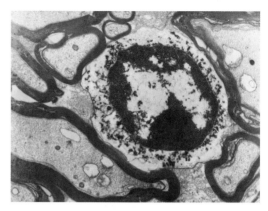

Figure 5–31. Another example of an apoptotic oligodendrocyte. This patient underwent a biopsy for acute MS. There is condensation of the nucleus. In this cell there is degeneration also in the cytoplasm. This cell shows a double membrane surrounding this cell, conclusively identifying the oligodendrocyte. The cell is in contact with multiple, relatively normal myelin sheaths. Some of the axons in this figure show intra-axonal evidence of vacuoles. These likely represent evidence of degenerating mitochondria within the axon, an early event prior to axonal injury.

noted ICAM-1–positive vessels exclusively in MS brains in contrast to control brain tissue with neurological disease. They detected LFA-1 on activated microglial cells close to the edge of demyelinating lesions. These results suggested a role for ICAM-1, ICAM-2, and LFA-1 in the transendothelial migration of leukocytes into MS brain and a role for these factors in the breakdown of the blood–brain barrier that leads to leukocyte infiltration in MS.

Monocytes and Macrophages

Investigators have looked at monocyte and macrophage differentiation in early MS lesions.[19] In biopsy material from MS lesions during the early course of disease, the pan-macrophage marker Ki-M1P revealed the highest numbers of macrophages in early and late active lesions, while lower numbers were present in inactive, demyelinated, or remyelinated lesions. MRP14 was found in early active lesions, whereas 27E10 was found in late active lesions. These specific immune markers on monocytes and macrophages have been helpful in determining lesion activity and lesion age in acute MS lesions.

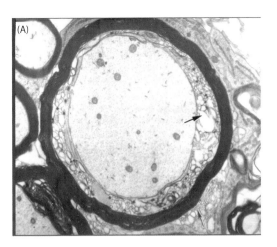

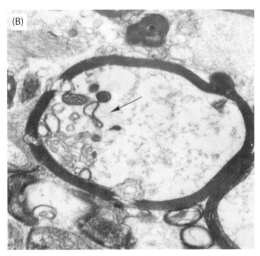

Figure 5–32. (**A**) Electron micrograph taken from a biopsy of a patient with acute MS showing regeneration of inner glial loops. This shows evidence of dying-back oligodendrogliopathy (pattern III lesion). Note the degeneration in the inner tongue of the myelin sheath. There is dissolution of the myelin sheath on the inside surface, while the outside surface of the myelin sheath remains relatively intact. This is a typical early finding of the dying-back oligodendrogliopathy concept. The injury occurs to the oligodendrocyte, which is outside of the field of this electron micrograph. As a result of injury to the oligodendrocyte, the most distal extension of that cell, which is the inner glial loop of this myelin sheath, begins to degenerate. Finally, as the cell has more difficulty maintaining its machinery and proteins down to these membranes, there is continued dissolution of myelin around the axon with complete demyelination. In addition, this figure shows evidence of axonal swelling, a characteristic feature of acute MS lesions with edema at times of biopsy, which are confused with brain tumors. (**B**) Dying-back oligodendrogliopathy in a pattern III lesion. The degeneration begins in the inner glial surfaces (*arrow*). Note that the outside of the myelin sheath is completely intact. In addition, there are no inflammatory cells that in any way attack the specific myelin sheath. The main attack actually occurs to oligodendrocytes outside of the viewing field. As a result of oligodendrocyte injury, the machinery of proteins is insufficient to maintain the status of the myelin surrounding the inner glial loop, which begins to degenerate immediately in the area surrounding the axons. However, the axon is completely intact, and there are multiple mitochondria with normal profiles, indicating that this axon is not undergoing a degenerative process at the present time. (Adapted from Rodriguez M, Scheithauer B. Ultrastructure of multiple sclerosis. Ultrastructural Pathol; 18:3–13, 1994.[30])

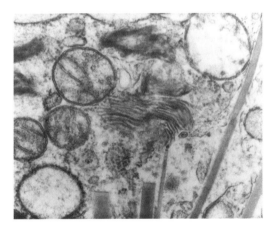

Figure 5–33. Abnormal mitochondria and fingerprint bodies. Electron micrograph of an acute biopsy from a patient with multiple sclerosis (MS) shows evidence of a typical fingerprint body within a macrophage in the lesion. In addition, there are number of normal mitochondria as well as swollen mitochondria with disruption of the cisternae. There are also characteristic pole-like bodies that have been described in some acute cases of MS.

Microglial cells apparently mediate damage and play a major role in clearing myelin debris from the CNS.[35,36] Investigators looked at T-cell infiltration, myelin clearance, microglial activation, and phagocytic activity distal to sites of axonal transection. Via double immunofluorescence and confocal microscopy, they demonstrated the presence of enhanced microglial response as a result of axonal transection. The microglial cells played a major role in phagocytosis of myelin debris during the degeneration of axons. This implied that some of the inflammatory response observed in the MS plaque may be protective rather than pathogenic because increased phagocytosis of myelin debris is necessary for repair.

Others have studied plasma cells in the perivascular components of chronic MS lesions for the presence of macrophages and lymphocytes.[37] This study involved CNS tissue from six MS patients and found cytoplasmic inclusions

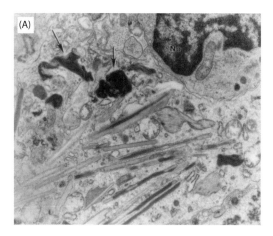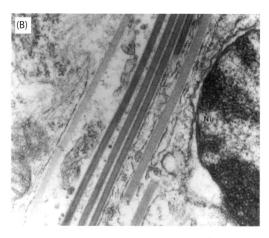

Figure 5–34. (**A**) Electron microscopy taken from a patient undergoing biopsy for fulminant MS. Shown is a macrophage at high magnification with multiple polelike bodies. In addition, there is dark osmophilic material, probably proteinaceous. The etiology of the polelike bodies is undetermined, but the structure is reminiscent of a proteinaceous material precipitated in the macrophage itself. These polelike bodies have not been described previously in MS lesions, but they represent some unclear aspects of the etiology. Similar polelike bodies have been observed in transgenic mice overexpressing specific interleukins. (**B**) This is an electron micrograph of a high-power image of a macrophage showing the unusual polelike bodies found in two acute cases of MS. These unusual polelike bodies were found exclusively in macrophages and not in other types of glial or neuronal cells. They were all intracytoplasmic. The appearance of the polelike bodies suggested precipitation of a proteinaceous material inside the macrophage. These polelike bodies had not been described previously in MS. Nu = nucleus. (**A, B**: Adapted from Rodriguez M, Scheithauer B. Ultrastructure of multiple sclerosis. Ultrastructural Pathol; 18:3–13, 1994.[30])

consisting of membrane-bound stacks of curved linear profiles, resembling myelin degradation, consistently in microglial cells. In addition, they found intense lymphocytes and plasma cells in the histologically normal white matter. The investigators considered whether two distinct types of phagocytic cells were necessary for the complete digestion of myelin in MS.[37] These two distinct types of macrophages and/ or microglial cells may have different sites of origin. One may be blood-borne, while the other may be present in CNS from birth. More recent evidence suggests that the blood-borne macrophages are cytopathic and seen primarily in pattern I and II lesions, while the more classical microglial cells are activated specifically in cases associated with oligodendrocyte injury in pattern III and IV lesions.

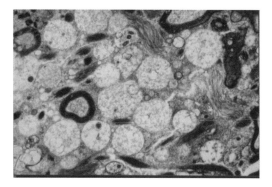

Figure 5–35. Electron micrograph showing multiple demyelinated axons in a field of acute MS. In the center of the field, there is a normally myelinated axon, and there are also normally myelinated axons in the edges of the field. However, the majority of the axons are demyelinated. In addition, there is darkly stained osmophilic material consisting of astroglial fibrils, which represent astrogliosis. There is axonal swelling characteristic of many acute lesions of MS, which show evidence of interstitial edema.

Dendritic Cells

Investigators have studied the maturation stages of dendritic cells in MS lesions.[38] To understand the role of dendritic cells in CNS inflammation, they performed detailed immunocytochemical analysis in maturating dendritic cells. They noted the presence of specific markers containing engulfed myelin components in both active and inactive MS lesions. Only 1 of 10 MS patients examined had evidence of perivascular CD1a+ dendritic cells in their active lesions. Although less numerous than DC-SIGN dendritic cells, cells expressing mature dendritic cell markers appeared consistently in the inflamed meninges and perivascular cuffs. Of interest, these investigators also found a close proximity between dendritic cells and CD8[+] T cells, indicating that dendritic cells recruited to the MS lesion make immunological synapses with CD8[+] T cells as they mature.

MHC Class I and Class II

The distribution of class I and class II MHC antigens is critical to the inflammatory response. Class I MHC antigens are expressed on all major cell types but not traditionally in CNS tissue. In contrast, antigen-presenting cells such as dendritic cells or macrophages primarily express class II MHC antigens, which are not constitutively expressed on other types of cells. Antigen distribution in the MS lesion is significant; class I MHC antigens facilitate engagement of CD8[+] T cells while class II MHC antigens play a critical role in engaging CD4[+] T cells. The presence of a large number of CD8[+] T cells in the MS lesion defies the traditional common wisdom that the nervous system does not express class I MHC antigens.

In 2004 investigators examined in detail the expression of MHC antigens in MS lesions.[20] They studied human autopsy material including 10 cases of acute MS, 10 cases of chronic active MS, 10 cases of chronic inactive MS, and 21 controls. Using quantitative immunohistochemical techniques, including double staining and confocal laser microscopy, to analyze the data, they found constitutive expression of MHC class I molecule on microglia and endothelial cells. A hierarchical upregulation of MHC class I appeared on astrocytes, oligodendrocytes, neurons, and axons, depending upon the severity of the disease and the activity of the lesions. In contrast, MHC class II molecules were expressed on microglia and macrophages but not on nervous system cells. These studies clearly suggest a key role for class I MHC-restricted cytotoxic CD8[+] T cells in the destructive process in MS lesions. The CD8 arm of the immune response may actively aid destruction rather than serve its classically perceived role as a "suppressive" cell that downregulates the function of CD4[+] T cells. The viral models of demyelination yield similar findings.[39–41]

Challenges to the Pathological Classification of Multiple Sclerosis

Recent papers have challenged the new classification of MS. In a well-described cohort of MS brains, investigators studied the four different demyelination patterns in active lesions.[42] They specifically looked for heterogeneity within their populations. The results demonstrated that complement and antibodies consistently correlated with macrophages in areas of active demyelination. They also observed preferential loss of myelin proteins and extensive hypoxia-like damage. Oligodendrocyte apoptosis was absent or rare. The immunopathological appearance was much more uniform and more characteristic of pattern II lesions rather than the four types of lesions described previously. However, the authors failed to prove that the analyzed lesions were still active. Lesions may become more homogeneous as the disease progresses. Whether the lesions are homogeneous from onset or whether they become so over time, the classical hypothesis of a CD4/TH1/TH17 T-cell–mediated disease similar to that observed in EAE deserves careful reconsideration with respect to MS.

Clearly there is evidence of complement and antibody deposition in the majority of acute lesions, as demonstrated by the response of more than 40% of patients to plasma exchange during acute devastating attacks unresponsive to high-dose methylprednisolone.[43,44] If further investigation supports this hypothesis, then investigators clearly should shift additional therapeutic emphasis to aggressive downregulation of immunoglobulins and complement activation rather than the current norm of targeting only T cells.

Cortical Demyelination

Cortical demyelination has recently become the focus of intense interest. Investigators have been aware of this process for over 100 years; almost all neuropathologists who have critically examined the MS lesion have described it. Some investigators observed more lesions in the cortex than in the periventricular white matter.[9] Cortical demyelinated lesions may be exceedingly small and difficult to observe even with current MRI technology. This may explain why investigators mostly ignored these lesions until recently, with the availability of higher-Tesla machines and new MRI techniques (see Chapter 4) better able to detect these lesions. These areas of subpial demyelination in the cerebral cortex correlate with disability, specifically cognitive disorders.

In a series of studies, investigators found extensive cerebral cortical demyelination in 78 tissue blocks from the brains of 20 MS patients but not in 28 tissue blocks from 7 healthy controls.[45] All the tissue blocks from MS patients contained cerebral cortex and periventricular or subcortical white matter. They identified 84% of the 109 demyelinating lesions in the cerebral cortex as purely intracortical, whereas 15% apparently extended through both white and gray matter. Of the 20 MS brains, subpial demyelination was extensive in the four widely spaced cortical areas studied. The percentage of demyelinated area was higher in the cerebral cortex than in other areas of white matter. Some cases of cortical demyelination exhibited atypical features, including absence of inflammation. The extent of cortical demyelination did not correlate with the duration of disease.

The clinical significance of cortical demyelination continues to be an area of extensive investigation, particularly as imaging techniques allow ever more detailed examination of cortical lesions over time. Cognitive impairment is apparently the most likely symptom associated with cortical demyelination.[46] However, general disability also appears to correlate with cortical lesions. Investigators have examined whether cortical lesion pathology differs from that of lesions of the noncortical white matter, comparing complement activation in white matter and cortical lesions.[47] They studied the brains of 22 MS patients and 5 nonneurological control patients obtained at autopsy. Deposition of the complement-activation products (membrane attack complex) was detected on and within macrophages/microglia and astrocytes and in blood vessel walls in white matter MS lesions. However, the gray matter portion of combined gray matter/white matter lesions showed less frequent complement activation but increased immunopositivity for C3d on blood vessels and for C3d and C4d on myelin in the border of the lesions compared to control areas. These studies suggested a location-dependent role of complement in MS pathogenesis.

Pathological changes in the cerebral cortex of patients with MS and PML based on autopsied brain tissue from 13 PML and 4 MS patients demonstrated leukocortical, intracortical, and subpial patterns of demyelination in the MS brain tissue.[48] The cortical lesions in PML and MS contained fewer inflammatory cells than the demyelinated region in other areas of the white matter, which again implies a less pronounced inflammatory response in cortical pathology than in white matter regardless of cause.

A group of investigators examined the propagation of depression as it correlates with cortical myelin content.[49] The authors found that CNS demyelinating disease severely affects cortical myelin. They went on to study the functional consequences of decreasing myelin content in the cortex. They studied cortical-spreading depression in a number of toxic and autoimmune models of cortical demyelination and demonstrated the correlation between cortical myelin loss and abnormalities in cortical physiology. Clearly, cortical myelin plays an increasingly active role in the stabilization and buffering of extracellular ion content that is decisive for cortical-spreading depression, propagation velocities, and cortical excitability. This provides strong evidence of marked clinical implications associated with demyelinating cortical lesions.

Of interest, cortical demyelination has not been observed in NMO.[8] A recent study of 19 autopsied patients with pathologically proven NMO noted preservation of aquaporin-4 in the normal distribution in the cerebrum and cerebellum but no evidence of cortical demyelination. Since cortical demyelination has been associated with a progressive course in MS and a progressive disease course does not occur in NMO, the absence of progression in NMO may be related to the absence of cortical demyelination.

SUMMARY

Understanding the pathology of MS is still a work in progress. Classical analyses described the lesion based on its inflammatory response and the presence of myelin debris detected as sudanophilic material in macrophages. More recent classifications of acute lesions have emphasized four distinct immunopathological patterns with clear therapeutic implications. The positive correlation with pattern II lesions in response to plasma exchange already offers evidence that treating the disease individually based on pathogenesis may improve the percentage of patients responding to a specific therapy.

REFERENCES

1. Piyasirisilp S, Schmeckpeper BJ, Chandanayingyong D, Hemachudha T, Griffin DE. Association of HLA and T-cell receptor gene polymorphisms with Semple rabies vaccine-induced autoimmune encephalomyelitis. Ann Neurol; 45:595–600, 1999.
2. Laureno R, Karp BI. Myelinolysis after correction of hyponatremia. Ann Intern Med; 126:57–62, 1997.
3. Gankam Kengne F, Soupart A, Pochet R, Brion JP, Decaux G. Re-induction of hyponatremia after rapid overcorrection of hyponatremia reduces mortality in rats. Kidney Int; 76:614–621, 2009.
4. Drobny M, Saniova B. Red wine drinkers' encephalopathy: Marchiafava Bignami disease. Neuroendocrinol Lett; 28 Suppl 4:17, 2007.
5. Wynn DR, Rodriguez M, O'Fallon WM, Kurland LT. Update on the epidemiology of multiple sclerosis. Mayo Clinic Proc; 64:808–817, 1989.
6. Wynn DR, Rodriguez M, O'Fallon WM, Kurland LT. A reappraisal of the epidemiology of multiple sclerosis in Olmsted County, Minnesota. Neurology; 40:780–786, 1990.
7. Filippi M, Rocca MA. MR imaging of gray matter involvement in multiple sclerosis: implications for understanding disease pathophysiology and monitoring treatment efficacy. AJNR Am J Neuroradiol; 31:1171–1177,
8. Lucchinetti CF, Popescu BF, Bunyan RF, et al. Inflammatory cortical demyelination in early multiple sclerosis. N Engl J Med; 365:2188–2197, 2011.
9. Lumsden CE, Properties and significance of the demyelinating antibody in multiple sclerosis. Int Arch Allergy Appl Immunol; 36(Suppl):247–275, 1969.
10. Marburg O. Die sogenannt "akute multiple sklerose" (Encephalomyelitis periaxialis scleroticans). Jhrd Psychiatr Neurol; 27:211–312, 1906.
11. Pittock SJ, McClelland RL, Achenbach SJ, et al. Clinical course, pathological correlations, and outcome of biopsy proved inflammatory demyelinating disease. J Neurol Neurosurg Psychiatry; 76:1693–1697, 2005.
12. Balo J. Encephalitis periaxialis concentrica. Arch Neurol Psychiat (Chic); 19:242–264, 1928.
13. Yao DL, Webster HD, Hudson LD, et al. Concentric sclerosis (Balo): morphometric and in situ hybridization study of lesions in six patients. Ann Neurol; 35:18–30, 1994.
14. Wingerchuk DM, Lennon VA, Pittock SJ, Lucchinetti CF, Weinshenker BG. Revised diagnostic criteria for neuromyelitis optica. Neurology; 66:1485–1489, 2006.
15. Pittock SJ, Weinshenker BG, Lucchinetti CF, Wingerchuk DM, Corboy JR, Lennon VA. Neuromyelitis optica brain lesions localized at sites of high aquaporin 4 expression. Arch Neurol; 63:964–968, 2006.
16. Roemer SF, Parisi JE, Lennon VA, et al. Pattern-specific loss of aquaporin-4 immunoreactivity distinguishes neuromyelitis optica from multiple sclerosis. Brain; 130:1194–1205, 2007.
17. Wingerchuk DM, Lucchinetti CF. Comparative immunopathogenesis of acute disseminated encephalomyelitis, neuromyelitis optica, and multiple sclerosis. Curr Opin Neurol; 20:343–350, 2007.
18. Wolswijk G. Chronic stage multiple sclerosis lesions contain a relatively quiescent population of oligodendrocyte precursor cells. J Neurosci; 18:601–609, 1998.
19. Bruck W, Porada P, Poser S, et al. Monocyte/macrophage differentiation in early multiple sclerosis lesions. Ann Neurol; 38:788–796, 1995.
20. Hoftberger R, Aboul-Enein F, Brueck W, et al. Expression of major histocompatibility complex class I molecules on the different cell types in multiple sclerosis lesions. Brain Pathol; 14:43–50, 2004.
21. Lucchinetti CF, Rodriguez M. The controversy surrounding the pathogenesis of the multiple sclerosis lesion. Mayo Clinic Proc; 72:665–678, 1997.
22. Lucchinetti CF, Brueck W, Rodriguez M, Lassmann H. Multiple sclerosis: lessons from neuropathology. Semin Neurol; 18:337–349, 1998.
23. Rodriguez M, Lucchinetti CF. Is apoptotic death of the oligodendrocyte a critical event in the pathogenesis of multiple sclerosis? Neurology; 53:1615–1616, 1999.
24. Lucchinetti C, Bruck W, Parisi J, Scheithauer B, Rodriguez M, Lassmann H. A quantitative analysis of oligodendrocytes in multiple sclerosis lesions. A study of 113 cases. Brain; 122 (Pt 12):2279–2295, 1999.
25. Lucchinetti C, Bruck W, Parisi J, Scheithauer B, Rodriguez M, Lassmann H. Heterogeneity of multiple sclerosis lesions: implications for the pathogenesis of demyelination. Ann Neurol; 47:707–717, 2000.
26. Tsunoda I, Kuang LQ, Theil DJ, Fujinami RS. Antibody association with a novel model for primary progressive multiple sclerosis: induction of relapsing-remitting and progressive forms of EAE in H2s mouse strains. Brain Pathol; 10:402–418, 2000.
27. Stefferl A, Brehm U, Linington C. The myelin oligodendrocyte glycoprotein (MOG): a model for antibody-mediated demyelination in experimental autoimmune encephalomyelitis and multiple sclerosis. J Neural Transm Suppl:123–133, 2000.
28. Keegan M, Konig F, McClelland R, et al. Relation between humoral pathological changes in multiple sclerosis and response to therapeutic plasma exchange. Lancet; 366:579–582, 2005.
29. Ludwin SK. The pathogenesis of multiple sclerosis: relating human pathology to experimental studies. J Neuropathol Exp Neurol; 65:305–318, 2006.
30. Rodriguez M, Scheithauer B. Ultrastructure of multiple sclerosis. Ultrastructural Pathol; 18:3–13, 1994.
31. Ludwin SK, Johnson ES. Evidence for a "dying-back" gliopathy in demyelinating disease. Ann Neurol; 9:301–305, 1981.
32. Hauser SL, Bhan AK, Gilles F, Kemp M, Kerr C, Weiner HL. Immunohistochemical analysis of the cellular infiltrate in multiple sclerosis lesions. Ann Neurol; 19:578–587, 1986.
33. Karaszewski JW, Reder AT, Anlar B, Arnason GW. Increased high affinity beta-adrenergic receptor

densities and cyclic AMP responses of CD8 cells in multiple sclerosis. J Neuroimmunol; 43:1–7, 1993.

34. Bo L, Peterson JW, Mork S, et al. Distribution of immunoglobulin superfamily members ICAM-1, -2, -3, and the beta 2 integrin LFA-1 in multiple sclerosis lesions. J Neuropathol Exp Neurol; 55:1060–1072, 1996.

35. Nielsen HH, Ladeby R, Fenger C, et al. Enhanced microglial clearance of myelin debris in T cell-infiltrated central nervous system. J Neuropathol Exp Neurol; 68:845–856, 2009.

36. Sriram S, Rodriguez M. Indictment of the microglia as the villain in multiple sclerosis. Neurology; 48:464–470, 1997.

37. Prineas JW, Wright RG. Macrophages, lymphocytes, and plasma cells in the perivascular compartment in chronic multiple sclerosis. Lab Invest; 38:409–421, 1978.

38. Serafini B, Rosicarelli B, Magliozzi R, et al. Dendritic cells in multiple sclerosis lesions: maturation stage, myelin uptake, and interaction with proliferating T cells. J Neuropathol Exp Neurol; 65:124–141, 2006.

39. Altintas A, Cai Z, Pease LR, Rodriguez M. Differential expression of H-2K and H-2D in the central nervous system of mice infected with Theiler's virus. J Immunol; 151:2803–2812, 1993.

40. Rodriguez M, David CS. Demyelination induced by Theiler's virus: influence of the H-2 haplotype. J Immunol; 135:2145–2148, 1985.

41. Rodriguez M, Leibowitz J, David CS. Susceptibility to Theiler's virus-induced demyelination. Mapping of the gene within the H-2D region. J Exp Med; 163:620–631, 1986.

42. Breij EC, Brink BP, Veerhuis R, et al. Homogeneity of active demyelinating lesions in established multiple sclerosis. Ann Neurol; 63:16–25, 2008.

43. Rodriguez M, Karnes WE, Bartleson JD, Pineda AA. Plasmapheresis in acute episodes of fulminant CNS inflammatory demyelination. Neurology; 43:1100–1104, 1993.

44. Weinshenker BG, O'Brien PC, Petterson TM, et al. A randomized trial of plasma exchange in acute central nervous system inflammatory demyelinating disease. Ann Neurol; 46:878–886, 1999.

45. Bo L, Vedeler CA, Nyland HI, Trapp BD, Mork SJ. Subpial demyelination in the cerebral cortex of multiple sclerosis patients. J Neuropathol Exp Neurol; 62:723–732, 2003.

46. Kutzelnigg A, Lucchinetti CF, Stadelmann C, et al. Cortical demyelination and diffuse white matter injury in multiple sclerosis. Brain; 128:2705–2712, 2005.

47. Brink BP, Veerhuis R, Breij EC, van der Valk P, Dijkstra CD, Bo L. The pathology of multiple sclerosis is location-dependent: no significant complement activation is detected in purely cortical lesions. J Neuropathol Exp Neurol; 64:147–155, 2005.

48. Moll NM, Rietsch AM, Ransohoff AJ, et al. Cortical demyelination in PML and MS: Similarities and differences. Neurology; 70:336–343, 2008.

49. Merkler D, Klinker F, Jurgens T, et al. Propagation of spreading depression inversely correlates with cortical myelin content. Ann Neurol; 66:355–365, 2009.

50. Rodriguez M, Scheithauer BW, Forbes G, Kelly PJ. Oligodendrocyte injury is an early event in lesions of multiple sclerosis. Mayo Clinic Proc; 68:627–636, 1993.

Chapter 6

What Has Immunology Taught Us About Multiple Sclerosis?

Abstract

There is strong evidence that MS is, at least in part, an immune-mediated disease. There is *less* evidence that MS is a classical autoimmune disease. Here we show the evidence that both supports and refutes the autoimmune hypothesis. We also discuss how different arms of the immune system may contribute to distinct aspects of the disease. It is seldom mentioned in textbooks that CD8[+] T cells make up the majority of the infiltrate in the MS plaque, irrespective of the acute pathology and the age of the lesion. We discuss the implication for CD8[+] T cells in association with upregulation of class I MHC on neural structures, with particular attention to the transection of axons and contribution to long-term disability. However, the activation of CD4[+] T cells to an autoantigen or to an exogenous antigen (possibly a virus) may occur early in the process, possibly even in the peripheral immune compartment rather than in the CNS. We also discuss how CD8[+] T cells are affected by partially effective, FDA-approved therapies and future "curative" therapies. Because interferon remains the cornerstone of effective therapy for most patients and viral examples of human and experimental demyelination exist naturally, there is ample rationale to continue searching for the infectious exogenous factor in MS. Thus, a preventive vaccine approach may eliminate the disease.

INTRODUCTION

Investigators and clinicians who have studied MS agree that the immune system plays a critical role in the development of lesions, especially during the acute early phases of the disease characterized by relapses. Relapses are fundamentally an inflammatory response occurring mostly in the white matter of the nervous system but possibly also within myelin tracts in the gray matter. Ultimately, this results in focal demyelination with relative axonal sparing. The best evidence for inflammation-induced relapses comes from work in MRI, which demonstrates the association of relapses with gadolinium enhancement—that is, disruption of the blood–brain barrier. Further, there is evidence of perivascular inflammation in biopsy specimens from patients experiencing an acute attack or at autopsy. As discussed in Chapter 5, the character of the immune response is similar in the four major patterns of acute MS lesion pathology. All of the acute pathological lesions show a marked predominance of CD8[+] T cells and a relative lack of CD4[+] T cells (ratios of 100:1 to 50:1).[1] In addition, there is a sea of macrophages, which plays a primary role in engulfing myelin debris, although their exact role in the disease process is still unknown. This has not been tested experimentally because there are no specific therapies to deplete macrophages, either in patients or experimental models. The contribution of the immune response to the more chronic neuronal degenerative phase of the disease is also unclear. Patients with primary progressive, nonrelapsing disease MRI studies have significantly fewer gadolinium-enhancing lesions as the disease evolves (Chapter 4). (Many consider these enhancing lesions to be the surrogate of inflammation in the CNS.) Not surprisingly, more published papers discuss the role of immune response in MS than any other aspect of the disease process. On many occasions, the findings *proposed* to occur in MS are findings that *actually* occur in the experimental model of autoimmune encephalomyelitis (EAE). Therefore, many studies and reviews are influenced by the frequent exchange of data between the human disease and the autoimmune model in animals.

FUNDAMENTAL QUESTION REGARDING THE IMMUNOLOGY OF MULTIPLE SCLEROSIS

A key issue is whether MS starts in the periphery or the interior of the CNS. That is, do inflammatory cells enter from lymph nodes, spleen, or blood through the blood–brain barrier to induce damage in the CNS, or does the disease occur inside the nervous system? Is the inciting event present in the CNS, which then recruits an inflammatory response to this exogenous or endogenous antigen? In addition, must inflammatory cells always undergo antigen presentation in the periphery, or can antigen presentation occur within the CNS as such, within inflammatory foci observed in the brain or, in particular, in the inflammatory follicles observed in the meninges, as they do in the lymph nodes or spleen? The answers to these questions are critical to determine treatment of the disease process. If the process begins in the periphery, then the current attempts to downregulate the inflammatory response in lymph tissue, by direct immunosuppression (cyclophosphamide [Cytoxan] or mitoxantrone), by inhibiting the outflow of cells from the lymph nodes (fingolamide), or by preventing the egress of cells through the blood–brain barrier (natalizumab), are logical and, ultimately, should prove curative. Indeed, the effectiveness of these agents over others (as discussed in Chapter 9) seems to suggest this. In contrast, if the process begins inside the CNS, the present approaches may have some palliative effect because the inflammatory response partially contributes to the disease process; however, unless the inciting agent is removed from the CNS, these approaches will not be curative. Some of the rebound effect observed after discontinuation of natalizumab suggests this. This is true of even the most aggressive form of immunosuppression, which is stem cell bone-marrow transplantation following complete ablation of the immune response. Current clinical experiments are testing this hypothesis by treating patients early in the disease course with very aggressive (but, at least for some patients, potentially lethal) treatments. If the process truly begins in the periphery and is mediated by peripheral immune cells, then those therapeutic processes will ultimately prove curative in nature.

IS MULTIPLE SCLEROSIS AN AUTOIMMUNE DISEASE?

Most textbooks and chapters about MS boldly state that MS is an autoimmune disease.

However, the evidence for such a statement is circumstantial at best, and there are defenders on both sides. We suggest revising the criteria for autoimmune diseases (Table 6.1).[2,3] We recommend that the reader contrast this with neuromyelitis optica (NMO), which is a proven autoimmune disease.

Immune Response to a Precise Autoantigen

The main criterion of a given autoimmune disease is that a precise autoantigen be present in all patients with the disease. Despite multiple attempts to identify potential MS antigens among various myelin proteins, lipids, and gangliosides, none have been proven or confirmed.

Reproduction of Lesion by Autoantibody or T Cell

Administration of autoantibody or T cells induces autoimmune disease in normal animals. Attempts to replicate these results in animal models of MS have been equivocal. An earlier study used mononuclear cells from the CSF of MS patients to induce MS-like lesions in animals with severe combined immunodeficiency.[4] MS patients, both during exacerbations and remissions, contributed the CSF used in these experiments. Animals with severe combined immunodeficiency received the collected CSF via intracisternal injection.

Table 6–1   **Criteria for Autoimmunity**

Revised Criteria for Determining Autoimmunity[3]	MS
1. Demonstration of an immune response to a precise autoantigen in all patients with the disease	No
2. Reproduction of the lesion by administration of autoantibody or T cells into a normal animal	No
3. Induction of lesion by immunizing an animal with relevant purified autoantigen	Possibly yes
4. Isolation or presence of autoantibody or autoreactive T cell from lesion (or serum)	Possibly yes
5. Correlation of autoantibody or autoreactive T cell with disease activity	No
6. Presence of other autoimmune disorders or autoantigens associated with disease	Possibly yes
7. Immune absorption with purified autoantigen abrogates pathogenic autoantibody or autoreactive T cell	No
8. Reduction of pathogenic autoantibody or T cell associated with clinical improvement	No

(Table adapted from Schwartz R, Datta S. Autoimmunity and autoimmune diseases. In: Paul W, ed. Fundamental immunology. 2nd ed. New York: Raven Press, Ltd., 1989: 819–866.[3])

The control animals received CSF samples from patients with cervical spondylosis or peripheral mononuclear cells from normal individuals. Within 4 to 6 weeks after transfer, the authors claimed that the majority of mice receiving CSF from MS patients showed disease exacerbation characterized by paralysis and ataxia. In addition, pathological evaluation of sacrificed mice revealed multiple scattered, discrete lesions localized in the white matter of the brainstem and spinal cords. The lesions were characterized by various amounts of inflammatory cell infiltrates. Most of the infiltrates were macrophages; however, granulocytes, albeit in small quantities, were also present. This is extremely unusual because granulocytes are seldom observed in the MS plaque. Furthermore, these lesions exhibited demyelination. In contrast, neither CSF of MS patients in remission, CSF cells from patients with cervical spondylosis, nor peripheral mononuclear cells from normal individuals resulted in disease in severe combined immunodeficiency mice. This potentially exciting paper was vigorously evaluated by the MS community, with many attempts to reproduce the findings. Investigators attempted to confirm the findings by injecting CSF cells donated by MS patients into the cisterna magna of laboratory animals.[5] They observed no neurological abnormalities and could reproduce none of the findings of demyelination via electron microscopy. A number of other laboratories worldwide performed the same studies, without success.

Lesion Induction by Autoantigen

The third major criterion for autoimmunity is the ability to induce lesions by immunizing animals with relevant autoantigen. Investigators focusing on the EAE models argue that this has been accomplished in MS, since a number of different antigens have been used and T cells transmit disease by adoptive transfer to other animals of the same species. In the autoimmune model, CD4+ T cells of the Th1/Th17 subgroup induce the disease. However, the results are ambiguous from the standpoint of identifying the "relevant" antigen in MS. While multiple different antigens can induce the disease process in the animal model, no one specific antigen has been shown to be superior to another.[6] Possibly, many antigens induce the

disease based on genetic subtype, which may make this criterion hard to fulfill in MS.

Isolation of Antibody or T Cells from Lesion or Serum

The fourth criterion is the ability to isolate autoantibody or autoreactive T cells from the lesion or serum. Multiple attempts have failed to identify autoreactive T cells from MS patients' blood or CSF.[7,8] Many investigators have suggested a higher precursor frequency of T cells, specifically of the CD4 subgroup, in patients with MS compared to healthy controls, which interact with myelin basic protein (MBP), proteolipid protein (PLP), myelin oligodendrocyte glycoprotein (MOG), or other such antigens from myelin. Unfortunately, because normal individuals have similar positive results, this criterion remains unproven. Some investigators have shown that MS serum reacts to a number of specific autoantigens, particularly MOG, MBP, PLP, and even other gangliosides.[9] Unfortunately, other investigators have repeated these studies without being able to discern a difference between MS patients and controls.[10,11]

Correlation of Autoantigen with Disease Activity

The fifth criterion is the correlation between the autoantigen and autoreactive T cells with disease activity. It is a consistent finding that autoreactive T cells occur with greater frequency in patients experiencing an exacerbation than in patients with progressive disease, which suggests a possible correlation between autoreactive T cells and disease activity. Even though the precursor frequency of autoreactive T cells is higher in MS than in normal controls, the presence of autoreactive T cells in normal controls casts doubt on the hypothesis that MS is an autoimmune disease.

Presence of Other Autoimmune Disorders

The sixth criterion is the presence of other autoimmune disorders or autoantigens associated with the disease. Many investigators have looked into this, and occasional case reports have demonstrated the presence of MS with other autoimmune diseases such as myasthenia gravis[12] and diabetes mellitus.[13] However, population-based cohort studies have failed to show an association between autoimmune diseases and MS.[14] The only possible increased odds ratio was found with thyroid disease, when hyperthyroidism and hypothyroidism were combined. In addition, there are documented, rare cases of patients having both MS and inflammatory bowel disease.[12,13] Multiple studies have also looked at the presence of autoantibodies, a characteristic of patients with autoimmune diseases, such as antibodies seen in Sjögren's syndrome, systemic lupus erythematosus (SLE), or myasthenia gravis, but to date no evidence indicates a higher concentration of these antibodies in MS patients than in normal controls. Of interest, this differs greatly from NMO,[15,16] which is notable for increased autoantibodies. The complexity of the disease process in MS may hamper the attempts to find an autoantibody association, but some population pockets of MS may be associated with increased autoimmunity.

Immune Absorption Abrogates Pathogen

An additional criterion is that immune absorption with purified autoantigen should abrogate the pathogenic autoantibody or autoreactive T cells. Since the putative autoantigen is not known in MS, these experiments cannot yield conclusive results. However, attempts to perform these experiments with specific antigens of myelin have shown that serum absorption with MBP does not prevent the antibodies from showing reactivity of to other myelin antigens.[17] Either there are multiple myelin antigens that can induce the disease process, or the findings are spurious. Clinical improvement should induce a reduction in the pathogenic autoantibody (on the T cell associated with the disease). Since the assays for reactivity against myelin antigens are observed not only in MS patients but also in neurological as well as healthy controls, it is difficult to correlate the clinical improvement with reduction of any kind of autoantibody or T-cell response to the myelin

antigen. Of interest, NMO, which closely mimics MS and is characterized by an immune response to aquaporin-4, appears to meet many criteria of an autoimmune disease.[2]

One disappointing aspect of this exercise has been the failure to demonstrate that MS is an autoimmune disease despite 50 years of work. All the other so-called "autoimmune disorders," such as myasthenia gravis, SLE, and Sjögren's syndrome, have definitive markers of the disease process against specific autoantigens, which can be used clinically to make the diagnosis and to follow the response to treatment. There still is not a definitive diagnostic test for MS utilizing a T cell, cytokine, or other immunological parameter against a myelin epitope. To date, it is still unclear whether a single autoantigen exists in MS.

CD8+ T Cells: Primary Mediator of Effector Function in the Multiple Sclerosis Plaque

The immune system is derived from bone marrow stem cells (Figs. 6.1 and 6.2). Pathological studies demonstrate that the CD8+ T cell is the most common T cell observed in the MS plaque. Conventional wisdom is that CD8+ T cells have two major functions: cytotoxicity and suppression. Because of the strong bias of the EAE models, the CD8+ T cell has been primarily thought to play a suppressive role in MS, since that has been the traditional role observed in EAE. In EAE, the CD4+ T cell, through its Th1 and Th17 function, mediates the disease and induces the inflammatory response, neurological deficits, paralysis, and histological findings. CD8+ T cells in EAE are associated with recovery of neurological function and have "suppressive" properties. In contrast, the CD8+ T cells appear to play a much more aggressive role in the MS plaque rather than just suppressing the inflammatory response. If this were not the case, then the CD8+ T cells would not be the most common T cell observed in the MS lesion. CD8+ T cells interact with major histocompatibility (MHC) class I antigens to induce their response[1] (Fig. 6.3A). In normal CNS, class I MHC is present only in vascular cells and rare meningeal cells. However, during the inflammatory phase of MS, class I MHC is present in astrocytes,

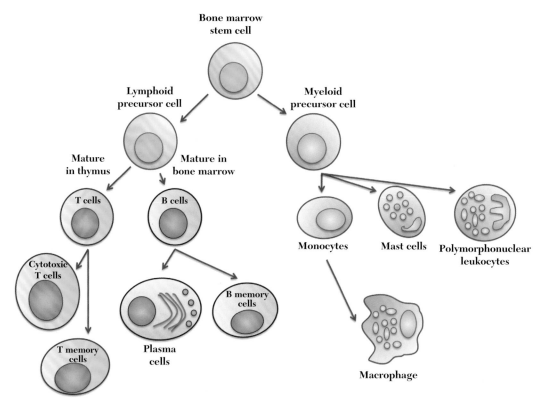

Figure 6–1. Development of bone marrow cells to mature T cells. The bone marrow cells divide into two major lines: (1) myeloid precursor line and (2) lymphoid precursor line. The myeloid precursor line ultimately leads to the development of macrophages, which are critical antigen-presenting cells in the MS lesion. This is the most common cell observed in MS plaques. It plays a major role in engulfing myelin debris and may actively strip off myelin sheaths as a result of capping immunoglobulins on its cell surface. Other myelin precursor cells, monocytes, mast cells, and polymorphonuclear cells are rarely observed in MS lesions except in very acute forms of demyelinating disease, such as Devic's disease or acute disseminated encephalomyelitis. Lymphoid precursor cell lines undergo two major divisions: one group develops in the thymus, and the second one in the bone marrow. Thymic cells develop into cytotoxic cells and memory T cells. These lines can differentiate further into cells with specific effector cell functions. The rest of the bone marrow line will form B cells, which ultimately develop into plasma cells, the cells that secrete immunoglobulins. Immunoglobulins are pathogenic in at least 50% of MS lesions. The patients with immunoglobulin deposition in their lesions respond dramatically to plasma-exchange therapy after acute devastating attacks that do not respond to high-dose methylprednisolone.

oligodendrocytes, and neurons, and even rarely on axons.[18] In addition, the CD8+ T cells appear to correlate with axonal injury, and there is strong evidence that CD8+ T cells play a major role in transecting axons *in vitro* (Fig. 6.3B).[19,20] Relapses of MS correlate with increased CD8+ T-cell cytotoxicity in the CSF.[21] Several clinical trials with monoclonal antibodies directed against CD4+ T cells failed to show any therapeutic benefit in MS.[22] In contrast, broader-spectrum antibodies (alemtuzumab CD52) can deplete all T cells,[23] including CD8+ T cells, which may play a critical role in MS pathogenesis. It is also noteworthy that CD8+ T cells play a major role in a number of proven autoimmune diseases including SLE, diabetes mellitus, Crohn's disease, Graves' disease, and autoimmune Addison's disease.[1]

Finally, unlike CD4+ T cells, CD8+ T cells show oligoclonal expansion in MS brains, blood, and CSF.[24–26] Some of the cytotoxic T cells react against autoantigens such as MBP.[6] If these cells traveled randomly in the CNS, then presumably their CD3 junctional region length would show a normal Gaussian distribution. In contrast, there appears to be skewing of the CDR3 junctional regions in MS, suggesting a selective infiltration or expansion of CD8+ T-cell clones into the CNS.[26] Moreover, the T-cell receptors of the CD8+ T cells

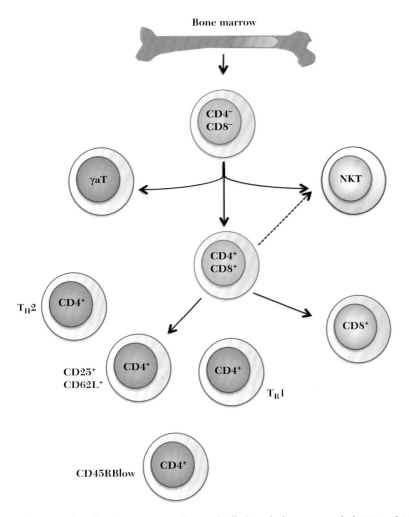

Figure 6–2. Development of T cells in bone marrow. The initial cells from the bone marrow lack CD4 and CD8 receptors. These cells will differentiate into three different types of cells: γΔ T cells, natural killer (NK) T cells, and cells that express both the CD4 and CD8 receptors on their surface. NK T cells are a unique T cell that recognizes glycolipids on the cell surface. Because glycolipids are common on the myelin sheaths, these cells may play a role in the pathogenesis of demyelination. Unfortunately, little work has been devoted to these cells. γΔ T cells are rare T cells that represent part of the immune response to virus infections. Double-positive CD4+/CD8+ T cells will differentiate into either single-positive CD8+ cells or CD4+ cells. The CD4+ cells then differentiate into a number of different populations, as shown in Figure 6.8.

demonstrate distinct CD8+ T cell clones with conserved specificity, implying recognition of an identical antigen that results in their proliferation in the CNS.

Much effort has focused on the potential role of interleukin (IL)-17 in the MS plaque, and given the bias of the EAE experiments, the CD4+ T cells have been proposed as the source. However, there is also evidence that CD8+ T cells make IL-17,[27] a point overlooked by most investigators viewing MS through the EAE model. Defining IL-17+ CD8+ T cells

opens up new avenues for future research and new immunotherapeutic targets.

CD8+ T cells secrete a number of molecules, including granzymes and perforin (Fig. 6.4). Strong evidence suggests that perforin contributes to axonal injury in the MS plaque (Fig. 6.5). Perforin appears to correlate with neurological disability and the presence of "black holes" on MRI. Therefore, CD8+ T cells may influence the acute inflammatory phase of the disease as well as the neurodegenerative phase. CD8+ T cells may account

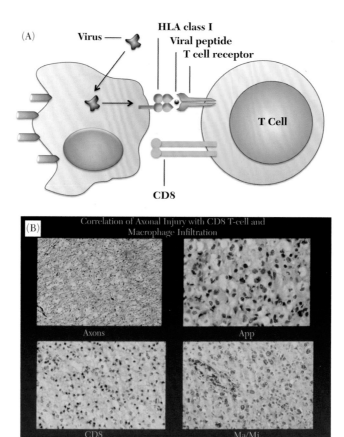

Figure 6–3. CD8+ T cells in the MS plaque. CD8+ T cells and macrophages are the primary effector cells for axonal injury in MS. (**A**) This panel, taken from an MS plaque, shows evidence of axonal loss stained with a silver stain (Bielschowsky). In addition, there is accumulation of amyloid precursor protein (APP) stained red by immunocytochemistry. APP is a normal component of neurons and axons that travels up and down the axon by axonal transport. When the axon is transected, the APP accumulates proximal to the site of injury. The red reaction product in this image signifies the number of dysfunctional axons in this MS lesion. (**B**) The next panel shows a large number of CD8+ T cells stained by immunocytochemistry. The CD8+ T cell is the most common T-cell subtype found in the MS lesion. In contrast, very few CD4+ T cells are seen in the typical plaque. In the same lesion, a marker for macrophages and microglial cells (Ma/Mi) shows an intense number of macrophages stained with a brown reaction product in this lesion, which shows axonal injury and accumulation of APP. (Adapted from Bitsch A, Schuchardt J, Bunkowski S, Kuhlmann T, Bruck W. Acute axonal injury in multiple sclerosis. Correlation with demyelination and inflammation. Brain; 123 (Pt 6):1174–1183, 2000.[110])

for axonal damage in MS as well as long-term neurological deficits.

It is also worthwhile to postulate a regulatory role for CD8+ T cells in MS. Investigators have identified CD8+/CD25+Foxp3+ as regulatory T cells in MS patients.[28] In these studies, they looked at peripheral blood, CSF, and CD8+ T-cell clones from patients with MS exacerbations, patients with remissions, healthy individuals, and patients with other inflammatory neurological diseases. The inhibition of CD4 self-reactive T-cell proliferation by CD8+ regulatory cells was mediated by IL-10 and transforming growth factor beta (TGF-β). Any attempt to delete CD8+ T cells from the MS lesion could potentially worsen the disease by eliminating regulatory cells. Therefore, caution is advisable in any effort to manipulate the CD8+ population.

CD8+ T cells may play a major role in the secondary progressive phase of the disease by secreting lymphotoxin.[29] Cytokine-secretion studies in patients with secondary progressive MS and normal controls revealed clear evidence of anti-CD3-stimulated CD8+ T cells in the patients with secondary progressive MS. These

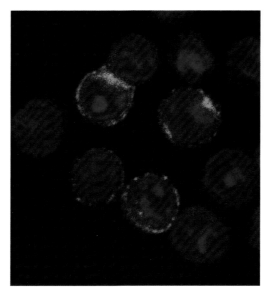

Figure 6–4. CD8⁺ T cells secrete perforin as a primary molecule to induce injury to their target cells. Perforin appears by Alexa Fluor 88 Green staining. The perforin is polarized to one side of CD8⁺ T cells, as shown in this figure. In contrast, the CD8 marker (Alexa 568 Red) completely surrounds the cells. Some cells in this figure are negative for the CD8 marker.

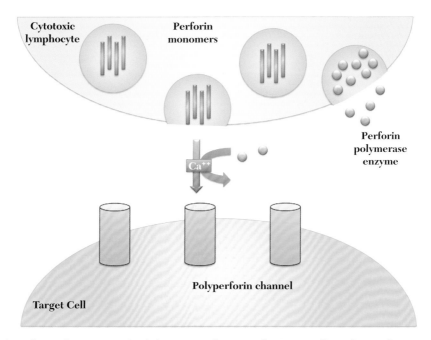

Figure 6–5. Perforin is the primary molecule known to mediate injury by CD8⁺ T cells. Perforin mediates axonal transection in MS and correlates with neurological disability. Cytotoxic T cells secrete perforin in the form of granules along with granzymes. This release activates calcium, which results in "poly-perforin" channels on the target cells. This results in holes in the membrane of the target cells, causing leakage of intracellular material, which results in cell death.

cells secrete lymphotoxin and other cytokines, which affect the progressive phase of the disease. This provides strong evidence of a role for CD8+ T cells in both the neurodegenerative aspect of the progressive phase of the disease and the early acute phase. It remains unclear whether MS represents a CD8-driven autoimmunity.

ROLE OF CYTOKINES AS SURROGATES FOR EXACERBATIONS OR PROGRESSION

Do cytokines predict exacerbations, and can they be targeted for immunotherapy? The discovery of new cytokines in immunology has been staggering. New cytokines or growth factors that play a major role in immune response are constantly being identified. In addition, the number of known CD antigens increases almost on a weekly basis. Therefore, it is not surprising that many have been investigated in MS, and some have been targeted for specific immunotherapy. Because many acute exacerbations are associated with aspects of inflammatory response, it is not surprising that many immune factors such as interferon-gamma (IFN-γ) and tumor necrosis factor (TNF), as well as other cytokines or lymphokines, are linked to acute exacerbations. In some studies, the presence of these factors precedes clinical exacerbations or MRI lesions or is associated with remission.[7] These factors play a critical role in the evolution of the disease process.[30]

Many investigators studied the secretion of IFN and TNF[31] longitudinally in MS patients. They demonstrated that both IFN-γ and TNF precede clinical symptoms by up to 2 weeks. In contrast, in benign cases, this increase in cytokine disappears rapidly, even before symptoms develop. These observations have led to the idea of therapeutically targeting these immune factors.

Because anti-TNF antibody-blocking therapy had proven effective in rheumatoid arthritis, similar studies were attempted in MS. Despite strong evidence that TNF prevents demyelination and promotes myelination in Theiler's murine encephalomyelitis virus (TMEV) models,[32] other experiments utilizing EAE found exactly the opposite: that is, anti-TNF therapy improved the function of EAE mice immunized with myelin antigens.[33] Anti-TNF therapy was then attempted in MS, but the study had to be terminated prematurely when the participants experienced significantly increased MRI lesions and neurological deficits.[34] This has led to an interesting scenario in which patients who received anti-TNF therapy for rheumatoid arthritis subsequently presenting with MS-like symptoms.[35] The frequency of these MS-like exacerbations is relatively low (2–3%) in patients receiving anti-TNF therapy, but the characteristics of the lesions are identical to those observed in conventional MS. However, the symptoms resolve shortly after discontinuing anti-TNF therapy, and the MRI lesions also improve. The current guidelines are to avoid prescribing anti-TNF therapy for any individual with a history of MS or demyelinating disease. Although the risk of an onset of demyelinating events is relatively small, this effect can be clinically "silent," making it difficult to assess the actual numbers of the affected individuals. The risk may increase with cumulative exposure.[36] This paradoxical result is exactly at odds with the findings in EAE but supports the finding in the TMEV model and raises important issues regarding the basic pathogenesis of MS. Using IFN-γ leads to a similar result.[37]

There has been much investigation into the immunological factors halting the evolution of a clinical relapse.[30] In EAE both IL-10 and TGF-β can arrest the evolution of EAE paralysis. Similarly, IL-10 appears to increase following an acute attack in human MS.[38,39] Thus, pro-inflammatory and anti-inflammatory cytokines appear to correlate with disease activity and remissions in MS. These correlations depend, in part, on the disease stage; IFN-γ and IL-12 have more impact in patients with active relapsing–remitting disease, whereas IL-10 decreases in patients with secondary progressive disease compared to controls,[39] suggesting and supporting the concept of a decreased role. In addition, IL-10 messenger RNA levels decrease 4 weeks before MRI activity and 6 weeks before relapses. The onset of secondary progressive disease coincides with low IL-10 messenger RNA levels constitutively, suggesting an important role for Th2-driven IL10 in controlling disease progression.[40] However, it is not clear if the decrease in "protective" cytokine levels is the result or cause of mechanisms that induce or propagate the "neurodegenerative" progression phenotype in MS. Certainly, it does not appear to be the cause.

As we discuss in subsequent chapters, the first-line disease-modifying medications that promote Th2-predominant cytokine profiles apparently do not prevent progressive disease in our experience.

ROLE OF CHEMOKINES IN MULTIPLE SCLEROSIS

Chemokines largely regulate the migration of immune cells. Studies in MS have shown that certain chemokines ($CXCL_{12}$ and $CXCL_{13}$) are up regulated differently dependent on CNS immune cell recruitment.[41] $CXCL_{12}$ is expressed in CNS parenchyma such as astrocytes and blood vessel walls, whereas $CXCL_{13}$ is located in perivascular infiltrates. Inflammatory diseases such as MS alter the display of chemokines along the blood brain barrier and may enable leukocytes to enter the CNS.[42]

ROLE OF PROTEINASES IN DISEASE PROGRESSION

Intense interest exists in a possible critical role for matrix metalloproteinases in inflammatory demyelination. Because these molecules degrade many components of the axonal matrix, they could be important targets for treatment. For that reason, they have been studied in a number of important conditions, including rheumatoid arthritis and tumor growth. In MS, matrix metalloproteinases[43] may be necessary for breaking down the blood–brain barrier, destroying myelin, and releasing disease-promoting cytokines. Investigating the role of kallikreins has also led to the discovery of a new set of proteases with a possible role in MS (Fig. 6.6).[44] The best-known of these is kallikrein-3 or "prostate-specific antigen," the cornerstone for the diagnosis of benign prostatic hypertrophy and prostatic carcinoma. Kallikrein-6, one of 15 kallikreins in the human genome, appears to be made exclusively in the CNS by oligodendrocytes. This led investigators to study the role of kallikreins in the evolution of MS lesions.[45] These kallikreins are also upregulated in immune cells[46] and activated by triggering the CD3 receptor. Thus, as a result of antigen stimulation, these factors may contribute significantly to demyelination. In addition, kallikrein-6 may play a critical role in spinal cord injury.[44] Various kallikreins are significant actors in the CNS.[47] To elucidate the potential kallikrein activity in MS, serum levels of kallikreins-1, -6, -7, -8, and -10 were measured in 35 MS patients and 66 controls by quantitative fluorometric enzyme-linked immunosorbent assays. Serum levels were measured against Expanded Disability Status Scale (EDSS) scores to determine the relationship between the serological sampling and functional status. MS patients had elevated serum levels of kallikreins-1 and -6 compared to controls. Patients with secondary progressive MS had the highest levels. Kallikrein-1 correlated with higher EDSS scores at the time of the serum sampling, whereas kallikrein-6 correlated with future EDSS worsening in relapsing–remitting patients. These studies support the concept that kallikreins, and potentially other serum metalloproteases, are associated

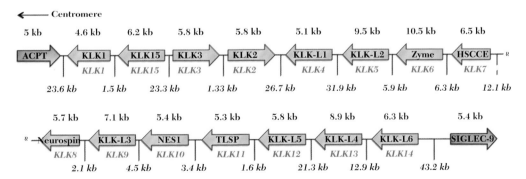

Figure 6–6. All of the identified kallikreins appear in line in the human genome. The kallikreins most important in MS are KLK1, KLK10, and KLK6. KLK6 is expressed on oligodendrocytes and neural cells, whereas many other kallikreins are expressed primarily on immune cells. KLK3, otherwise known as prostate-specific antigen, is a known marker for prostate cancer and benign prostatic hypertrophy. Further investigation as to the role of kallikreins in MS may lead to a reliable diagnostic test for MS.

with the progressive aspects of MS. These novel proteases may serve as serological markers of disease progression and may contribute directly[48] to neurological disability by promoting axonal injury and neuronal cell death.

PERSISTENT VIRUS INFECTION AS A CAUSE OF MULTIPLE SCLEROSIS?

A persistent virus infection may be the pathogenic mechanism of MS.[49] The evidence of a role for virus in MS development also comes from work in experimental animals, in which viruses from a large number of subgroups and families have induced MS-like diseases or are associated with human demyelination, such as the picornavirus group,[50,51] the coronavirus,[52,53] mouse hepatitis virus,[54] herpes virus, type 6[55–57] (Fig. 6.7), and retrovirus HTLV1.[58] Intrathecal Epstein-Barr virus antibodies are also part of the polyspecific immune response in MS.[59] The viral hypothesis receives additional support because independent MHC class I genes contribute to susceptibility.[60] One potential avenue of investigation in this area is the natural killer (NK) cell, since NK cells are the

primary effectors that eliminate viruses from the CNS prior to the development of the adaptive immune response.

NATURAL KILLER CELLS

Investigators have studied the function of NK cells in MS (Fig. 6.8).[61,62] Compared to age- and sex-matched controls, MS patients had less natural killing activity than the control population, suggesting that fewer NK cells may predispose them to virus infections. Other investigators have independently confirmed the paucity of NK cells in MS. This defect may be selective and may predispose to specific virus infection in the CNS. In addition, investigators examined NK-cell activity in 12 patients receiving IFN-γ[63] and demonstrated an increase in NK cell activity following IFN-γ therapy. This was performed using NK-cell–mediated lysis of Cr-labeled-K-562 cells. The NK cell activity was normal after treatment and reached baseline within 1 week despite continuous IFN-γ administration over the next 6 months. *In vitro* augmentation of NK cells by IFN-γ also appears to prevent the infection of

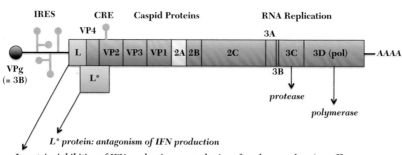

Figure 6–7. Theiler's virus genome. Theiler's virus is an RNA picornavirus similar to the poliovirus that is an excellent model for human MS. The virus is injected directly into the CNS of particular genetic strains of mice. Depending on the strain, animals develop acute encephalitis and clear the virus, or mice develop persistent infection with demyelination in the spinal cord. In the B6 strain, the majority of CD8+ T cells are directed against an antigen on VP2 capsid proteins of the virus (VP2$_{121-130}$). The genetic size of this virus is approximately 9 Kb, which is small (pico). This virus is approximately 28 nm; therefore, it is impossible to distinguish the virus from a normal ribosome by electron microscopy. It is not possible to distinguish lesions caused by Theiler's virus from lesions caused by inflammatory diseases such as EAE. However, by *in situ* hybridization, all Theiler's virus lesions show infectious RNA.

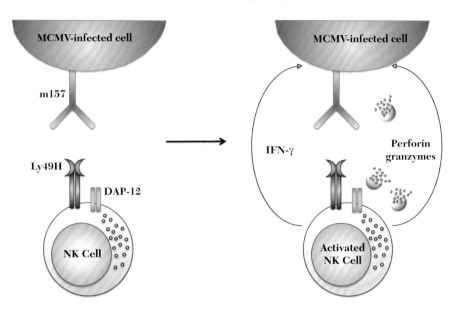

Figure 6–8. Activation of NK cells by virus. NK cells are the primary cells mediating the early immune response to viral infection. Prior to development of the adaptive immune response, NK cells enter the lesion and begin to kill virus-infected cells. These cells are unique in that they do not recognize MHC; in contrast, they recognize the absence of MHC. Therefore, those cells that do not have MHC on their cell surface are more likely to be lysed by NK cells. The NK cells express ly49h receptor, which recognizes m157 receptor on the surface of the infected cell. This interaction causes activated NK cells to release perforin and granzymes to kill infected cells. The ultimate effector function of NK cells is similar to that of CD8+ T cells, in that both secrete perforin and granzymes. The difference is that CD8+ T cells recognize the processed viral peptide. In contrast, NK cells do not have to recognize any viral peptide but will kill the virus-infected cells in the absence of antigen processing and peptide recognition.

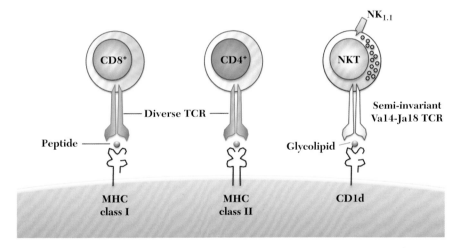

Figure 6–9. NK T cells recognize glycolipids. Each different type of T cells recognizes specific receptors on the antigen-presenting cells. Antigen-presenting cells can either be macrophages or dendritic cells. In the nervous system, astrocytes or microglial cells may also present antigen. CD8+ T cells recognize peptides in the context of class I MHC. Class I MHC is present on all cells and is upregulated in neurons, axons, astrocytes, and oligodendrocytes in the MS plaque. CD4+ T cells recognize class II MHC antigens on their surface. Those cells that express class II antigens are primarily dendritic cells and macrophages. In contrast, NK T cells recognize glycolipids through the CD1 D-receptor on the surface. This is a unique cell that downregulates the immune response in MS.

other viruses, including measles viruses; thus, retaining the normality of NK cell function by IFN may result in nonspecific antiviral defense in the CNS of MS patients. In contrast, NK T cells recognize a glycolipid in association with CD1don the target cell (Fig. 6.9). Their function in MS may be relevant because glycolipids are expressed on myelin and oligodendrocytes.

CSF, IGG, AND OLIGOCLONAL BANDS

CSF IgG and oligoclonal bands (Fig. 6.10) remain the most predictive immunological test for the diagnosis of MS. All immunoglobulin subtypes have been implicated in MS (Fig. 6.11). It is possible to elute oligoclonal IgG bands from MS plaques.[64] Investigators have studied oligoclonal IgG patterns from individual unbound plaque extracts from autopsied MS brains by post-isoelectric focused immunofixation. They demonstrated the presence of distinct oligoclonal bands. Different sections of a single MS brain had similar banding profiles, which implied a common immunological response.[65] Because an elevated CSF IgG index, as well as the presence of oligoclonal bands in the CSF not present in the serum, remains the most reliable test for the diagnosis of MS, it is difficult to understand why MS immunology research has focused more on the role of CD4 T cells rather than the role of an unidentified antibody. This may be another manifestation of the influence of the EAE model on the investigation of MS. Clearly, CD4 T cells mediate the pathology and the effector functions in the experimental model, but their role in the human disease remains speculative.

As discussed in earlier chapters, there have been multiple attempts to identify the source of the antibody response in patients with MS.[66] This has ranged from looking at a number of myelin antigens to potential etiological factors such as viruses. CSF IgG in patients with MS clearly does react with a very large number of virus proteins.[67] However, most of this response apparently targets the Epstein-Barr virus, the virus considered to be the most likely infectious factor increasing the risk of MS. (See discussion in Chapter 3.) Immune responses to other viruses have also been described, including varicella zoster, rubella, vaccinia viruses, and measles viruses.

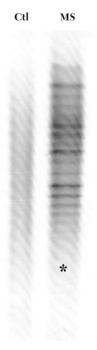

Ctl   MS

*

Figure 6–10. The presence of oligoclonal bands in the CSF is the most specific test for the diagnosis of MS.[65] The specificity of these bands is not known, although some target viral proteins and some are directed against myelin antigens. The diagnostic test used is the presence of oligoclonal bands that are not present in the serum. In control CSF, no banding occurs, and the gel shows as a smear. In contrast, discrete banding is present in MS. The pattern of banding is distinct for each individual patient. The banding pattern is constant throughout the patient's disease course, indicating that the pattern results from VDJ rearrangements of the immunoglobulin genes at the onset of disease. Approximately 95% of MS patients have oligoclonal bands or an increase in the CSF IgG index.

Because immunoglobulins target many viruses, the antibody response in MS may be a so-called "nonsense antibody," as proposed by Mattson in 1980.[17] Investigators attempted to elute the IgG from CSF and tissue of MS patients and compare it to patients with subacute sclerosing panencephalitis (SSPE). SSPE is a CNS response to persistent measles infection and, therefore, provided an important control for MS IgG. The results, using isoelectric-focusing techniques, demonstrated that the IgG eluted from CSF or tissue of MS patients reacted against a wide variety of different antigens. However, the IgG isolated from SSPE reacted specifically to measles virus. It is important, however, to note that elution taken from individual patients elicited a distinct IgG

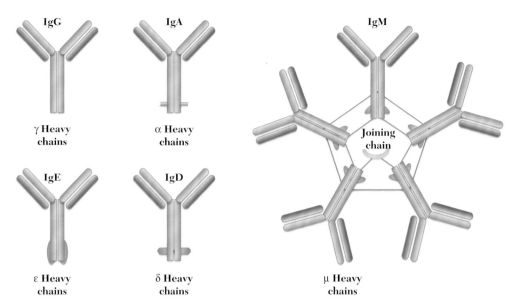

Figure 6–11. Different forms of immunoglobulins are present in the human repertoire. Immunoglobulin IgGs are the presumptive immunoglobulins pathogenic in MS and may be directed against autoantigens or against viral antigens. IgA antibodies are found primarily in the gut of patients with MS. IgE antibodies are usually a response to an allergic reaction and are rarely elevated in MS. Some IgM antibodies are part of the reparative response. Human monoclonal antibodies of the IgM isotype have been shown to be directed against either oligodendrocytes or neurons. When these antibodies are injected into animals with demyelinating disease, they show evidence of CNS repair with either remyelination or preservation of axons.

pattern in MS patients. The same experiment done with separate SSPE samples taken from different brain areas from individual patients showed an identical banding, pattern. An identical IgG pattern from different areas of SSPE brain suggests a common response to the same antigen (measles virus). An identical IgG response among different MS plaques of the individual, but a different response in control patients, suggests a variable response to the same antigen as a result of unique aspects of the genetics of individuals to raise an immune response. The other possibility is that each patient has different MS antigens. The last possibility is that these responses are part of the so-called "nonsense antibody response," which some investigators call the "natural autoantibody response." Of interest, some studies have shown part of this natural antibody response to play a role in the reparative aspect of demyelinating lesions.[68] Investigators have cloned and sequenced a human antibody (antibody 22) for phase I clinical trials.[69] This natural autoantibody stimulates oligodendrocytes *in vivo* to promote CNS remyelination in various experimental animal models of MS.[69] The clinical

trial will determine whether the antibody does, indeed, enhance CNS remyelination and result in functional improvement in MS. This immunoglobulin may be a unique, repair-inducing response to the CNS.[68–73]

To test the autoimmune hypothesis, investigators have tried to determine whether antibodies found in the CSF or serum of MS patients target specific myelin antigens.[9] Unfortunately, the results of these experiments have been extremely variable, with outcomes ranging from positive to no response. For example, some laboratories have obtained antibody responses against MOG using recombinant human extracellular immunoglobulin domains of MOG.[9] These investigators screened serum and CSF in 130 MS patients, 32 patients with other inflammatory diseases, and 30 patients with noninflammatory neurological disorders. They demonstrated seropositivity directed against a MOG–Ig complex in a small percentage of MS patients. Approximately one third of patients responded to MBP. There was a smaller response in patients with other neurological diseases and in patients with rheumatoid arthritis. The investigators demonstrated that part of the intrathecal synthesis of IgG in MS patients targets the MOG–Ig complex.[9] However, the presence of a response in normal controls precludes using this assay as a diagnostic test in MS. One can conclude from these experiments that there are elevated immunoglobulin responses against CNS antigens; however, this response is also present in controls.

Antibodies produced in the CSF of MS patients come from cloned, expanded plasma cells.[10] These investigators produced 53 human IgG1 human monoclonal recombinant proteins that expressed heavy- and light-chain variable regions from 51 plasma-cell clones from MS CSF cells. The investigators tested these responses against a number of different myelin components and concluded that the oligoclonal B-cell response in MS CSF does not target any well-characterized myelin antigens such as MBP, PLP, or MOG. These experiments provide the strongest refutation of the hypothesis that the antibody response in MS CSF targets myelin antigens.

Others have tested whether antibody responses in MS targeted specific antigens on oligodendrocytes such as oligodendrocyte-specific protein (OSP).[11] They tested serum and CSF samples from MS patients with relapsing–remitting disease and compared them to controls; they determined that a percentage of MS patients had an immune response against a region of the OSP molecule and that this antibody also cross-reacts with several common viral peptides. This supports the occurrence of molecular mimicry in the CSF immunoglobulin response and suggests links between CSF IgG and viral and myelin antigens. This hypothesis states that, following viral infection, "molecular mimicry" mechanisms amplify the cross-reactivity response to myelin antigens.[74]

Because plasma exchange is beneficial in patients with acute fulminant attacks of MS, immunoglobulins in the lesions may play a pathogenic role in the disease process.[48] A positive response to plasma exchange correlated precisely with patients with biopsy-proven pattern II-type lesions, in which IgG and the terminal component of complement actively engaged to destroy myelin sheaths.[75] Other investigators tested whether the terminal component of complement is present in the CSF of MS patients and plays a role in the disease process.[76] Investigators using an immunoradiometric assay measured the terminal component of complement (C9) in the CSF of 35 MS patients as well as 55 neurological controls. There was a highly significant reduction of CSF C9 concentration in MS patients compared to controls. Reduced C9 concentration in MS patients led investigators to suggest that C9 consumption was a result of membrane attack complex-induced myelin damage. Other investigators repeated experiments to confirm these results.[77] They tested 93 consecutive patients referred for CSF examination in the outpatient clinic; unfortunately, these studies showed no differences in CSF C9 or C9 index between MS patients and neurological controls.

Clearly, the immunoglobulin in MS lesions induces injury.[78] Some findings may be relevant to the immunopathology of secondary progressive MS.[79] In these experiments, the investigators looked at macrophages from MS tissue and demonstrated a cap in the surface IgG on the poles of macrophages. There was no such staining for albumin on macrophages. The capping implied the presence of a multivalent ligand close to the cell surface. Because the cap formation was observed only in macrophages contacting myelin sheaths, it suggested that a cytophilic antimyelin antibody was present in the CNS of MS patients. It implied that immune-mediated ligand cytolysis is an early event in the breakdown of myelin in the disease process, which is consistent with the observations demonstrating the presence of IgG in specific forms of MS.[80] The presence of CD3, an opsinin formed during the complement activation, associates with destructive myelin. CD3 coupling increases the immunogenicity of specific antigens. It suggested the disruptive myelin close to plaques as the possible source of the putative MS antigen. This provides further evidence that immunoglobulin-plus-complement deposition injures MS lesions.

IMMUNOGLOBULINS AS A HINDRANCE TO OLIGODENDROCYTE PROGENITOR DIFFERENTIATION AND REMYELINATION

Can immunoglobulins prevent oligodendrocyte progenitor (OPC) differentiation (and thus remyelination)? In a series of experiments, investigators asked whether antibody diminished remyelination of demyelinated lesions.[81] They specifically looked for antibodies directed against antigens on OPCs. In myelinated cultures, they demonstrated cell lysis with an antibody that recognized OPC surface antigens (AN2) and suppressed the synthesis of myelin proteins. CSF from patients with active relapsing–remitting MS generated antibodies against AN2; however, CSF from patients with nonactive disease did not mount this response. This provided initial evidence that antibodies in the MS lesion actually inhibit the development and propagation of remyelination and may lead to the cascade of events presenting as a relapse with poor recovery.

Other investigators have demonstrated increased circulating antiganglioside antibodies in both primary and secondary progressive MS.[82] In these studies, plasma samples from 70 MS patients were compared to samples from 41 patients with other neurological diseases and 38 normal subjects. Samples were tested against various gangliosides, including GM1, GM3, GD1a, GD1b and GD3, using enzyme-linked immunosorbent assays. They demonstrated that patients with primary progressive MS and secondary progressive MS, compared to patients with relapsing–remitting MS or healthy controls, had a higher percentage of antibodies against GM3. The elevated antiganglioside antibodies may be secondary to axonal damage or may directly reduce axonal damage. This suggests that antibodies contribute directly to the progressive phases of MS lesions by binding to gangliosides on axons and neurons.

B CELLS AS ANTIGEN-PRESENTING CELLS

B cells are traditionally thought to be the primary source of antibody in the CNS. Can B cells also act as antigen-presenting cells and thus contribute to the pathogenesis of MS? Traditionally, microglia, macrophages, or even astrocytes were considered candidates for antigen-presenting cells in the CNS that contribute to pathogenesis. However, more recent data also suggest B cells as an important source of antigen presentation, specifically from the standpoint of generating antibody responses detrimental to the disease process.[83] B cells have long been known as enigmatic actors in MS pathogenesis. Evidence supports each immunoglobulin produced in the CNS as the result of B cells proliferating in the CNS during the course of the disease. These B-lineage cells are long-lived, especially as plasma cells that can survive for many years, even for the lifespan of the individual. This offers a possible explanation for CSF oligoclonal bands that persist throughout the disease course. The pattern of CSF IgG oligoclonal banding does not change in a unique patient;[65] however, the banding pattern differs between patients.[17] This suggests that individual genetics or early environment determines oligoclonal band patterning. In contrast, if the CSF IgG bands were the result of a common antigen, one would expect the oligoclonal banding pattern to be similar among all patients. Unique oligoclonal banding patterns among patients suggest that genes within B cells or plasma cells critically affect some aspect of the pathogenesis or "repair" because the CSF IgG oligoclonal bands are present in over 95% of patients with MS.[84]

B cells may also secrete abnormal cytokines, which could, in themselves, trigger the T-cell–mediated disease. Experiments using B cells from MS patients exhibited aberrant, inflammatory cytokines, including lymphotoxin and TNF secretion, in the context of pathogen-associated toll-like receptor (TLR) nonligand CPG DNA. B-cell depletion, either *ex vivo* or *in vivo*, yielded diminished putative inflammatory cytokines of the Th1 and Th17 pattern, which could affect both CD4 and CD8+ T cells. These soluble products appear largely mediated by activated B cells. These findings point to a possible association between infections and new MS relapses, since TLR appears to be the pathogen-associated ligand on B cells. This may explain the therapeutic properties of immune depletion of B cells with rituximab, an anti-CD20 antibody.[85]

TEARS AS A SOURCE OF OLIGOCLONAL IGG IN MULTIPLE SCLEROSIS PATIENTS

Sometimes it is difficult to persuade patients to undergo CSF examination because they fear persistent headache or pain from having a needle in the back. However, studies suggest that oligoclonal bands are present in the tears as well as in the CSF of MS patients.[86] Investigators found IgG banding patterns in tears from 28 MS patients and 4 patients with optic neuritis. In contrast, patients with systemic inflammatory or other neurological diseases did not exhibit this characteristic. Tears provide an easily available source for studying abnormal oligoclonal band response in MS. The presence of oligoclonal bands in tears challenges the hypothesis that oligoclonal bands are unique to the CSF and are uniquely made by B cells in the CNS and CSF. Their presence in tears suggests that B cells travel to other organs and supports the hypothesis that MS is not a totally CNS-specific disease but may be a manifestation of a more broadly defined systemic disease with predominant abnormalities in the CNS. A recent French study confirms these findings.[87]

ROLE OF CD4+ T CELLS AS INITIATORS OF DISEASE VERSUS EFFECTORS IN DESTRUCTION OF MYELIN

The area of greatest confusion in the MS literature is the role of CD4+ T cells in disease pathogenesis. As mentioned previously, CD8+ T cells are the most common cells found in the MS plaque. However, CD4 cells predominate in EAE as the effectors of disease and myelin destruction. Many investigators influenced by the experimental model have attempted to show a pathogenic role for CD4+ T cells in the evolution of MS. While many findings regarding the role of CD4+ T cells reported cannot be reproduced elsewhere,[88] there is strong experimental evidence that the immune response begins through the engagement of antigen recognized by receptors on CD4+ T cells. In concept, dendritic cells, both outside and inside the CNS, take up the exogenous or endogenous antigen and present it to CD4+ T cells. As a result, these CD4+ T cells differentiate into four distinct subtypes, depending on the inflammatory milieu (Fig. 6.12). The first is the Th1-type CD4+ T cell, which primarily secretes IFN-γ and TNF-α. The second CD4+ T cell, frequently called Th2, secretes primarily TGF-β and IL-10. The third is a CD4+ T$_{REG}$ cell

that performs a regulatory function.[89] These T cells express a number of transcription factors, including FoxP3[90,91] and other molecules, which play a major role in downregulating the immune response.[92] Finally, CD4+ T cells that primarily secrete IL-17 are called Th17 cells. Th17 cells induce most of the pathology in EAE. They may be present in the MS plaque, where they preferentially recruit IFN-γ.[93] Data strongly suggest that CD4+ T cells from MS patients use unique human T-cell beta receptors.[94] In these studies, the investigators used T-cell lines from MS patients as well as healthy controls and showed that these CD4+ T-cell lines reacted against certain human MBPs, specifically residues 84–102 and 143–168. They showed that the CD4+ T-cell receptors used were primarily of the Vβ17 and Vβ12 family. Vβ12 receptors were used frequently in recognition with MBP 84–102, while Vβ17 mostly reacted against MBP 143–168.

The presence of unique T-cell receptor Vβ gene usage has generated a series of experimental animal trials as well as early human trials with the goal of deleting specific Vβ T cells in MS patients.[95] These experiments have been relatively successful in EAE; however, the approach has been less effective in MS. Of interest, investigators have also isolated MBP-reactive CD4+ T-cell lines from normal human blood.[96] The fact that these T-cell lines respond to MBP,[97] similar to the response observed in MS patients, raises major questions as to the specificity of the response of CD4+ T-cell lines to myelin antigen in MS patients.[98] The CD4+ T-cell lines obtained from non-MS patients secrete IL-2 similar to that seen with MS patients. All of the T-cell lines isolated from the peripheral blood were of the CD4 phenotype.[99]

Investigators have examined peripheral blood lymphocytes from MS patients and other neurological controls in effort to study specific T-cell populations against purified human MBP and other brain antigens.[100] Lymphocytes from MS patients were more likely to react against MBP. Unfortunately, they discerned only minor differences between MS patients and normal controls as to the specificity of the response to any brain-tissue antigens. Most responses were found in patients with chronic progressive MS, a phase when T cells are least active in the disease. These results also raise concerns about the specificity of the T-cell immune response to myelin antigens in MS patients, given the very subtle differences between MS patients

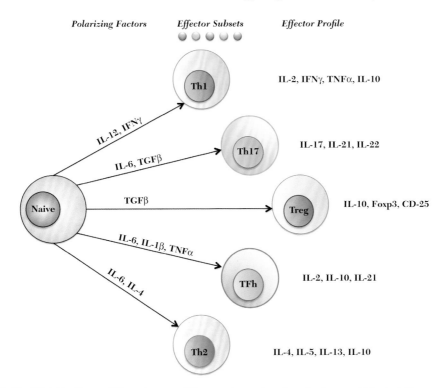

Figure 6–12. CD4⁺ T cells can differentiate into different subtypes based on the factors within the inflammatory milieu with which T cells come into contact. Th1⁺ cells secrete IFN-γ and TNF and mediate the pathology in EAE. Many of the results previously attributed to Th1⁺ cells are actually mediated by Th17⁺ cells. Th17⁺ cells secrete IL-17, IL-21, and IL-22. These cells have been identified in MS lesions, where they may serve as important effectors. As a result of TGF-β stimulation, CD4⁺ T cells develop into T-regulatory cells. These cells downregulate the immune response and express FOXP3, CD25, and IL10. The mechanism of suppression is by the secretion of factors such as IL-10. Th-helper cells provide "help" to other T cells, such as CD8⁺ T cells or B cells. Th-helper cells secrete IL-2, IL-10, and IL-21. Th2⁺ cells downregulate the immune response and are associated with recovery from acute attacks in EAE and, possibly, MS. The cytokines that mediate the downregulation of the immune response are IL-4 and IL-10, in addition to IL-13 and IL-5.

and normal individuals. Even those investigators claiming a positive, "statistically significant" response show enough overlap in results between patients and controls to make these assays unfeasible as a diagnostic test for MS.[101]

An interesting attempt was made to study T-cell receptor (TCR) usage in genetically identical twins with MS.[102] Monozygotic twin pairs in MS have ~26% concordance with disease, in contrast to dizygotic twins (0–5%). Epidemiological studies suggest environmental triggers in addition to genetic factors to explain these differences. Investigators compared TCR usages in concordant versus discordant monozygotic twins to assess their response to self and foreign antigens. They demonstrated that, after stimulation with MBP or tetanus toxoids, both control and concordant twin sets selected similar V_α chains. However, only discordant twin

sets selected different V_β TCRs after antigen stimulation. Because the twins are genetically identical, this proves definitively that exogenous factors or other aspects of disease shape the TCR repertoire in MS patients in comparison with unaffected but genetically identical individuals. This indicates that skewing the TCR repertoire could affect the pathogenesis of MS or other T-cell–mediated diseases. From these experiments, one might conclude that the T-cell response to MBP or other myelin antigens is a feature of MS. However, it may not be the primary, disease-inducing event.

Other investigators examined the selection of TCR β-V-D-J gene rearrangements with specificity for MBP peptides in brain lesions of MS.[103,104] They analyzed TCR gene rearrangements directly for MS brain plaques using the polymerase chain reaction with transcribed messenger RNA. They concluded that the TCRs previously described in MBP T-cell clones from MS patients or in the EAE model were most abundantly used by CD4+ T cells. They found rearrangements of Vβ 5.2 genes in the brains of patients with certain specific HLA haplotypes. Common, identical motifs appeared in various T-cell clones at the VDJ region. Some clones were cytotoxic against targets containing MBP peptide 89–106. Of interest, the same deduced amino-acid sequence of rearrangement was also described in rat T cells cloned from animals with EAE specific to peptide 87–99. The results clearly demonstrated the presence of CD4+ T cells directed to MBP in the periphery and plaques of MS patients. However, their precise role in disease pathogenesis remains unclear, particularly since these CD4+ T cells are so rare in pathological specimens and depletion of CD4+ T cells had no positive effect on the disease course; in fact, it may have worsened the disease in some individuals.[105]

Recent work has focused on Th17+ cells in MS.[106,107] Investigators looked at evidence implicating IFN-γ–producing hybrid T cells (so-called Th1 cells) as well as IL17+ lymphocytes (Th17+ cells) in MS. They compared this to animals with EAE and demonstrated expansion of Th17 lymphocytes from the blood of healthy controls as well as from patients with relapsing MS. In response to IL-23, which is known to expand the Th17 phenotype, they showed simultaneous expressions of IFN-γ and IL-17. They noted that patients with relapsing–remitting MS had increased production of IFN-γ by Th17 cells. The same findings were also present in the experimental model. Both these datasets support the hypothesis that Th17 cells affect the pathology of MS and EAE. However, the presence of Th17 cells in MS does not automatically prove that they play a role in pathogenesis.[108] No known data demonstrate that Th17 cell deletion improves MS or that elevated TH17 cells in lesions correlate with disability. In contrast, the work done on CD8+ T cells reveals a strong correlation between CD8+ T cells, perforin, and other CD8+ T-cell–secreted molecules with disease disability. Some cytotoxic T cells even react to autoantigens like MBP.[109] The correlation between CD8+ T cells and "black holes" by MRI (linked to poor outcome) is well established, and there is ample evidence that cytotoxic T cells from MS patients transect axons *in vivo* and *in vitro*. All these facts provide direct proof that CD8+ T cells, in contrast to CD4+ T cells, affect the destruction of myelin and axons in the MS plaque.

SUMMARY

The immunology of MS continues to be an area of intense investigation. A possible model for the role of immune cells is provided (Fig. 6.13). More papers deal with this issue than with any other area of investigation in MS. At the same time, no area of MS research has had the greatest number of misleading "definitive," subsequently disproven conclusions regarding MS pathogenesis. This highlights the heterogeneity of MS immunopathogenesis once the disease is established. Immunomodulatory and immunosuppressive therapies do decrease relapses and the number of gadolinium-enhancing lesions in MS brain. However, the long-term consequences of immunosuppression on disease course are unknown because most published clinical trials last less than 5 years, an insufficient period of time to address the long-term consequences of these treatments.

It is increasingly evident that CD8+ T cells and their effector molecules directly affect the disease process. Unfortunately, despite documented involvement of CD8+ T cells in MS lesions, there has been little experimentation. This is probably due to the CD4+ T-cell bias of the EAE experimental model. However, in human disease, the MHC class II CD4+ T-cell immune response yields less critical data than similar aspects of the MHC class I CD8+ T-cell immune response. This is likely because CD4+ T cells may not be as important during the manifestation of MS symptoms as they were during the biological induction phase of the disease. The role of CD8+ T cells certainly merits more attention.

The most important diagnostic test for MS continues to be the presence of increased CSF IgG and specific oligoclonal bands in the CSF but not in the serum. Therefore, it is critical to identify the specificity of these bands. Ultimately, we may even discover that CSF oligoclonal IgG bands play a neuroprotective rather than a pathological role.

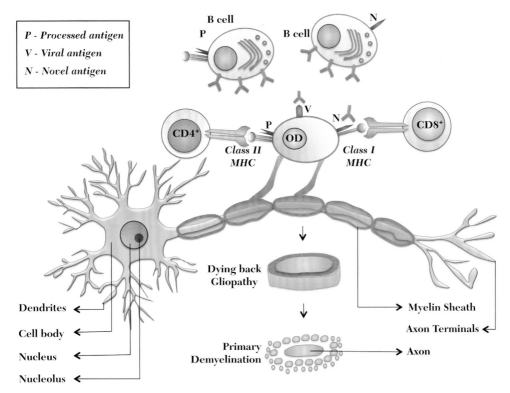

Figure 6–13. This conceptual figure demonstrates how injury to the oligodendrocyte may result in demyelination. For the oligodendrocyte to be injured by inflammatory cells, it must express MHC class I or class II genes. *N* stands for a novel protein that is expressed in the context of class I MHC. Each class I MHC molecule can then be engaged by CD8⁺ T cells. CD8⁺ T cells can then secrete perforin, granzyme, or other factors that may directly injure or kill the oligodendrocyte, resulting in demyelination. The oligodendrocyte can also be injured by antibodies. Antibodies are secreted by plasma cells and B cells. B cells would secrete antibodies, as shown by *Y*. Antibodies can bind to the surface of the cell and, in association with complement, may induce direct injury to myelin or the oligodendrocytes. This is potentially the mechanism of demyelination seen in pattern II lesions in human MS. The B cells may also present virus antigens in the context of class II MHC molecules.. Viral proteins shown are also a blue triangle as *V*. The B cells may present antigens in context of class II MHC, and then the B cells can interact directly with oligodendrocytes or myelin to induce injury. The oligodendrocyte itself may also express class II MHC. This presentation of the viral protein (as denoted by the triangle *P*) must be processed, which allows the CD4⁺ T cells to be engaged with class II MHC to induce injury, the common mechanism of injury presumed to be present in EAE, and may be the pattern of injury in MS in pattern I lesions. The oligodendrocyte may itself die as a consequence of direct virus infection. This is shown by the letter *V*. The virus may enter the oligodendrocyte and directly result in the death of the oligodendrocyte. This is ultimately manifested by dying-back oligodendrogliopathy. Degeneration is first observed in the inner glial loop, and then the myelin unravels from the axon. Primary demyelination is shown at the bottom of the figure. This is the pattern of pathology observed in pattern III or IV lesions in human MS. These mechanisms of injury may be independent or occur concurrently in each brain. The data, however, suggest that each lesion behaves as its own internal universe, but one pattern of pathology predominates. Most data suggest that the pattern of pathology observed among lesions in individual brains is similar. Another possibility is that the mechanisms of injury may relate to stages of progression of demyelinating disease. At present, there is no clear evidence that these patterns of injury relate to various stages of the disease course, and they do not correlate with the clinical subtypes of relapsing–remitting MS, secondary progressive MS, or primary progressive MS, although this is yet to be completely determined. However, what has become more apparent is that the dying-back oligodendrogliopathy is the mechanism of death in primary progressive MS, a disease without exacerbation or remission. In pattern IV lesions, oligodendrocytes are dying in the center of the lesion but also show evidence of apoptosis outside in the normal-appearing white matter.

REFERENCES

1. Friese MA, Fugger L. Pathogenic CD8(+) T cells in multiple sclerosis. Ann Neurol; 66:132–141, 2009.
2. Rodriguez M. Have we finally identified an autoimmune demyelinating disease? Ann Neurol; 66:572–573, 2009.
3. Schwartz R, Datta S. Autoimmunity and autoimmune diseases. In: Paul W, ed. *Fundamental Immunology*. New York: Raven Press, Ltd.; 819–866, 1989.
4. Saeki Y, Mima T, Sakoda S, et al. Transfer of multiple sclerosis into severe combined immunodeficiency mice by mononuclear cells from cerebrospinal fluid of the patients. Proc Natl Acad Sci USA; 89:6157–6161, 1992.

5. Hao Q, Saida T, Nishimura M, Ozawa K, Saida K. Failure to transfer multiple sclerosis into severe combined immunodeficiency mice by mononuclear cells from CSF of patients. Neurology; 44:163–165, 1994.

6. Richert JR, Robinson ED, Deibler GE, Martenson RE, Dragovic LJ, Kies MW. Human cytotoxic T-cell recognition of a synthetic peptide of myelin basic protein. Ann Neurol; 26:342–346, 1989.

7. Araki M, Kondo T, Gumperz JE, Brenner MB, Miyake S, Yamamura T. Th2 bias of CD4+ NKT cells derived from multiple sclerosis in remission. Int Immunol; 15:279–288, 2003.

8. Correale J, Villa A. Role of CD8+ CD25+ Foxp3+ regulatory T cells in multiple sclerosis. Ann Neurol; 67:625–638, 2010.

9. Reindl M, Linington C, Brehm U, et al. Antibodies against the myelin oligodendrocyte glycoprotein and the myelin basic protein in multiple sclerosis and other neurological diseases: a comparative study. Brain; 122 (Pt 11):2047–2056, 1999.

10. Owens GP, Bennett JL, Lassmann H, et al. Antibodies produced by clonally expanded plasma cells in multiple sclerosis cerebrospinal fluid. Ann Neurol; 65:639–649, 2009.

11. Bronstein JM, Lallone RL, Seitz RS, Ellison GW, Myers LW. A humoral response to oligodendrocyte-specific protein in MS: a potential molecular mimic. Neurology; 53:154–161, 1999.

12. Lo R, Feasby TE. Multiple sclerosis and autoimmune diseases. Neurology; 33:97–98, 1983.

13. Warren S, Warren KG. Multiple sclerosis and associated diseases: a relationship to diabetes mellitus. Can J Neurol Sci; 8:35–39, 1981.

14. Wynn DR, Rodriguez M, O'Fallon WM, Kurland LT. A reappraisal of the epidemiology of multiple sclerosis in Olmsted County, Minnesota. Neurology; 40:780–786, 1990.

15. Pittock SJ, Lennon VA, de Seze J, et al. Neuromyelitis optica and non organ-specific autoimmunity. Arch Neurol; 65:78–83, 2008.

16. Wingerchuk DM. Evidence for humoral autoimmunity in neuromyelitis optica. Neurol Res; 28:348–353, 2006.

17. Mattson DH, Roos RP, Arnason BG. Isoelectric focusing of IgG eluted from multiple sclerosis and subacute sclerosing panencephalitis brains. Nature; 287:335–337, 1980.

18. Hoftberger R, Aboul-Enein F, Brueck W, et al. Expression of major histocompatibility complex class I molecules on the different cell types in multiple sclerosis lesions. Brain Pathol; 14:43–50, 2004.

19. McDole J, Johnson AJ, Pirko I. The role of CD8+ T-cells in lesion formation and axonal dysfunction in multiple sclerosis. Neurol Res; 28:256–261, 2006.

20. Melzer N, Meuth SG, Wiendl H. CD8+ T cells and neuronal damage: direct and collateral mechanisms of cytotoxicity and impaired electrical excitability. Faseb J; 23:3659–3673, 2009.

21. Malmestrom C, Lycke J, Haghighi S, et al. Relapses in multiple sclerosis are associated with increased CD8+ T-cell mediated cytotoxicity in CSF. J Neuroimmunol; 196:159–165, 2008.

22. van Oosten BW, Lai M, Hodgkinson S, et al. Treatment of multiple sclerosis with the monoclonal anti-CD4 antibody cM-T412: results of a randomized, double-blind, placebo-controlled, MR-monitored phase II trial. Neurology; 49:351–357, 1997.

23. Moreau T, Coles A, Wing M, et al. CAMPATH-IH in multiple sclerosis. Mult Scler; 1:357–365, 1996.

24. Jacobsen M, Cepok S, Quak E, et al. Oligoclonal expansion of memory CD8+ T cells in cerebrospinal fluid from multiple sclerosis patients. Brain; 125:538–550, 2002.

25. Junker A, Ivanidze J, Malotka J, et al. Multiple sclerosis: T-cell receptor expression in distinct brain regions. Brain; 130:2789–2799, 2007.

26. Skulina C, Schmidt S, Dornmair K, et al. Multiple sclerosis: brain-infiltrating CD8+ T cells persist as clonal expansions in the cerebrospinal fluid and blood. Proc Natl Acad Sci USA; 101:2428–2433, 2004.

27. Tzartos JS, Friese MA, Craner MJ, et al. Interleukin-17 production in central nervous system-infiltrating T cells and glial cells is associated with active disease in multiple sclerosis. Am J Pathol; 172:146–155, 2008.

28. Correale J, Villa A. Role of CD8+ CD25+ Foxp3+ regulatory T cells in multiple sclerosis. Ann Neurol; 67:625–638,

29. Buckle GJ, Hollsberg P, Hafler DA. Activated CD8+ T cells in secondary progressive MS secrete lymphotoxin. Neurology; 60:702–705, 2003.

30. Beck J, Rondot P, Catinot L, Falcoff E, Kirchner H, Wietzerbin J. Increased production of interferon gamma and tumor necrosis factor precedes clinical manifestation in multiple sclerosis: do cytokines trigger off exacerbations? Acta Neurol Scand; 78:318–323, 1988.

31. Rieckmann P, Albrecht M, Kitze B, et al. Tumor necrosis factor-alpha messenger RNA expression in patients with relapsing-remitting multiple sclerosis is associated with disease activity. Ann Neurol; 37:82–88, 1995.

32. Paya CV, Leibson PJ, Patick AK, Rodriguez M. Inhibition of Theiler's virus-induced demyelination in vivo by tumor necrosis factor alpha. Int Immunol; 2:909–913, 1990.

33. Selmaj K, Raine CS, Cross AH. Anti-tumor necrosis factor therapy abrogates autoimmune demyelination. Ann Neurol; 30:694–700, 1991.

34. van Oosten BW, Barkhof F, Truyen L, et al. Increased MRI activity and immune activation in two multiple sclerosis patients treated with the monoclonal anti-tumor necrosis factor antibody cA2. Neurology; 47:1531–1534, 1996.

35. Fromont A, De Seze J, Fleury MC, Maillefert JF, Moreau T. Inflammatory demyelinating events following treatment with anti-tumor necrosis factor. Cytokine; 45:55–57, 2009.

36. Sicotte NL, Voskuhl RR. Onset of multiple sclerosis associated with anti-TNF therapy. Neurology; 57:1885–1888, 2001.

37. Panitch HS, Hirsch RL, Schindler J, Johnson KP. Treatment of multiple sclerosis with gamma interferon: exacerbations associated with activation of the immune system. Neurology; 37:1097–1102, 1987.

38. de Jong BA, Schrijver HM, Huizinga TW, et al. Innate production of interleukin-10 and tumor necrosis factor affects the risk of multiple sclerosis. Ann Neurol; 48:641–646, 2000.

39. van Boxel-Dezaire AH, Hoff SC, van Oosten BW, et al. Decreased interleukin-10 and increased interleukin-12p40 mRNA are associated with disease

activity and characterize different disease stages in multiple sclerosis. Ann Neurol; 45:695–703, 1999.

40. Balashov KE, Comabella M, Ohashi T, Khoury SJ, Weiner HL. Defective regulation of IFNgamma and IL-12 by endogenous IL-10 in progressive MS. Neurology; 55:192–198, 2000.

41. *Brain* 129:200–211, 2005.

42. *Biochimica et Biophysica Acta,* Molecular Basis of Disease 1812:220–230, 2011

43. Kieseier BC, Seifert T, Giovannoni G, Hartung HP. Matrix metalloproteinases in inflammatory demyelination: targets for treatment. Neurology; 53:20–25, 1999.

44. Scarisbrick IA, Sabharwal P, Cruz H, et al. Dynamic role of kallikrein 6 in traumatic spinal cord injury. Eur J Neurosci; 24:1457–1469, 2006.

45. Scarisbrick IA, Blaber SI, Tingling JT, Rodriguez M, Blaber M, Christophi GP. Potential scope of action of tissue kallikreins in CNS immune-mediated disease. J Neuroimmunol; 178:167–176, 2006.

46. Sotiropoulou G, Pampalakis G. Kallikrein-related peptidases: bridges between immune functions and extracellular matrix degradation. Biol Chem; 391:321–331,

47. Scarisbrick IA, Linbo R, Vandell AG, et al. Kallikreins are associated with secondary progressive multiple sclerosis and promote neurodegeneration. Biol Chem; 389:739–745, 2008.

48. Rodriguez M, Karnes WE, Bartleson JD, Pineda AA. Plasmapheresis in acute episodes of fulminant CNS inflammatory demyelination. Neurology; 43:1100–1104, 1993.

49. Brahic M. Multiple sclerosis and viruses. Ann Neurol; 68:6–8, 2010.

50. Njenga MK, Rodriguez M. Animal models of demyelination. Curr Opin Neurol; 9:159–164, 1996.

51. Rodriguez M. Central nervous system demyelination and remyelination in multiple sclerosis and viral models of disease. J Neuroimmunol; 40:255–263, 1992.

52. Bender SJ, Weiss SR. Pathogenesis of murine coronavirus in the central nervous system. J Neuroimmune Pharmacol; 5:336–354,

53. Lane TE, Hosking MP. The pathogenesis of murine coronavirus infection of the central nervous system. Crit Rev Immunol; 30:119–130, 2010.

54. Rodriguez M. Mechanisms of virus-induced demyelination and remyelination. Ann NY Acad Sci; 540:240–251, 1988.

55. Berti R, Brennan MB, Soldan SS, et al. Increased detection of serum HHV-6 DNA sequences during multiple sclerosis (MS) exacerbations and correlation with parameters of MS disease progression. J Neurovirol; 8:250–256, 2002.

56. Riverol M, Sepulcre J, Fernandez-Diez B, et al. Antibodies against Epstein-Barr virus and herpesvirus type 6 are associated with the early phases of multiple sclerosis. J Neuroimmunol; 192:184–185, 2007.

57. Voumvourakis KI, Kitsos DK, Tsiodras S, Petrikkos G, Stamboulis E. Human herpesvirus 6 infection as a trigger of multiple sclerosis. Mayo Clin Proc; 85:1023–1030,2010.

58. Hollsberg P. Pathogenesis of chronic progressive myelopathy associated with human T-cell lymphotropic virus type I. Acta Neurol Scand Suppl; 169:86–93, 1997.

59. Otto C, Oltmann A, Stein A, et al. Intrathecal EBV antibodies are part of the polyspecific immune response in multiple sclerosis. Neurology; 76:1316–1321, 2011.

60. Cree BA, Rioux JD, McCauley JL, et al. A major histocompatibility Class I locus contributes to multiple sclerosis susceptibility independently from HLA-DRB1°15:01. PloS one; 5:e11296, 2010.

61. Hauser SL, Ault KA, Levin MJ, Garovoy MR, Weiner HL. Natural killer cell activity in multiple sclerosis. J Immunol; 127:1114–1117, 1981.

62. Sakuishi K, Miyake S, Yamamura T. Role of NK cells and invariant NKT cells in multiple sclerosis. Results Probl Cell Differ; 51:127–147, 2010.

63. Rice GP, Casali P, Merigan TC, Oldstone MB. Natural killer cell activity in patients with multiple sclerosis given alpha interferon. Ann Neurol; 14:333–338, 1983.

64. Mehta PD, Miller JA, Tourtellotte WW. Oligoclonal IgG bands in plaques from multiple sclerosis brains. Neurology; 32:372–376, 1982.

65. Walsh MJ, Tourtellotte WW. Temporal invariance and clonal uniformity of brain and cerebrospinal IgG, IgA, and IgM in multiple sclerosis. J Exp Med; 163:41–53, 1986.

66 .Lipton HL. The specificity of oligoclonal bands in multiple sclerosis. Ann Neurol; 65:621–622, 2009.

67. Shirodaria PV, Haire M, Fleming E, Merrett JD, Hawkins SA, Roberts SD. Viral antibody titers. Comparison in patients with multiple sclerosis and rheumatoid arthritis. Arch Neurol; 44:1237–1241, 1987.

68. Rodriguez M. Effectors of demyelination and remyelination in the CNS: implications for multiple sclerosis. Brain Pathol; 17:219–229, 2007.

69. Rodriguez M, Warrington AE, Pease LR. Invited article: human natural autoantibodies in the treatment of neurologic disease. Neurology; 72:1269–1276, 2009.

70. Bieber AJ, Ure DR, Rodriguez M. Genetically dominant spinal cord repair in a murine model of chronic progressive multiple sclerosis. J Neuropathol Exp Neurol; 64:46–57, 2005.

71. Bieber AJ, Warrington A, Asakura K, et al. Human antibodies accelerate the rate of remyelination following lysolecithin-induced demyelination in mice. Glia; 37:241–249, 2002.

72. Rodriguez M. A function of myelin is to protect axons from subsequent injury: implications for deficits in multiple sclerosis. Brain; 126:751–752, 2003.

73. Warrington AE, Bieber AJ, Ciric B, Pease LR, Van Keulen V, Rodriguez M. A recombinant human IgM promotes myelin repair after a single, very low dose. J Neurosci Res; 85:967–976, 2007.

74. Scarisbrick IA, Rodriguez M. Hit-Hit and hit-Run: viruses in the playing field of multiple sclerosis. Curr Neurol Neurosci Reports; 3:265–271, 2003.

75. Keegan M, Konig F, McClelland R, et al. Relation between humoral pathological changes in multiple sclerosis and response to therapeutic plasma exchange. Lancet; 366:579–582, 2005.

76. Morgan BP, Campbell AK, Compston DA. Terminal component of complement (C9) in cerebrospinal fluid of patients with multiple sclerosis. Lancet; 2:251–254, 1984.

77. Rodriguez M, Wynn DR, Kimlinger TK, Katzmann JA. Terminal component of complement (C9) in the

cerebrospinal fluid of patients with multiple sclerosis and neurologic controls. Neurology; 40:855–857, 1990.

78. Prineas JW, Graham JS. Multiple sclerosis: capping of surface immunoglobulin G on macrophages engaged in myelin breakdown. Ann Neurol; 10:149–158, 1981.

79. Prineas JW, Kwon EE, Cho ES, et al. Immunopathology of secondary-progressive multiple sclerosis. Ann Neurol; 50:646–657, 2001.

80. Lucchinetti CF, Noseworthy JH, Rodriguez M. Promotion of endogenous remyelination in multiple sclerosis. Mult Scler; 3:71–75, 1997.

81. Niehaus A, Shi J, Grzenkowski M, et al. Patients with active relapsing-remitting multiple sclerosis synthesize antibodies recognizing oligodendrocyte progenitor cell surface protein: implications for remyelination. Ann Neurol; 48:362–371, 2000.

82. Sadatipour BT, Greer JM, Pender MP. Increased circulating antiganglioside antibodies in primary and secondary progressive multiple sclerosis. Ann Neurol; 44:980–983, 1998.

83. Meinl E, Krumbholz M, Hohlfeld R. B lineage cells in the inflammatory central nervous system environment: migration, maintenance, local antibody production, and therapeutic modulation. Ann Neurol; 59:880–892, 2006.

84. Bar-Or A, Fawaz L, Fan B, et al. Abnormal B-cell cytokine responses a trigger of T-cell-mediated disease in MS? Ann Neurol; 67:452–461, 2010.

85. Hauser SL, Waubant E, Arnold DL, et al. B-cell depletion with rituximab in relapsing-remitting multiple sclerosis. N Engl J Med; 358:676–688, 2008.

86. Mavra M, Thompson EJ, Nikolic J, et al. The occurrence of oligoclonal IgG in tears from patients with MS and systemic immune disorders. Neurology; 40:1259–1262, 1990.

87. Calais G, Forzy G, Crinquette C, et al. Tear analysis in clinically isolated syndrome as new multiple sclerosis criterion. Multiple Sclerosis; 16:87–92, 2010.

88. Sriram S and Steiner I: Experimental allergic encephalomyelitis: a misleading model of multiple sclerosis. Ann Neurol; 58:939–945, 2005.

89. Costantino CM, Baecher-Allan C, Hafler DA. Multiple sclerosis and regulatory T cells. J Clin Immunol; 28:697–706, 2008.

90. Huan J, Culbertson N, Spencer L, et al. Decreased FOXP3 levels in multiple sclerosis patients. J Neurosci Res; 81:45–52, 2005.

91. Sakaguchi S, Miyara M, Costantino CM, Hafler DA. FOXP3+ regulatory T cells in the human immune system. Nature Rev; 10:490–500, 2010.

92. Cvetanovich GL and Hafler DA: Human regulatory T cells in autoimmune diseases. Curr Opin Immunol; 22:753–760, 2010.

93. Lovett-Racke AE, Yang Y, Racke MK. Th1 versus Th17: are T cell cytokines relevant in multiple sclerosis? Biochim Biophys Acta; 1812:246–251, 2011.,

94. Wucherpfennig KW, Ota K, Endo N, et al. Shared human T cell receptor V beta usage to immunodominant regions of myelin basic protein. Science; 248:1016–1019, 1990.

95. Hafler DA, Saadeh MG, Kuchroo VK, Milford E, Steinman L. TCR usage in human and experimental demyelinating disease. Immunol Today; 17:152–159, 1996.

96. Burns J, Rosenzweig A, Zweiman B, Lisak RP. Isolation of myelin basic protein-reactive T-cell lines from normal human blood. Cell Immunol; 81:435–440, 1983.

97. McLaurin JA, Hafler DA, Antel JP. Reactivity of normal T-cell lines to MBP isolated from normal and multiple sclerosis white matter. J Neurol Sci; 128:205–211, 1995.

98. Li Y, Huang Y, Lue J, Quandt JA, Martin R, Mariuzza RA. Structure of a human autoimmune TCR bound to a myelin basic protein self-peptide and a multiple sclerosis-associated MHC class II molecule. Embo J; 24:2968–2979, 2005.

99. Brinkman CJ, Nillesen WM, Hommes OR, Lamers KJ, de Pauw BE, Delmotte P. Cell-mediated immunity in multiple sclerosis as determined by sensitivity of different lymphocyte populations to various brain tissue antigens. Ann Neurol; 11:450–455, 1982.

100. Wucherpfennig KW, Hafler DA, Strominger JL. Structure of human T-cell receptors specific for an immunodominant myelin basic protein peptide: positioning of T-cell receptors on HLA-DR2/peptide complexes. Proc Natl Acad Sci USA; 92:8896–8900, 1995.

101. Severson C, Hafler DA. T-cells in multiple sclerosis. Results Probl Cell Differ; 51:75–98, 2010.

102. Utz U, Biddison WE, McFarland HF, McFarlin DE, Flerlage M, Martin R. Skewed T-cell receptor repertoire in genetically identical twins correlates with multiple sclerosis. Nature; 364:243–247, 1993.

103. Oksenberg JR, Panzara MA, Begovich AB, et al. Selection for T-cell receptor V beta-D beta-J beta gene rearrangements with specificity for a myelin basic protein peptide in brain lesions of multiple sclerosis. Nature; 362:68–70, 1993.

104. Steinman L, Zamvil SS. How to successfully apply animal studies in experimental allergic encephalomyelitis to research on multiple sclerosis. Ann Neurol; 60:12–21, 2006.

105. Wiendl H, Hohlfeld R. Therapeutic approaches in multiple sclerosis: lessons from failed and interrupted treatment trials. BioDrugs; 16:183–200, 2002.

106. Kebir H, Ifergan I, Alvarez JI, et al. Preferential recruitment of interferon-gamma-expressing TH17 cells in multiple sclerosis. Ann Neurol; 66:390–402, 2009.

107. Sinha S, Subramanian S, Proctor TM, et al. A promising therapeutic approach for multiple sclerosis: recombinant T-cell receptor ligands modulate experimental autoimmune encephalomyelitis by reducing interleukin-17 production and inhibiting migration of encephalitogenic cells into the CNS. J Neurosci; 27:12531–12539, 2007.

108. Montes M, Zhang X, Berthelot L, et al. Oligoclonal myelin-reactive T-cell infiltrates derived from multiple sclerosis lesions are enriched in Th17 cells. Clin Immunol; 130:133–144, 2009.

109. Martin R, Jaraquemada D, Flerlage M, et al. Fine specificity and HLA restriction of myelin basic protein-specific cytotoxic T cell lines from multiple sclerosis patients and healthy individuals. J Immunol; 145:540–548, 1990.

110. Bitsch A, Schuchardt J, Bunkowski S, Kuhlmann T, Bruck W. Acute axonal injury in multiple sclerosis. Correlation with demyelination and inflammation. Brain; 123 (Pt 6):1174–1183, 2000.

Chapter 7

Neural Degeneration and Potential Novel Treatments

Abstract

Whereas scientists once thought of MS as a disease of myelin and, possibly, oligodendrocytes, many now consider it to be a disease where neuronal and axonal injury occurs simultaneously with demyelination. Both pathological and imaging studies lead to many of the same conclusions: that is, the effects of the disease extend far beyond what is observed in the well-demarcated plaques. Disability correlates better with the neuronal and axonal loss than with the number or distribution of demyelinated, inflammatory plaques. Evidence for lower motor neuron involvement early in the disease course has come to light in recent reports. Therefore, therapeutic approaches must account for gray matter abnormalities. The *innate* immune response (activated microglia and dendritic cells), rather than the *adaptive* immune response (T and B cells), may be more relevant to gray matter injury. Targeting structures in the CNS (neurons, axons, microglia, astrocytes, and oligodendrocytes) instead of the adaptive immune response may be a more rational approach to a sustained cure. This chapter provides some of the recent data implicating injury to neuronal structure early in the evolution of the MS paradigm and provides a theoretical framework to change the focus of curative therapy.

INTRODUCTION

The classical definition of MS as a demyelinating disease of myelin with relative preservation of axons has given way as investigators focus more attention on axonal and neuronal loss. The original intention of the classical definition was to distinguish MS from other disorders of the CNS; for example, in cerebral infarction, myelin loss occurs as a secondary consequence of the ischemic event, whose primary consequence is neuronal loss and axonal degeneration. In MS, despite current data supporting a process that begins at the level of oligodendrocytes or myelin, the actual site of primary etiological injury may, in fact, be vulnerable axons or neurons. In other words, the vulnerability of the axon may result in injury or loss of the neuron supplying the axon prior to demyelination. This is clearly an area of intense research and, obviously, much controversy. Imaging studies have increasingly supported the hypothesis that abnormal axons are present in the normal-appearing white matter prior to the initiation of the demyelinating event (see Chapter 4). MRI can provide serial measurements of the same lesion, which obviously cannot be performed with pathological specimens. Nevertheless, increasing data in the pathological literature also indicate axonal injury and neuronal degeneration as hallmarks of this disease process.[1]

AXONAL LOSS IN NORMAL-APPEARING WHITE MATTER

There is evidence of axonal loss in the plaque.[2] This may appear early in the disease course and, depending on the type of lesion, may be relatively scant (as in primarily inflammatory plaques) or severe (large tumefactive lesions).[3,4] Less apparent is the demonstration of axonal loss in normal-appearing white matter,[5,6] which may predispose to a plaque-inducing demyelinating event. Evidence gathered from cerebral lesions increasingly supports a correlation between the number of transected axons[7] and the degree of inflammation, and this may occur early in the disease course.[8] In spinal cord lesions from patients with disease of long duration,[9] the total axon numbers may be reduced by as much as 80%. *In vivo* spectroscopy (MRS), primarily investigating a neuron-specific marker in N-acetyl aspartate (NAA), has provided new insights into neural damage. Decreases in NAA in patients with MS correlate strongly with disability and increased disease duration. In addition, chronic MS lesions with decreased NAA correlate powerfully with axonal loss at autopsy.

It is clear that axons undergo irreversible degeneration distal to the site of transection (Fig. 7.1).[10] In contrast, myelin internodes surrounding degenerating axons persist long after injury. They may appear histologically or pathologically normal. Therefore, it is possible for NAA reductions observed in normal-appearing white matter to represent axonal degeneration distal to the MS lesion. However, abnormalities in axons can appear remote from MS lesions and resolve with time. The subsequent improvement of NAA reflects a reversal of axonal dysfunction or a transient metabolic change occurring in the axon.[11]

RELATIONSHIP BETWEEN AXONAL TRANSECTION AND INFLAMMATION

Several studies have demonstrated that transecting apoptotic neurons may be influenced by inflammation in MS lesions (Fig. 7.2); many of these transected neurons appear in the cortex.[7,12] The authors investigated

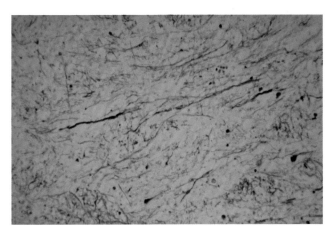

Figure 7–1. Abnormal axon profile. This sample is taken from an acute MS plaque, stereotactically biopsied. It is apparent that the axons are undergoing severe degeneration. This paraffin-embedded material has been processed with Bielschowsky silver stain. In the center of the figure are multiple degenerating axons with abnormal axon profiles. The number of axons in this field is remarkably reduced compared to what would be seen in a normal field of white matter. Many of the axon profiles are seen on end (they look like small black dots). These are likely manifestations of transected axons, as there is accumulation of axon material at the edge of the transection.

demyelinating lesions in the cortex of MS patients. They identified 112 cortical lesions from 50 patients that demonstrated three patterns of cortical demyelination. Type I lesions were contiguous with subcortical white matter lesions; type II lesions were small, confined to the cortex and often perivascular; type III lesions extended from the pial surface to cortical layers 3 and 4. The investigators found cortical lesions to contain fewer of the CD3+ lymphocytes that mark all T-cell subsets. All transected neurons occurred at greater density in the key cortical lesions. They also demonstrated that activated microglia closely opposed the destroyed neurites and perikarya. Thus, MS brains are identifiable not only by demyelination but also by axonal transection, dendritic transection, neuronal death by apoptosis, and, at times, inflammatory cell infiltrates, specifically and more commonly in deep gray matter structures and in cortical lesions. The findings of potentially irreversible neuronal damage, typically in the cortex, call into question the precise etiology of neurological deficits in MS.

NEURONAL AND AXONAL DEATH

Neuronal and axonal death may be very common in MS.[13] Newer MRI technology better visualizes these lesions *in vivo*. Areas of dendritic loss, previously unrecognized as a pathological change in MS, may contribute to neurological disability as a result of decreasing input into the cortex. In addition, axons aligned from distant neurons may sprout at the union of the postsynaptic densities. However, when these neurons lose their sustaining elements (axons and dendrites), they eventually die from deprivation of critical nutrients provided by neurites.

Neuronal death appears to be relatively common in MS in areas not in direct continuity with white matter tracts.[14] The presence of classical inflammatory infiltrates surrounding degenerating neurons suggests microglial activation as the predominant immunopathological cause of the destruction of neurons and neurites in these areas. These cells appear to be activated in areas of apoptotic neuronal cell death. The microglia appear morphologically similar to the microglia observed following experimental transection of specific nerve tracts or nuclei in animals. Whether this relationship between microglia and neurons destroys or ultimately protects neurons is unknown. In any event, it is likely that microglia-targeted neurons are functionally impaired. The findings are somewhat reminiscent of neuropathological findings in classical noninflammatory diseases such as Alzheimer's disease and amyotrophic lateral sclerosis (ALS). Thus, future effective neuroprotective treatments against the classical neurodegenerative disorders may also be effective

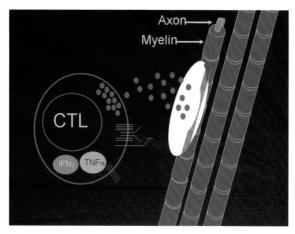

Figure 7–2. Potential molecules that injure the axon after demyelination. It is proposed that demyelination predisposes the axon to cytotoxic injury by CD8+ T cells. The CD8+ T cells are the most common and predominant T cells found in the MS CNS. CD8+ T cells can directly release perforin, which directly induces holes in the membrane of axons and destroys axonal function. The CD8+ T cells engage through their receptor with class I MHC molecules; however, it is difficult to demonstrate the expression of MHC molecules on axons. This has been observed on occasion, but it is relatively rare. More commonly in MS, class I MHC is expressed on the surface of the neuronal body, which is not shown in this figure. CD8+ T cells may also release other factors, such as tumor necrosis factors (TNF) or interferon (IFN)-γ, both of which may play a role in the final destruction or possibly in helping to preserve myelin or promote axon extension after injury. Studies in MS indicate that IFN-γ may be toxic because treatment with IFN-γ resulted in increased exacerbations in MS patients. In contrast, experiments have shown that treatment with an anti-TNF antibody, which was found to be extremely effective in patients with rheumatoid arthritis, was deleterious in MS patients, resulting in increased inflammatory lesions and exacerbations. These data are consistent with experiments in the Theiler's model system in which anti-TNF antibodies make the animals worse, while treatment with TNF molecule results in less inflammation and demyelination. In contrast, in the EAE model, anti-TNF antibodies were beneficial. That was the reason why this antibody treatment was tried in human MS. Of interest, patients with rheumatoid arthritis who benefited from anti-TNF antibodies are now being seen with new onset of MS-like disease. These patients present with multiple lesions on MRI as well as inflammatory neurological deficits. If the TNF antibody is removed from their medical regimen, then many of these lesions improve and the patients also recover. This provides strong evidence that TNF antibodies can worsen MS and that TNF might be one of the protective, repair-promoting, anti-inflammatory factors secreted by T cells, as supported by the findings in the TMEV model. CTL = cytotoxic T lymphocyte.

in combating MS, especially the progressive disease course (see Chapter 1).

Wallerian Degeneration

Wallerian degeneration is another relatively common pattern of axonal destruction in MS. It occurs early in the disease course.[15] Most autopsy-based pathological studies have focused on Wallerian degeneration in chronic lesions. However, investigations in the corticospinal tracts of patients with relatively acute lesions show Wallerian degeneration even at the initial stages of the disease course.[15]

Studies of Wallerian degeneration suggest that this type of axonal injury occurs as sequelae to demyelinating lesions in patients presenting with early symptoms of MS. Therefore, developing an axon-regenerating method during the Wallerian degeneration process may prevent

progressive disability in MS during the early phase of disease.

Myelin as a Protective Barrier to Axons

An important but often-ignored concept is the possibility that oligodendrocytes and myelin serve as a protective shield against neurotoxins or inflammatory toxins that may injure either the axon or neuron.[16] In animals with myelin mutations, for example, mutations of MBP in *shiverer*[17] mice or PLP mutations in *jimpy* mice, axons appear to shrink as disease progresses. Similar observations have been made in patients with PMP22 duplication.[18] However, in some lesions, the diameter of demyelinated axons increases[19] due to increased permeability of the demyelinated axolemma. Also, axon numbers decrease dramatically as a function of time, even though these disorders are the result of a defect that only fully involves the oligodendrocyte and myelin sheath. Thus, oligodendrocytes and myelin must provide either nutritive or protective factors to prevent axonal atrophy. This may have particular relevance to MS, in which myelin and oligodendrocytes die rapidly and, at times, simultaneously.

To determine whether these processes occur early in the disease course or only as a phenomenon of late disease, investigators have examined macroscopically normal-appearing white matter in the brain in cases of mild or spinal MS.[20] By studying brains of patients with mild (13) and spinal (17) cases of MS, investigators found evidence of abnormality in macroscopically normal white matter in 70% of the samples. Problems such as gliosis appear in normal-appearing white matter with a nodular, pericapillary, or diffuse pattern of "arborization" in many specimens. Venular inflammation was also observed but was a much less constant finding. Perivascular deposits of lipofuscin were also observed. The authors proposed a diffuse abnormality in the blood–brain barrier in MS that produces astrocytic activation in areas away from the plaques. Perivascular inflammation in MS, although not a constant finding, may activate astrocytes. In contrast, this astrocytic proliferation may be the primary feature of the disease process, resulting in the secondary activation of lymphocytes.

GRAY MATTER INVOLVEMENT IN MULTIPLE SCLEROSIS

Most investigators consider MS as a white matter disease, but increasing evidence supports gray matter involvement also.[21] It is important to recognize that the gray matter contains oligodendrocytes, most of which produce myelin connections. The concept of a nonmyelinating perineural oligodendrocyte may be rare, since many oligodendrocytes in the gray matter show myelination by electron microscopy. Therefore, gray matter involvement in MS is not surprising. Its occurrence, however, highlights an important question regarding the pathogenesis of the disease: Do gray matter lesions differ fundamentally from white matter lesions?[22] To start, effector cells of ramified microglial cells predominate in the inflammation of gray matter. This implies that many MS lesions are independent of T-cell or B-cell inflammation coming from the periphery. Investigators have observed apoptotic neurons in many gray matter structures in MS. Again, imaging studies have led the way in this arena because it is possible to obtain serial images of the same brain over time.[23] As imaging technology has improved, the number of visualized cortical lesions increases, and abnormalities in the gray matter are more easily appreciated. Usually, large-scale studies of gray matter lesions have demonstrated a consistent loss of gray matter volume involving a number of different nuclei, suggesting gray matter changes as a fundamental hallmark of the disease process.[24]

Clinical Relevance of Gray Matter Disease in Multiple Sclerosis

If gray matter involvement is a predominant feature of MS, then what is its clinical relevance? These abnormalities could result in cognitive impairment related to cortical gray matter involvement. There are strong statistical correlations of gray matter injury with impaired verbal memory, verbal fluency, attention, and concentration,[25] all worrisome symptoms in MS patients. In addition, gray matter involvement may also affect general physical disability. Further, the Expanded Disability Severity Scale (EDSS), a scale consistently and clinically associated with white matter disease, appears to correlate better with spinal cord disease than brain disease and gray matter lesions than white matter lesions.[26]

Could Gray Matter Injury Be an Initial Event in Multiple Sclerosis?

Could involvement of the gray matter be the primary event or initiator of the disease process, leading to axonal degeneration and subsequent demyelination? This is considered the "inside-out" model of MS; that is, the process begins at the level of neurons and axons, and then myelin injury occurs as a consequence of disrupted connectivity between axon membranes and oligodendrocytes. This model also has been proposed in the viral murine model of demyelination (i.e., Theiler's murine encephalomyelitis virus [TMEV] infection.[27] However, the pathological patterns in MS and TMEV infection do not support this model; MS lesions do not follow typical patterns observed with neurodegenerative "tract" disorders, which affect specific fiber tracts or cortical structures. Neurodegenerative diseases such as ALS, in which neuron and axon injury precedes demyelination, affect entire structures; for example, the corticospinal tracts may be demyelinated from the cortex down to the spinal cord. In contrast, MS presents as a patchy loss of normal structures in the form of well-demarcated plaques with sharp borders interspersed with normal areas along the corticospinal tract. This better supports the hypothesis of initial myelin or oligodendrocyte injury with subsequent axonal degeneration. However, unknown mechanisms may injure or protect specific areas of the axon tract such that the macroscopic appearance of lesions is of a focal patchy nature but the intrinsic process involves the entire axon or neuronal structures along the tract. This possibility would be most likely if genetic, metabolic, or toxic effects were the initiating events in MS, which would first target the neuron or axon. The relatively disappointing results of immunomodulatory therapies in preventing MS disease progression support this hypothesis. The degeneration occurring in the deep gray matter structures appears not to be mediated by classical T cells coming from the periphery but instead by endogenous microglial cells.

BIPHASIC DISEASE: INFLAMMATORY DEMYELINATION FOLLOWED BY AXONAL PATHOLOGY

Many investigators consider MS as a biphasic disease with two distinct time frames (Fig. 7.3), the first involving inflammatory mechanisms, which primarily affect the white matter, and the second involving axons and gray matter structures. Supporting this concept is the observation that patients early in the disease course have attacks resulting from inflammatory lesions that demyelinate white matter tracts. For many patients, this period may last 5 to 10 years. Most lesions resolve, thereby implying some element of repair, either by remyelination or resolution of inflammation surrounding the conduction block or slowing in demyelinated fibers. The disease then evolves until relapses are infrequent and then slowly progresses to a chronic condition with the phenotypic features of a neurodegenerative disease (i.e., progressive MS). During this phase, neurons and axons are presumably the target and the cause of disability. Inflammation also resolves during this phase, and immunomodulatory therapy has no effect. However, the pathological data do not support such a strict concept of a biphasic disease. Neuronal injury and neural loss occur not only in the secondary progressive phase of disease, but simultaneously with the onset of the inflammatory phases of the disease.[28] Recent studies support aging as a key factor in this transition, but there clearly are clinical and subclinical overlaps[29] (also see Chapter 1).

Neuronal loss early in the process is an attractive hypothesis because many patients apparently have inflammatory lesions associated with neurological relapses followed by secondary axonal progression. Some patients with primary progressive disease do not experience the early inflammatory phase of the disease and present only with the degenerative process. Given that inflammation and neural degeneration occur simultaneously, neuroprotective treatments are indicated early in the disease course.

WHY DO NEURONS AND AXONS NOT REGENERATE IN MULTIPLE SCLEROSIS?

The failure of neurons and axons to survive or regenerate is a critical question in MS. Not all MS pathologies are associated with irreversible neuronal loss mediated by either cytotoxic or hypertoxic mechanisms. Some patients have relapses, recover completely, and never develop permanent disability or even a progressive disease course[29–31] (see discussion in Chapter 1). However, many pathological and MRI studies indicate that patients do have relapses and that cumulative neurological dysfunction eventually results in permanent abnormalities. Factors such as chemokines, cytokines, and changing receptors on target cells result in reversible axonal injury, which, on occasion, responds to anti-inflammatory therapy. However, the process

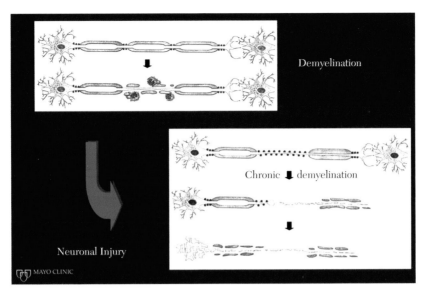

Figure 7–3. Process of demyelination followed by neuronal injury. The defining event in MS is demyelination of the axon. This demyelination is suspected to begin with inflammatory cells invading the CNS. These inflammatory cells come in contact with the myelin and begin to destroy the myelin at the internodes. This results in severe slowing of the action potential and, ultimately, conduction block. Following chronic demyelination, there is reorganization of sodium channels, as demonstrated by the black dots in the figure. This reorganization of sodium channels is later followed by the process of Wallerian degeneration, where the axon distal to the demyelinating lesion begins to degenerate prior to the axon closest to the neuronal body. However, as the disease progresses, there is death of the proximal axon and, ultimately, death of the neuron supplying the axon. Therefore, although MS is a primary demyelinating disorder, the ultimate consequence of demyelination is axonal and neuronal injury. It is the axonal and neuronal injury that ultimately correlates with long-term neurological deficits.

is complex because certain inflammatory mediators, such as interleukin (IL)-6 and TGF-β, have regenerative potential. IL-6, for example, protects neurons from death in both *in vivo* and *in vitro* models.[32] TGF-β modulates the inflammatory response and prevents myelin injury.[33] Therefore, reducing the entire inflammatory response may actually inhibit the regenerative potential of these molecules and other potentially beneficial inflammatory mediators. The only strategy to address this paradox is to design very specific inhibitors of cytokines or chemokines so that treatment during the various phases of degeneration and regeneration can be deciphered. The complexity of the inflammatory response and, specifically, its relevance to axonal loss, neuronal death, and oligodendrocyte survival needs further elucidation.[10,22,28]

DEMYELINATION WITHIN DEEP GRAY MATTER STRUCTURE

In 2005 a group studied the extent and distribution of gray matter demyelinating lesions in MS.[22] They examined coronal sections of six MS brains and six control brains and performed immunocytochemistry for myelin gene products, neurofilaments, synaptophysin, and caspase-3. Demyelinating lesions were observed in many deep gray matter structures, including the cerebral cortex, thalamus, basal ganglia, and hippocampus. Many lesions demonstrated significantly reduced neuronal density. In addition, rare apoptotic neurons that expressed caspase-3 were present in the demyelinated deep gray matter structures as well as the normal-appearing cortex. Cortical lesions also demonstrated decreased optical density of synaptophysin staining. These findings all support the concept that gray matter demyelination and injury are consistent features of MS.

WHAT IS THE MECHANISM THAT INJURES AXONS AND NEURONS?

One hypothesis regarding the ultimate mechanism of axonal and neuronal injury in MS implicates mediation through some aspect of mitochondrial dysfunction. A study demonstrates ultrastructural changes that support calcium-mediated destruction of chronically demyelinated axons.[34] The authors compared the expression of 33,000 genes in postmortem motor cortex from six control and six MS brains. The majority of the genes identified in the comparison between MS brains and controls were involved with energy metabolism and calcium-mediated axonal regeneration. Of the genes identified, 26 were involved with mitochondrial gene expression. Mitochondrial respiratory chain complexes I and III were decreased in the MS motor cortex. This, plus reduced mitochondrial gene expression, was specific for neurons. Presynaptic and postsynaptic components of GABAergic neurotransmissions and the density of inhibitory interneuron processes were also decreased in the MS neuronal structures. These studies support a possible abnormality in energy metabolism, such as ATP production, that may be critical in ion homeostasis in MS and may induce pathologically observed axonal degeneration and neuronal loss.

In addition, electron microscopy studies have demonstrated a dramatic increase in axonal mitochrondria prior to axonal injury.[35] Along with axonal swelling prior to axonal shrinkage and, finally, axonal death, this observation suggests that the axons are in a state of energy hyperactivity, which could contribute to the calcium-mediated axonal degeneration.

DOES INFLAMMATION CONTRIBUTE TO NEURONAL AND AXONAL DEATH?

What are the immunological mediators of axonal injury in MS? Axonal loss results in spinal cord atrophy and electrophysiological abnormalities following demyelination in viral models of MS.[36] Similar findings appear in chronic demyelinated cervical spinal cord plaques in MS.[37] Clearly, the previously mentioned CD8+ T cells in the CNS predominate as the principal T cell infiltrating both the cerebral white matter as well as the cortical and deep gray matter structures. Then, it is possible that these CD8+ T cells play a major role in inducing direct injury to neurons.[38] The CD8+ T cells express perforin and constitutively also express granzymes,

which could be the principal mediators of axonal injury.[39] CD8+ T cells have been demonstrated to transect axons[40] *in vitro*; moreover, class I MHC was found to be expressed in neurons and axons in MS lesions.[41] This finding suggests a working hypothesis for demyelination and the neuronal consequences of MS. It predisposes the axons and neurons to destruction in an MHC class I-restricted, CD8-mediated, perforin-dependent mechanism.[42]

In perforin-deficient mice in the context of various animal models of MS, animals failing to express class I MHC do not manifest neurological injury despite extensive demyelination.[43,44] Similarly, CD8-deficient mice have much less axonal loss and motor dysfunction compared to animals deleted of other T-cell subtypes.[45,46]

Finally, perforin-deficient mice with normal numbers of CD8+ T cells and normal granzymes were completely protected from virus-induced demyelinating axonal injury.[46] Even though virus continued as a result of the CD8 depletion and demyelination was prominent, these animals continued to behave normally in a paradigm using a rotarod, which measures the motor performance of mice similar to a human treadmill. These studies indicate that demyelination, in the absence of perforin, is insufficient to cause axonal injury. Clearly, perforin is the key mediator of axonal injury, and this lends support to the hypothesis that CD8+ T cells are primarily responsible for the axon damage occurring in MS.[39,47,48] Therefore, perforin is a critical target for future therapies in MS.

LOWER MOTOR NEURON LOSS OCCURS IN MULTIPLE SCLEROSIS

All studies to date have focused primarily on the presence of axonal and neuronal loss in the brain. What has been completely unexpected is the finding that lower motor neurons are lost in both MS and the experimental autoimmune encephalomyelitis (EAE) model of MS.[49] Investigators studied 69 MS patients and 75 healthy controls using established techniques of electrophysiology to examine motor unit number estimates. The results indicated extensive lower motor neuron loss in MS patients, which was highly significant ($p < .001$) compared to healthy controls. Many patients showed markedly decreased compound muscle action potential (CMAP) amplitudes (below the 10th percentile). Of interest, the patients with electrophysiological evidence of lower motor neuron loss were more severely disabled and showed reduced walking distance. The investigators also studied the pathology from nine MS patients and nine age-to-sex-matched controls. Using a recently established high-precision computer-based stereology system, they detected an overall loss of neurons (~25% in MS patients), which was statistically significant ($p < .001$), including a 48% decrease in α-motor neurons, an 81% loss in γ-motor neurons, and a 67% loss in interneurons from the lumbar spinal cord. A remarkable loss of motor neurons in MS raises important implications for the pathogenesis of neurological deficits, specifically gait disorders in MS. The findings were similar to the typical early course of a classical neurodegenerative disorder such as ALS. MS patients typically do not present with clinical signs of lower motor neuron loss characterized by loss of deep tendon reflexes or fasciculations, although the findings more closely resemble those observed in some poliomyelitis survivors (motor neuron loss, secondary to an aspect of axonal pathology), where the primary event is the axon as the disease progresses. The fact that lower motor neuron loss is also observed in EAE, in which the only pathogenic antigens are directed against myelin, suggests that the loss of motor neurons is a secondary phenomenon resulting from demyelination and axonal loss. Data reveal extensive early neurodegeneration in the spinal cord in the face of neuroinflammation. Investigators demonstrated that the death-like TRAIL (tumor necrosis factor-related apoptosis-inducing ligand) is an important contributor to this neuronal cell death, at least in the experimental model. The prominent role of lower motor neuron cell loss in MS pathology argues strongly for the identification and development of novel therapeutic strategies with neuroprotective potential.[49]

One group of investigators examined the spinal cord of 30 clinically well-characterized MS patients compared to ALS patients.[50] They found evidence of early neuronal stress and damage in MS patients, with a significant loss of intraspinal neurons in the cervical and lumbar levels already in the early stages of lesion development. This strongly indicates that the process of neuronal loss and axonal degeneration in MS is an early event and not an occurrence secondary to other factors as the disease progresses. This study of neuronal loss did not include histological lesion stage or duration or age of patients; therefore, the acute inflammatory process apparently implicates both the gray matter and the white matter as contributing to the neuronal damage. Of interest, there is no evidence that degenerative events are a result of GAP43 loss and newly forming synapses. These findings support the concept that neurons in early MS require timely protection through a combination of both anti-inflammatory and neuroprotective strategies.

SUMMARY

Currently, MS is considered a disease of myelin and oligodendrocytes. However, even pathological studies from 100 years ago demonstrated cortical lesions, gray matter lesions, and abnormalities in the so-called "normal-appearing white matter." If this is true, then we must reconsider the evolution of the disease as we attempt to develop rational therapies based on pathogenesis. All efforts to date have focused on downregulating the immune response in the hope that this drives all subsequent events, thus making the treatment curative. Unfortunately, numerous clinical trials to test this hypothesis with various immunosuppressive and immunomodulatory strategies have not yielded a major inroad to understanding pathogenesis or therapy. Given the possibility that axonal loss and neuronal injury occur simultaneously and either dependently or independently of demyelination, we need to explore other aspects of pathogenesis and, finally, etiology. Therefore, an attempt to target the cells included in the CNS (neurons, axons, oligodendrocytes, microglia, astrocytes) must become the new frontier of therapy. If the process begins in the CNS and inflammatory cells are attracted to the injury either specifically or nonspecifically, then targeting inflammation will likely never be definitive curative therapy. The experimental models that best mimic these processes are induced by toxins, viruses, and genetic/metabolic abnormalities. As we learn more from pathological analysis and imaging of structures not previously considered important in MS, we expand our knowledge of etiology, which allows us to develop novel therapies targeting structures other than inflammation.

REFERENCES

1. Barnes D, Munro PM, Youl BD, Prineas JW, McDonald WI. The longstanding MS lesion. A quantitative MRI and electron microscopic study. Brain; 114 (Pt 3):1271–1280, 1991.
2. Ferguson B, Matyszak MK, Esiri MM, Perry VH. Axonal damage in acute multiple sclerosis lesions. Brain; 120 (Pt 3):393–399, 1997.
3. Marburg O. Die sogenannt "akute multiple sklerose" (Encephalomyelitis periaxialis scleroticans). Jhrd Psychiatr Neurol; 27:211–312, 1906.
4. Nesbit GM, Forbes GS, Scheithauer BW, Okazaki H, Rodriguez M. Multiple sclerosis: histopathologic and MR and/or CT correlation in 37 cases at biopsy and three cases at autopsy. Radiology; 180:467–474, 1991.
5. Bjartmar C, Kinkel RP, Kidd G, Rudick RA, Trapp BD. Axonal loss in normal-appearing white matter in a patient with acute MS. Neurology; 57:1248–1252, 2001.
6. Fu L, Matthews PM, De Stefano N, et al. Imaging axonal damage of normal-appearing white matter in multiple sclerosis. Brain; 121 (Pt 1):103–113, 1998.
7. Trapp BD, Peterson J, Ransohoff RM, Rudick R, Mork S, Bo L. Axonal transection in the lesions of multiple sclerosis. N Engl J Med; 338:278–285, 1998.
8. Proceedings of a meeting to discuss neurodegeneration, neuroprotection and repair, and the interrelated issues of glial cells and myelin in multiple sclerosis. May 24, 2006. Geneva, Switzerland. Neurology; 68:S2–S96, 2007.
9. De Stefano N, Matthews PM, Arnold DL. Reversible decreases in N-acetylaspartate after acute brain injury. Magn Reson Med; 34:721–727, 1995.
10. Lisak RP. Neurodegeneration in multiple sclerosis: defining the problem. Neurology; 68:S5–S12; discussion S43–54, 2007.
11. Arnold DL. Reversible reduction of N-acetylaspartate after acute central nervous system damage [abstract]. Paper presented at: Proceedings of the Eleventh Annual Meeting of the Society for Magnetic Resonance in Medicine, 1992.
12. Peterson JW, Bo L, Mork S, Chang A, Trapp BD. Transected neurites, apoptotic neurons, and reduced inflammation in cortical multiple sclerosis lesions. Ann Neurol; 50:389–400, 2001.
13. Wegner C, Esiri MM, Chance SA, Palace J, Matthews PM. Neocortical neuronal, synaptic, and glial loss in multiple sclerosis. Neurology; 67:960–967, 2006.
14. Seewann A, Vrenken H, van der Valk P, et al. Diffusely abnormal white matter in chronic multiple sclerosis: imaging and histopathologic analysis. Arch Neurol; 66:601–609, 2009.
15. Simon JH, Kinkel RP, Jacobs L, Bub L, Simonian N. A Wallerian degeneration pattern in patients at risk for MS. Neurology; 54:1155–1160, 2000.
16. Rodriguez M. A function of myelin is to protect axons from subsequent injury: implications for deficits in multiple sclerosis. Brain; 126:751–752, 2003.
17. Pitt D, Gonzales E, Cross AH, Goldberg MP. Dysmyelinated axons in shiverer mice are highly vulnerable to alpha-amino-3-hydroxy-5-methylisoxazole-4-propionic acid (AMPA) receptor-mediated toxicity. Brain Res; 1309:146–154, 2010.
18. Sahenk Z, Chen L, Mendell JR. Effects of PMP22 duplication and deletions on the axonal cytoskeleton. Ann Neurol; 45:16–24, 1999.
19. Shintaku M, Hirano A, Llena JF. Increased diameter of demyelinated axons in chronic multiple sclerosis of the spinal cord. Neuropathol Appl Neurobiol; 14:505–510, 1988.
20. Allen IV, Glover G, Anderson R. Abnormalities in the macroscopically normal white matter in cases of mild or spinal multiple sclerosis (MS). Acta Neuropathol; 7:176–178, 1981.
21. Pascual AM, Martinez-Bisbal MC, Bosca I, et al. Axonal loss is progressive and partly dissociated from lesion load in early multiple sclerosis. Neurology; 69:63–67, 2007.
22. Vercellino M, Plano F, Votta B, Mutani R, Giordana MT, Cavalla P. Grey matter pathology in multiple sclerosis. J Neuropathol Exp Neurol; 64:1101–1107, 2005.
23. Wylezinska M, Cifelli A, Jezzard P, Palace J, Alecci M, Matthews PM. Thalamic neurodegeneration in relapsing-remitting multiple sclerosis. Neurology; 60:1949–1954, 2003.
24. Cifelli A, Arridge M, Jezzard P, Esiri MM, Palace J, Matthews PM. Thalamic neurodegeneration in multiple sclerosis. Ann Neurol; 52:650–653, 2002.
25. Pirko I, Lucchinetti CF, Sriram S, Bakshi R. Gray matter involvement in multiple sclerosis. Neurology; 68:634–642, 2007.
26. Fisher E, Lee JC, Nakamura K, Rudick RA. Gray matter atrophy in multiple sclerosis: a longitudinal study. Ann Neurol; 64:255–265, 2008.
27. Tsunoda I, Fujinami RS: Inside-out versus outside-in models for virus induced demyelination: axonal damage triggering demyelination. Springer Seminars in Immunopathology; 24:105–125, 2002.
28. Dutta R, Trapp BD. Pathogenesis of axonal and neuronal damage in multiple sclerosis. Neurology; 68:S22–S31; discussion S43–54, 2007.
29. Tutuncu M, Tang J, Zeid NA, et al. Onset of progressive phase is an age-dependent clinical milestone in multiple sclerosis. Mult Scler, 2012 June 26 [E-pub ahead of print].
30. Pittock SJ, Mayr WT, McClelland RL, et al. Change in MS-related disability in a population-based cohort: a 10-year follow-up study. Neurology; 62:51–59, 2004.
31. Pittock SJ, McClelland RL, Mayr WT, et al. Clinical implications of benign multiple sclerosis: a 20-year population-based follow-up study. Ann Neurol; 56:303–306, 2004.
32. Pavelko KD, Howe CL, Drescher KM, et al. Interleukin-6 protects anterior horn neurons from lethal virus-induced injury. J Neurosci; 23:481–492, 2003.
33. Drescher KM, Murray PD, Lin X, Carlino JA, Rodriguez M. TGF-beta 2 reduces demyelination, virus antigen expression, and macrophage recruitment in a viral model of multiple sclerosis. J Immunol; 164:3207–3213, 2000.
34. Dutta R, McDonough J, Yin X, et al. Mitochondrial dysfunction as a cause of axonal degeneration in multiple sclerosis patients. Ann Neurol; 59:478–489, 2006.
35. Sathornsumetee S, McGavern DB, Ure DR, Rodriguez M. Quantitative ultrastructural analysis of a single spinal cord demyelinated lesion predicts total lesion load,

axonal loss, and neurological dysfunction in a murine model of multiple sclerosis. Am J Pathol; 157:1365–1376, 2000.

36. McGavern DB, Murray PD, Rivera-Quinones C, Schmelzer JD, Low PA, Rodriguez M. Axonal loss results in spinal cord atrophy, electrophysiological abnormalities and neurological deficits following demyelination in a chronic inflammatory model of multiple sclerosis. Brain; 123 Pt 3:519–531, 2000.

37. Lovas G, Szilagyi N, Majtenyi K, Palkovits M, Komoly S. Axonal changes in chronic demyelinated cervical spinal cord plaques. Brain; 123 (Pt 2):308–317, 2000.

38. Neumann H. Molecular mechanisms of axonal damage in inflammatory central nervous system diseases. Curr Opin Neurol; 16:267–273, 2003.

39. Deb C, Lafrance-Corey RG, Zoecklein L, Papke L, Rodriguez M, Howe CL. Demyelinated axons and motor function are protected by genetic deletion of perforin in a mouse model of multiple sclerosis. J Neuropathol Exp Neurol; 68:1037–1048, 2009.

40. Medana I, Martinic MA, Wekerle H, Neumann H. Transection of major histocompatibility complex class I-induced neurites by cytotoxic T lymphocytes. Am J Pathol; 159:809–815, 2001.

41. Hoftberger R, Aboul-Enein F, Brueck W, et al. Expression of major histocompatibility complex class I molecules on the different cell types in multiple sclerosis lesions. Brain Pathol; 14:43–50, 2004.

42. Bitsch A, Schuchardt J, Bunkowski S, Kuhlmann T, Bruck W. Acute axonal injury in multiple sclerosis. Correlation with demyelination and inflammation. Brain; 123 (Pt 6):1174–1183, 2000.

43. Rivera-Quinones C, McGavern D, Schmelzer JD, Hunter SF, Low PA, Rodriguez M. Absence of neurological deficits following extensive demyelination in a class I-deficient murine model of multiple sclerosis. Nature Med; 4:187–193, 1998.

44. Ure DR, Rodriguez M. Preservation of neurologic function during inflammatory demyelination correlates with axon sparing in a mouse model of multiple sclerosis. Neuroscience; 111:399–411, 2002.

45. Deb C, Lafrance-Corey RG, Schmalstieg WF, et al. CD8+ T cells cause disability and axon loss in a mouse model of multiple sclerosis. PloS One; 5:e12478, 2010.

46. Murray PD, Pavelko KD, Leibowitz J, Lin X, Rodriguez M. CD4(+) and CD8(+) T cells make discrete contributions to demyelination and neurologic disease in a viral model of multiple sclerosis. J Virol; 72:7320–7329, 1998.

47. Kivisakk P, Stawiarz L, Matusevicius D, et al. High numbers of perforin mRNA expressing CSF cells in multiple sclerosis patients with gadolinium-enhancing brain MRI lesions. Acta Neurol Scand; 100:18–24, 1999.

48. Rubesa G, Podack ER, Sepcic J, Rukavina D. Increased perforin expression in multiple sclerosis patients during exacerbation of disease in peripheral blood lymphocytes. J Neuroimmunol; 74:198–204, 1997.

49. Vogt J, Paul F, Aktas O, et al. Lower motor neuron loss in multiple sclerosis and experimental autoimmune encephalomyelitis. Ann Neurol; 66:310–322, 2009.

50. Schirmer L, Albert M, Buss A, et al. Substantial early, but nonprogressive neuronal loss in multiple sclerosis (MS) spinal cord. Ann Neurol; 66:698–704, 2009.

SECTION **2**

TREATMENT

Chapter 8

Treatment of Acute Exacerbations of Multiple Sclerosis

Abstract

Over the past two decades, the available treatment options for MS have multiplied, and several partially effective treatment modalities are now available to address various aspects of this disease. There are four aspects of MS that respond to pharmacotherapy: treatment of new attacks, prevention of relapses, symptomatic treatment, and tissue restoration (remyelination, axonal/neuronal recovery). While there are approved treatment modalities to address the first three of these aspects, we are only beginning to understand how to address the issue of tissue restoration. In this chapter, we will focus on the treatment of acute attacks.

INTRODUCTION

Relapses are defined as the development of new neurological symptoms lasting at least 24 hours, for which no other cause can be identified. Patients should be free of infection and afebrile. Relapses typically evolve over hours or days, followed by a plateau stage that persists for several days or for 2 to 6 weeks and, finally, partial or complete recovery. While MS can cause almost

135

any CNS-related neurological symptoms, a few clinical syndromes are particularly suggestive of MS. These include monocular, often painful, vision loss suggestive of optic neuritis, unilateral facial or extremity numbness and/or paresthesias, weakness of one or more limbs, gait or limb ataxia, partial or complete Brown-Séquard syndrome, and diplopia, especially in the context of internuclear ophthalmoplegia.

Since 80% of MS cases fall into the relapsing–remitting category, this is a very common clinical scenario.[1] Steroids have been established as an effective treatment for MS relapses for several decades. However, before considering such treatment, it is important to clarify whether the presenting neurological symptom complex truly represents a new attack. Several features can help distinguish true attacks from pseudo-recurrences (Table 8.1), which can also be labeled as Uhthoff-like phenomena. (Uhthoff's original description related to the optic nerve, but the same mechanism can lead to symptomatic worsening in other white matter pathways as well.) The most relevant distinguishing feature of a true relapse is the presence of any truly *new* symptom. Partial recurrences of *previous* symptoms are more typical of pseudo-recurrences and are related to heat-induced conduction delay in white matter fibers. Several sources also emphasize the significance of duration, namely that pseudo-recurrences are generally short-lived (<24 hours). However, when a persistent condition gives rise to conduction delay (such as low-grade fever related to an infection, etc.), then the pseudo-event lasts as long as the provoking factor is present. Perhaps the most common example would be the persistent symptoms of a urinary tract infection. Such infections are very common in MS due to urinary retention. Further, typical urinary tract infection symptoms of dysuria or burning sensations may not be perceived in the context of MS due to sensory involvement.

In general, it is best to start with a basic workup to rule out infections (Table 8.2). In more advanced cases, it may be necessary to look for less common causes of inflammation, such as decubitus ulcers or ingrown toenails. MRI is the *non plus ultra* method in distinguishing attack from pseudo-attack; new attacks can be accompanied by new lesion formation, which should be captured as lesional gadolinium enhancement, as discussed in Chapter 4, if the timing of the MRI is right. If no enhancing lesion is found and the patient's symptoms are actually recurrences of previously existing symptom(s), the likelihood that the symptoms are related to a new attack is decreased, and a pseudo-relapse seems more likely. Some types of symptoms might also require scanning the spinal cord; a negative brain MRI obviously does not rule out new spinal cord attacks.

SHOULD ALL MULTIPLE SCLEROSIS ATTACKS BE TREATED?

Once it is clear that the symptoms truly represent a new attack, one can consider treatment.

Table 8–1 Differences Between Relapses and Pseudo-attacks (Uhthoff's-like Phenomena)

	Pseudo-relapse	Relapse
Temporal course	Often short-lived (up to 24–28 hours), but may be longer if precipitating factor persists	Subacute onset, 2–6 weeks in duration
Type of symptom	Partial or complete recurrence of former symptom(s)	New symptom not experienced before
Trigger factors	Anything that results in elevated core temperature (stress, overheating, fever, infections, lack of sleep, ingrown toenail, decubitus ulcer, etc.)	Usually no identifiable trigger; infections or major stressors may precede relapses
MRI findings	No new or enhancing lesions	New lesion, typically enhancing for 2–4 weeks
Response to steroids	No response, or partial response due to nonspecific boost effect	Most relapses respond to steroids

Table 8–2 Workup Before Steroid Treatment

Basic workup before steroid treatment:
Complete blood count with differential
Urinalysis, with Gram stain and cultures
Chest x-ray (if applicable)
Comprehensive workup (to differentiate relapse from pseudo-relapse if clinically ambiguous):
MRI to look for new lesions
Detailed skin and dental exam (abscesses, ulcers, ingrown toenails)

However, treatment of relapses is not a "must do," as summarized in Table 8.3. For example, mild sensory events typically neither lead to long-term disability nor respond well to treatment. In general, it is best to treat only attacks that are potentially associated with an unfavorable long-term disability profile. Mild attacks can respond to rest and resolve completely with time. We recommend ruling out infections prior to treatment, even in the absence of obvious symptoms. This will prevent worsening of the infection if it is present and also will differentiate pseudo-attacks from real ones, as summarized above.

TREATMENT MODALITIES TO ADDRESS MULTIPLE SCLEROSIS RELAPSES: STEROIDS

Treatment of relapses typically means intravenous steroid treatment, with the goal of hastening recovery from bothersome, potentially disabling symptoms. Conventional wisdom holds that steroids do not improve long-term recovery; they simply make recovery faster. Some more recent observations may challenge this assumption, but overall beneficial long-term effects were reported in only one trial as per a recent Cochrane Library review.[2] The typical treatment involves 3 to 5 days of intravenous methylprednisolone, 1,000 mg per day. In our experience, this is best infused slowly, over 90 minutes. We do not generally recommend premedication or an oral-steroid taper following intravenous treatment. Some groups may prefer to extend the treatment duration 7 to 10 days. There is insufficient evidence to suggest that a longer course is better, but we do extend treatment in some cases depending on the perceived and documented severity of the relapse. Lasting suppression of the suprarenal glands is highly unlikely with the proposed brief high-dose pulsed treatment. Oral steroids can be used in place of intravenous treatment, but one would need to give the clinically unfeasible dose of 1,250 mg of prednisone per day to accomplish the same dose equivalent as with intravenous treatment. Absorption and bioavailability are also suboptimal with the oral formulation. The Optic Neuritis Treatment Trial suggested that oral steroids given without prior intravenous steroids increase the risk of attacks in the ensuing 3 years.[3,4–8] For this reason, intravenous steroids are preferred in most practice settings; they may have complementary effects to ongoing immunomodulation in "prevention of relapses."

In terms of adverse effects, the treatment generally is well tolerated.[9] The universally known side effects of steroids are most commonly seen

Table 8–3 When to Offer Steroid Treatment

Symptoms where treatment should be considered	Symptoms that may not need treatment
Severe motor weakness	Mild sensory symptoms that don't result in ataxia or sensory useless hand
Ataxia	Mild blurry vision as a result of optic neuritis
Incontinence (bowel and/or bladder)	
Moderate to severe vision loss due to optic neuritis	
Diplopia	
Sensory symptoms associated with sensory useless hands, ataxia, and/or other forms of posterior column dysfunction	
Cognitive dysfunction, moderate to severe, with associated enhancing lesions	

with long-term oral treatment as opposed to short-term intravenous use. *Insomnia* may occur during the days of treatment but rarely requires intervention. The patients and, more importantly, their relatives need to be aware of possible *mania and behavioral changes*. Short-term steroid courses occasionally result in *acne* and *bruising*, but these are much more common with prolonged steroid use. *Peptic ulcer disease and/or worsening of gastroesophageal reflux disease* may occur, and individuals prone to these symptoms should receive appropriate treatment such as proton-pump inhibitors or H2 blockers. A metallic taste often accompanies the use of intravenous steroids, related to the excretion of steroids through the salivary glands. *Osteoporosis* can worsen with intravenous steroid treatment, especially when used monthly or every 3 months. Supplementary calcium and vitamin D are essential, along with regular screening with DEXA scans to monitor bone density.

In an idiosyncratic manner, high-dose steroid treatment may cause *osteonecrosis of the femur head*, which is a severe complication requiring hip prosthesis implantation in most cases. Inherited thrombophilia, such as factor V Leiden or prothrombin mutation, may predispose patients to this, but appropriate treatment may prevent these events,[10,11] although this remains controversial.[12] Liver cirrhosis is also a potential risk factor,[13] and VEGF receptor polymorphism also increases the likelihood of this severe complication.[14,15]

Do Steroids Always Work?

While intravenous steroids have a reasonably high success rate, they are ineffective in approximately 15% of cases. One consideration is delay between symptom onset and treatment initiation. In general, earlier treatment is preferable, but anecdotally steroids may work up to 8 to 12 weeks after a relapse. It is important to remember that the effects of steroids are typically delayed; following a 5-day course, peak effect should occur between days 7 and 10. Therefore, in general, one should wait at least 2 weeks after initiation to decide whether treatment has been successful. In cases of a moderate steroid-unresponsive, nonsensory deficit, rescue therapies are an option. The first-line treatment in that setting is plasma exchange, as

established via an NIH-funded, randomized, placebo-controlled clinical trial (PLEX).[16,17]

TREATING STEROID-UNRESPONSIVE ATTACKS: PLASMAPHERESIS

It is important to note that the original PLEX trial[17] enrolled patients with severe and fixed deficits; several of the cases were many weeks to a few months after the attack. In other words, these were the so-called "hopeless cases." A patient was considered a responder if only he or she demonstrated a clinically meaningful improvement following plasma exchange. Approximately 42% of steroid failure cases responded to plasma exchange in the trial. The responders often had a rather dramatic response; some became fully ambulatory after weeks of paralysis. For details of the PLEX protocol, please see Table 8.4.

As established in *post hoc* analyses and extensions to our initial trial, meaningful improvement is unlikely if it does not occur by the fourth exchange.[18] If improvement is noticeable, then the full seven-session course should be completed. Male sex, preserved reflexes, and early initiation of treatment were markers of moderate to marked improvement following plasma exchange. Ring enhancement and mass effect also predicted a beneficial response.[18,19]

Why Does Plasma Exchange Work in Steroid-Unresponsive Cases?

The concept behind the use of plasma exchange is relatively simple: steroids can efficiently

Table 8–4 Plasma Exchange Protocol Used in PLEX Trial

Use either peripheral vein (often possible) or central line.
Exchange 1.1 plasma volume units at each exchange.
One exchange every other day
A total of seven exchanges (over 2 weeks)
Heparin/citrate mixture or heparin alone for anticoagulation
Close monitoring for line complications (if applicable)

address cell-mediated immune responses but have relatively minimal impact on antibody-mediated immunity. While plasma exchange has multiple potential mechanisms for immunomodulation, the most likely mechanism in the treatment of MS relapses is the rapid removal of pathogenic antibodies or cytokines from the circulation and from the tissue itself via equilibration. The fact that plasma exchange works very efficiently in neuromyelitis optica (NMO) exacerbations is another indirect proof that the mechanism of action is related to antibody removal, because NMO has been shown to be an antibody-mediated disease.[2] In addition, it is noteworthy that in a biopsy-proven cohort of MS patients, only those with pattern II MS responded. Pattern II represents an antibody- and complement-mediated pathomechanism[20] (see Chapter 5, Figs. 5.22 and 5.23).

The question often arises whether IVIG has the same effects as plasma exchange. Extrapolating from other neurological diseases, such as myasthenia gravis or Guillain-Barré syndrome, one could conclude that the two work equally well. However, this has never been systematically studied in MS. Most IVIG studies investigated its impact on relapse prevention rather than acute attacks.[21,22]

Side Effects and Complications of Plasma Exchange

Plasma exchange seldom has serious adverse effects; however, in most cases, it requires line placement, which does have potential adverse effects. Furthermore, citrate toxicity occasionally occurs because citrate is often used to prevent clot formation during plasma exchange. This can result in perioral and acral paresthesias, which may be mistaken for new MS attacks. Patients undergoing plasma exchange also need to be monitored for anemia.

TREATMENT OF FULMINANT MULTIPLE SCLEROSIS ATTACKS

MS may occasionally present with very severe attacks that do not respond to steroids or plasma exchange. Some of these cases represent the unipolar acute progressive Marburg's variant, which usually leads to death within a few months. There are no well-performed clinical trials for rare situations like these; however, the prevailing opinion is to utilize strong immunosuppressive therapies. In these cases, we often utilize cyclophosphamide with steroids, as per the established protocol,[23–26] which can be found at http://www.partnersmscenter.org/index.php?id=45&mn=5&sm=5-4.

Alemtuzumab (Campath) treatment is also an option in these situations, but the treatment has significant risk for side effects, including the development of MS-unrelated autoimmune conditions, such as autoimmune thyroiditis.[27–31] The dosing scheme of alemtuzumab in the original British studies was a daily intravenous dose of 12, 20, 24, or 30 mg for 5 consecutive days, along with 1 g methylprednisolone concurrently for the first 3 days of treatment. In the CAMMS trial, a daily dose of 12 and 24 mg for 5 days was utilized, with the same methylprednisolone dose as above.[32] In this trial, there was no difference between the 12-mg and 24-mg doses in terms of treatment outcome.[32] Natalizumab (Tysabri) is another option for these patients, although no established acute treatment protocol exists.

SUMMARY

Over the past two decades, several partially effective treatment modalities have become available to treat new attacks and prevent relapses. While the treatment of catastrophic attacks expected to lead to persistent disability is especially important, in general mild attacks may not require treatment. Even when treated, faster recovery does not generally translate to more complete recovery in the long term. After ruling out pseudo-attacks, in most cases intravenous steroid administration is sufficient to address the relapse, with escalation to plasma exchange for severe steroid-unresponsive attacks. We find that other treatment modalities are only very rarely required.

REFERENCES

1. Noseworthy JH, Lucchinetti C, Rodriguez M, Weinshenker BG. Multiple sclerosis. N Engl J Med; 343:938–952, 2000.

2. Ciccone A, Beretta S, Brusaferri F, Galea I, Protti A, Spreafico C. Corticosteroids for the long-term treatment in multiple sclerosis. Cochrane Database Syst Rev:CD006264, 2008.

3. Beck RW, Cleary PA, Anderson MM, Jr., et al. A randomized, controlled trial of corticosteroids in the treatment of acute optic neuritis. The Optic Neuritis Study Group. N Engl J Med; 326:581–588, 1992.

4. Beck RW, Gal RL. Treatment of acute optic neuritis: a summary of findings from the optic neuritis treatment trial. Arch Ophthalmol; 126:994–995, 2008.

5. Katz B, Trobe JD, Beck RW. The Optic Neuritis Treatment Trial: implications for clinicians. Semin Ophthalmol; 10:214–220, 1995.

6. Corbett JJ. What have the Optic Neuritis Treatment Trial and the Longitudinal Optic Neuritis Study shown us? J Neurol Sci; 125:1–2, 1994.

7. Beck RW, Cleary PA. Optic Neuritis Treatment Trial. One-year follow-up results. Arch Ophthalmol; 111:773–775, 1993.

8. Beck RW. The Optic Neuritis Treatment Trial. Implications for clinical practice. Optic Neuritis Study Group. Arch Ophthalmol; 110:331–332, 1992.

9. Chrousos GA, Kattah JC, Beck RW, Cleary PA. Side effects of glucocorticoid treatment. Experience of the Optic Neuritis Treatment Trial. JAMA; 269:2110–2112, 1993.

10. Omeroglu H, Inan U. Inherited thrombophilia may be a causative factor for osteonecrosis of femoral head in male patients with developmental dysplasia of the hip: a case series. Arch Orthop Trauma Surg; 132(9):1281–1285, 2012.

11. Glueck CJ, Freiberg RA, Boppana S, Wang P. Thrombophilia, hypofibrinolysis, the eNOS T-786C polymorphism, and multifocal osteonecrosis. J Bone Joint Surg Am; 90:2220–2229, 2008.

12. Seguin C, Kassis J, Busque L, et al. Non-traumatic necrosis of bone (osteonecrosis) is associated with endothelial cell activation but not thrombophilia. Rheumatology (Oxford); 47:1151–1155, 2008.

13. Hung TH, Hsieh YH, Tsai CC, Tseng CW, Tseng KC. Is liver cirrhosis a risk factor for osteonecrosis of the femoral head in adults? A population-based 3-year follow-up study. Intern Med; 50:2563–2568, 2011.

14. Li W, Sakai T, Nishii T, et al. Distribution of TRAP-positive cells and expression of HIF-1alpha, VEGF, and FGF-2 in the reparative reaction in patients with osteonecrosis of the femoral head. J Orthop Res; 27:694–700, 2009.

15. Radke S, Battmann A, Jatzke S, Eulert J, Jakob F, Schutze N. Expression of the angiomatrix and angiogenic proteins CYR61, CTGF, and VEGF in osteonecrosis of the femoral head. J Orthop Res; 24:945–952, 2006.

16. Rodriguez M, Karnes WE, Bartleson JD, Pineda AA. Plasmapheresis in acute episodes of fulminant CNS inflammatory demyelination. Neurology; 43:1100–1104, 1993.

17. Weinshenker BG, O'Brien PC, Petterson TM, et al. A randomized trial of plasma exchange in acute central nervous system inflammatory demyelinating disease. Ann Neurol; 46:878–886, 1999.

18. Keegan M, Pineda AA, McClelland RL, Darby CH, Rodriguez M, Weinshenker BG. Plasma exchange for severe attacks of CNS demyelination: predictors of response. Neurology; 58:143–146, 2002.

19. Magana SM, Keegan BM, Weinshenker BG, et al. Beneficial plasma exchange response in central nervous system inflammatory demyelination. Arch Neurol; 68:870–878, 2011.

20. Keegan M, Konig F, McClelland R, et al. Relation between humoral pathological changes in multiple sclerosis and response to therapeutic plasma exchange. Lancet; 366:579–582, 2005.

21. Strasser-Fuchs S, Fazekas F, Deisenhammer F, Nahler G, Mamoli B. The Austrian Immunoglobulin in MS (AIMS) study: final analysis. Mult Scler; 6 Suppl 2:S9–S13, 2000.

22. Fazekas F, Strasser-Fuchs S, Hommes OR. Intravenous immunoglobulin in MS: promise or failure? J Neurol Sci; 259:61–66, 2007.

23. Elkhalifa A, Weiner H. Cyclophosphamide treatment of MS: Current therapeutic approaches and treatment regimens. Int Mult Scler J; 17:12–18, 2010.

24. Gauthier SA, Weiner HL. Cyclophosphamide therapy for MS. Int Mult Scler J; 12:52–58, 2005.

25. Weiner HL, Mackin GA, Orav EJ, et al. Intermittent cyclophosphamide pulse therapy in progressive multiple sclerosis: final report of the Northeast Cooperative Multiple Sclerosis Treatment Group. Neurology; 43:910–918, 1993.

26. Weiner HL, Hauser SL, Hafler DA, Fallis RJ, Lehrich JR, Dawson DM. The use of cyclophosphamide in the treatment of multiple sclerosis. Ann NY Acad Sci; 436:373–381, 1984.

27. Costelloe L, Jones J, Coles A. Secondary autoimmune diseases following alemtuzumab therapy for multiple sclerosis. Expert Rev Neurother; 12:335–341, 2012.

28. Perumal JS, Foo F, Cook P, Khan O. Subcutaneous administration of alemtuzumab in patients with highly active multiple sclerosis. Mult Scler; 18:1197–1199, 2012.

29. Fox EJ, Sullivan HC, Gazda SK, et al. A single-arm, open-label study of alemtuzumab in treatment-refractory patients with multiple sclerosis. Eur J Neurol; 19:307–311, 2012.

30. Wood H. Multiple sclerosis: Benefits of alemtuzumab in MS. Nat Rev Neurol; 7:245, 2011.

31. Minagar A, Alexander JS, Sahraian MA, Zivadinov R. Alemtuzumab and multiple sclerosis: therapeutic application. Expert Opin Biol Ther; 10:421–429, 2010.

32. Coles AJ, Compston DA, Selmaj KW, et al. Alemtuzumab vs. interferon beta-1a in early multiple sclerosis. N Engl J Med; 359:1786–1801, 2008.

Chapter 9

Disease-Modifying Therapies in Multiple Sclerosis

Abstract

Several recently available medications offer preventive treatment in MS. The primary goal is to alter the natural course of the disease by reducing the frequency and severity of relapses and by preventing or slowing the progression of disability. Seven FDA-approved, disease-modifying medications are available in the United States at the time of writing this chapter: four injectable products, two intravenous medications, and one oral medication. Of note, the percentages quoted (i.e., relapse rate reduction by 60%) reflect group data. In other words, the treated group on average experienced 60% fewer relapses, but both treatment and control groups included both individuals who did very well or very poorly. Therefore, the group data do not apply to every individual case.

Also of note, most clinical trials rely on MRI-proven disease activity as a secondary or even primary outcome. However, conventional, clinically derived MRI measures tend to correlate imperfectly with clinical outcome. Despite substantial progress in addressing the relapsing–remitting or highly inflammatory stages of MS, currently available treatment modalities fail to address the disabling progressive form of MS. Successful modification of the disease course is most likely to occur in three patient groups: those with clinically isolated syndromes, those with relapsing–remitting MS, and those with "highly inflammatory" forms of secondary or primary progressive MS, as discussed later.

ASSESSING MAGNITUDE OF TREATMENT EFFECT

Before we discuss specific data, it is useful to review the most important evidence-based medicine statistics used to assess the magnitude of treatment effect. Relative risk reduction (RRR) is the metric most commonly cited in publications and promotional materials about clinical trials. The RRR is the degree to which treatment reduces the frequency of the outcome measure (experimental event rate; e.g., relapse, progression) compared with the control treatment (control event rate). The RRR is a ratio, not an absolute number, and is calculated as follows:

RRR = (Control event rate – Experimental event rate)/Control event rate

If the control event rate is low (making the denominator smaller), it will obviously inflate the RRR. An "impressive" 50% RRR may have low biological significance if the outcome occurs infrequently. Therefore, the absolute risk reduction (ARR) should be calculated to correct for the frequency of the outcome.

ARR = Control event rate – Experimental event rate

For most approved MS agents, the calculated ARR is considerably less (and therefore less impressive) than RRR. Most reports and publications of clinical trials of disease-modifying agents do not cite this metric. Calculation of risk reduction requires access to the data citing comparisons of proportions (ratios), and the required "raw data" are not always immediately available in publications.

Another useful measure of treatment effect is the "number needed to treat" (NNT). It is calculated as the inverse of the ARR: **NNT = 1/ARR**.

Overall, the NNTs for the disease-modifying agents in MS are approximately in the 4-to-14 range for 2- to 3-year treatment periods. However, these NNTs are often for outcome measures with limited predictive value for long-term outcomes. For example, relapse behavior does not generally reflect long-term disability except in patients with high early relapse rate with limited recovery (see Chapter 1). Furthermore, the agents are expensive, may pose various risks, and are often inconvenient to use. We must also remember that clinical trials typically enroll patients with very restricted eligibility criteria (often a history of significant recent disease activity and/or disability progression), and trial coordinators exert considerable effort to optimize compliance with the treatment plan. As such, the NNT experienced in a trial setting (effectiveness) may considerably exceed what is observed in the average practice setting. In some practice settings, however, the NNT may actually be stronger than the trial (e.g., patients with very high relapse and MRI activity).

USE OF DISEASE-MODIFYING AGENTS IN CLINICALLY ISOLATED SYNDROME

A central question about disease-modifying therapies is when to initiate treatment. There are many vocal advocates of early treatment, even at the clinically isolated syndrome (CIS) stage. However, early treatment may obscure whether the disease-modifying agents actually prevent relapse or MRI progression or whether the natural history of MS in that given individual has just resolved to a stable clinical picture.[1,2] This becomes especially problematic if a CIS patient receives early treatment and, after years of inactive disease, wishes to stop taking disease-modifying agents. As discussed in Chapter 1, this is further complicated by population-based epidemiology studies indicating that approximately 20% of patients with MS do not develop long-term disability even without using disease-modifying agents.

Two classic multicenter studies have addressed disease-modifying agent use in persons at high risk of developing MS (high-risk CIS cases). In the CHAMPS study,[3] 383 patients with an initial episode of presumed demyelinating disease ("CIS"), in the setting of an abnormal, asymptomatic baseline cranial MRI scan, were randomized to receive either weekly interferon beta-1a, 30 mcg given intramuscularly, or placebo after an initial course of steroid therapy. Investigators terminated this study early because a greater number of placebo-treated patients reached the primary outcome measure of conversion to "clinically definite MS" (CDMS) status. Although not unexpected given the known effect of interferons on reduced relapse rate, these findings do provide support for early treatment. The duration of follow-up in this study (71% 1 year, 34% 2 years, 16% 3 years) was insufficient to determine long-term benefit from early intervention. It is also clear that the treatment is only partially effective because 50% of interferon-treated patients in the CHAMPS trial had clinical or MRI evidence of recurrent disease within 18 months of starting treatment.[4] The analysis of treatment effect related to the CHAMPS trial revealed a RRR of 38%, an ARR of 14.6%, and an NNT of seven patients over 2 years to prevent one conversion to CDMS. It is also worth mentioning that by the most recent MS criteria (2010 modifications to the McDonald criteria), many cases enrolled in this and other "CIS" trials actually should be classified as having MS rather than CIS (see extensive discussion in Chapter 1). This will definitely affect which data to quote when counseling patients and how clinicians use the available CIS data. In our practice, explaining the changing definition and discussing the previous knowledge base of CIS as "early MS" seems reasonable. As discussed in Chapter 1, one way to improve the odds of NNT in this trial is to look at subgroups. It is clear that patients with transverse myelitis *and* brainstem syndromes are more likely to benefit from early treatment than those with optic neuritis (Fig. 9.1).

In the second placebo-controlled study published to date, enrolling 309 patients with either monosymptomatic (61%) or multifocal-onset (39%) early demyelinating disease, early treatment with interferon beta-1a in an unusually low dose (22 mcg given subcutaneously once weekly) reduced conversion to CDMS (34% vs. 45%) at 2 years.[5] Again, no data exist on whether these treatments offer long-term benefit. The evidence-based medicine calculations for this trial show an RRR of 24% and an ARR of 11% and require an NNT of nine patients over 2 years to prevent one conversion to "CDMS." These two studies provide support for initiating treatment in patients presenting with first attack (mainly with brainstem, cerebellar, or spinal cord syndrome) *and* multiple asymptomatic MRI lesions.

The most recent addition to the CIS studies is the PreCISe study,[6] which analyzed the use of glatiramer acetate as a disease-modifying

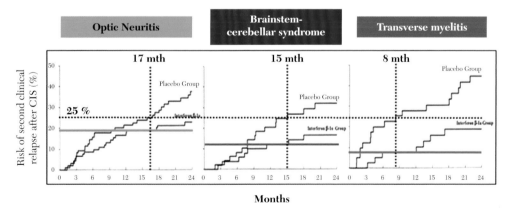

Figure 9–1. Risk of second demyelinating attack (clinically definite MS by Poser criteria) following a clinically isolated syndrome in patients treated with interferon γ1a versus patients who have received placebo.[4] It takes about 17 months for 25% of patients with isolated optic neuritis to develop a new relapse, while it takes 15 months for patients with an isolated brainstem syndrome and 8 months for patients with an isolated transverse myelitis to reach the same target. It is clear that patients with transverse myelitis *and* brainstem syndromes are more likely to benefit from early treatment than those with optic neuritis.

agent. Investigators studied 482 patients on a standard glatiramer dose (n = 243) or placebo (n = 238). Glatiramer acetate reduced the risk of CDMS by 45% compared with placebo (hazard ratio 0.55, 95% CI 0.40–0.77; p = .0005). Raw data are not available to permit accurate evidence-based medicine calculations; based on approximate values from the provided survival curves, the approximate RRR was 40%, while the ARR was 10% at 1 year and the NNT was ~10 over 1 year.

It is important to note that these studies offer no guidance when patients with CIS present with a brain MRI that is not suggestive of MS (i.e., only one optic nerve, brainstem, or cord lesion explaining the CIS symptoms). We currently do not recommend interferon treatment for CIS patients with less than two asymptomatic MRI lesions. Please see "Summary of RRMS Treatments" below for patient counseling advice regarding the use of disease-modifying medications, as well as Chapter 1.

ALTERING THE COURSE OF RELAPSING–REMITTING MULTIPLE SCLEROSIS

Tier 1 Medications

BETA-INTERFERONS

Interferons are peptides with antiviral and immunoregulatory properties. Interferon beta-1b (Betaseron) was the first drug approved by the FDA specifically for the treatment of MS. A large clinical study in relapsing–remitting MS (RRMS) demonstrated that patients receiving a subcutaneous injection every other day had a reduced frequency of relapses by about one third.[7] The severity of relapses was also decreased. Interferon beta-1b had a striking effect on MRI measures of disease activity, such as the frequency of new lesion formation. The placebo-control group continued to accumulate white matter lesions, whereas patients in the high-dose arm (8 million IU) had stabilized MRI lesion loads. Interestingly, there was no significant difference in disability levels between treated patients and controls. Side effects included injection-site reactions, flu-like symptoms (low-grade fever, myalgias, headache; these lessen in frequency after a few months of

treatment), mild liver enzyme elevation, and lymphopenia. Depression and attempted suicide were more common in the treated groups. Evidence-based medicine calculations revealed an RRR of 18% and an ARR of 15%; the NNT analysis showed that seven patients must be treated over 3 years to increase the relapse-free number by one patient.

INTERFERON BETA-1A (AVONEX)

Interferon beta-1a (Avonex) has the same amino acid sequence as natural interferon beta and differs from interferon beta-1b by one amino acid as well as by the presence of carbohydrate moieties. Once-weekly intramuscular interferon beta-1a has a similar efficacy to interferon beta-1b in reducing the frequency of MS relapses. In addition, it decreases disability and has fewer side effects. In the original interferon beta 1-a I.M. trial, the primary outcome measure was time to Expanded Disability Severity Scale (EDSS) progression. The RRR was 37%, the ARR was 13%, and NNT was eight for 2 years to prevent one patient from developing EDSS progression. The calculations for "proportion relapse free" showed an RRR of 16%, an ARR of 12%, and an NNT of eight over 2 years (eight patients need treatment for 2 years to increase the number of relapse-free patients by one). Neutralizing autoantibodies (NAbs) occurred half as often as with interferon beta-1b (approximately 40% vs. 20%). The FDA has approved interferon beta-1a for "relapsing MS."[8]

The "correct" dose of interferon continues to be debated. In a more recent placebo-controlled trial, patients randomized to receive a high dose of interferon beta-1a (44 mcg three times a week) did better than those receiving half this weekly dose. Both groups outperformed the placebo group. The high dose seemed more effective in limiting relapse severity, hospitalizations, MRI activity, lesion-volume accumulation, and, possibly, disability in the most severely disabled patients. At the end of 2 years of follow-up, placebo-treated patients were randomized to receive 22 or 44 mcg given subcutaneously three times weekly; patients on active treatment remained at their original dose.[9] The authors reported a benefit for the higher dose and for those treated for the full 4 years, again suggesting that early treatment and, perhaps, higher doses of interferons may be beneficial.

The primary outcome, however, was relapse count per patient per 4 years, and patients treated early had an advantage in terms of this outcome measure. Trends favoring the higher dose included relapse rate and MRI volumes but not time to first confirmed disability progression (not to be confused with progressive disease; see Chapter 1). The evidence-based medicine calculations based on the "proportion relapse free" data for the original interferon beta-1a (Rebif) study showed an RRR of 19%, an ARR of 16%, and an NNT of six over 2 years to increase the relapse-free number by one. Investigators are still trying to establish relative treatment advantages of interferon beta-1a and -1b.[10–12] Higher-dose interferon beta-1a is slightly more advantageous than low-dose interferon beta-1a or -1b. A pilot study in RRMS patients suggests that interferon-alpha also has a therapeutic effect.[13] A study of interferon responders showed that younger patients with frequent relapses and higher EDSS scores upon entry may achieve a better response.[14] This is expected, since the RRR will be easier to detect in these groups.

One disturbing aspect of interferon therapy is the appearance of NAbs in ~40% of patients after 3 years of interferon beta-1b treatment. Not only do patients with these antibodies fail thereafter to respond to this drug, but the NAbs may also cross-react with natural interferon beta to interfere with its function. All positive sera for NAbs seem to cross-react with both interferon beta-1a and -1b. Switching from one preparation to the other does not change the pattern of antibody response.[9] The long-term effects of NAbs are unknown. Recent studies seem to suggest that NAb formation reduces clinical and MRI effects, although NAb formation often subsides with time. There are no firm guidelines for monitoring NAb formation. Most physicians do not measure NAbs but instead change therapies empirically when treatment appears unsuccessful. Low-titer NAbs may be just a transient phenomenon related to interferon treatment; persistent high-titer NAbs on two consecutive tests at least 6 months apart may correlate with a poor treatment response to INF. In our practice, we test NAbs in patients who have severe recurrences or unexpected increases in MRI activity in the setting of previous stability on interferons. If NAbs are positive, we consider switching to glatiramer acetate in the same tier or consider stronger tier 2 medications such as fingolimod or natalizumab in severe cases. If there are no NAbs (true failure of interferon), then we consider trying fingolimod or natalizumab as of this writing. As other medications become available and longer-term safety data permit, more treatment options will be available in both tier 1 and tier 2.

Even though interferon products are generally safe to use, they can lead to potentially harmful adverse reactions. We recommend obtaining a baseline complete blood count, liver function test, and thyroid-stimulating hormone (TSH) test for each patient prior to treatment. The liver function tests and blood counts should be repeated after 1 week, 1 month, and every 3 months thereafter; the TSH should be repeated every 6 to 12 months.

GLATIRAMER ACETATE

Glatiramer acetate (Copaxone) is a synthetic mixture of polypeptides produced by the random combinations of the four most common amino acids in myelin basic protein (MBP). Of note, there is little evidence that MBP is an important target antigen in MS. After a preliminary study suggested efficacy,[15] a phase III randomized, double-blind, placebo-controlled, multicenter trial showed a 29% reduction in relapse rate.[16] The FDA has approved this medication for use in RRMS. Even though this disease-modifying therapy requires daily subcutaneous administration, there are several advantages; the side effects are relatively minor compared to interferons, patients do not need regular laboratory monitoring, and NAb formation is not a problem.

Glatiramer acetate reduces new lesion formation, the number of T2-enhancing lesions, lesion volumes, and the percentage of new lesions evolving into T1 "black holes," although the MRI effect may be less pronounced compared to the interferon products and is not apparent until the agent has been used for at least 6 months.[17–19] The evidence-based medicine calculations for glatiramer acetate using the "proportion relapse free" data from the original trial showed an RRR of 10%, an ARR of 7%, and an NNT of 14 over 2 years to increase the relapse-free number by one.

Tier 2 Medications

NATALIZUMAB

In late 2004, natalizumab (Tysabri) was approved for the treatment of RRMS.[20] Natalizumab is a humanized alpha-4 integrin antibody that inhibits the migration of all leukocytes (except for neutrophils) to target organs. A phase II study established[21] that a 300-mg monthly dose reduced the number of gadolinium-enhancing lesions by 90% and the clinical relapse rate by over 50% compared to placebo. This study was followed by the AFFIRM and SENTINEL phase III studies. The AFFIRM study enrolled over 900 patients with RRMS; none had been on other approved immunomodulators for longer than 6 months. The annualized relapse rate at 1 year was reduced from 0.74 in the placebo group to 0.25 in the treated group (66% relative reduction, $p < .0001$). The proportion of relapse-free patients was 76% in the treated group and 53% in the placebo group. The number of enhancing lesions was reduced by 92%, and the number of new or newly enlarging T2 lesions was reduced by 80%. The proportion of patients without clinical and MRI activity was 46% in the natalizumab group and 14% in the placebo group. In the SENTINEL trial, the combination of intramuscular interferon beta-1a and natalizumab was studied against intramuscular interferon beta-1a and placebo in patients who had demonstrated an incomplete response (relapse suppression) to interferon therapy. The evidence-based medicine calculations of the AFFIRM data based on proportion with relapses suggested an RRR of 49%, an ARR of 23%, and an NNT of four over 1 year to increase the relapse-free proportion by one. The SENTINEL data showed an RRR of 31%, an ARR of 17%, and an NNT of six over one year to increase the relapse-free proportion by one. The original pilot-trial data showed an RRR of 50% and an ARR of 19%, with an NNT of five over 6 months to increase the relapse-free proportion by one. Based on these data, the FDA granted expedited approval of natalizumab on November 23, 2004. Natalizumab appears more effective than all the previously discussed tier 1 medications.

However, on February 28, 2005, the sponsor (Biogen-Elan) voluntarily withdrew the medication from the market after two cases of progressive multifocal leukoencephalopathy (PML) were reported in the SENTINEL study cohort.[22,23] Both patients were in the combined interferon-and-natalizumab arm. A third PML case later presented from one of the phase III inflammatory bowel trials of this agent. Based on the best evidence now available, we do not recommend using natalizumab in combination with interferon or other disease-modifying agents. In June 2006, after careful review of all available data and analysis of risk–benefit ratios, an expert panel recommended the reintroduction of natalizumab, which the FDA approved. Natalizumab is available only through the TOUCH prescribing program, which is meant to provide a company-sponsored safety-monitoring system as well as a partial standardization of the frequency and nature of follow-up visits for patients taking natalizumab.

In our view, natalizumab is not indicated in patients with relatively stable cases of MS who respond to tier 1 medications. As demonstrated during the early years of natalizumab use, the combination of potent immunomodulators may result in unpredictable adverse outcomes. Many MS experts anticipate that future MS therapies will be administered in combination to optimize therapeutic benefit. However, the exact effect of these combinations on the highly complex immune system is difficult, if not impossible, to predict. In any case, as evidenced by the autologous bone marrow transplantation studies, our inability to treat MS more effectively does not stem from our inability to provide powerful immunosuppression. While MS is a complex disease with a prominent inflammatory component, increasing evidence suggests that the neurodegenerative component of this illness is partially independent of the inflammatory component (but occurs only in an inflammatory milieu) and is more important in determining long-term disability.

The frequency of PML occurrence was ~1/1,000 in the early studies. Newer observations suggested that the risk can be stratified: in patients with anti-JCV antibodies and a history of prior immunosuppressant use (e.g., azathioprine, methotrexate, mitoxantrone, cyclophosphamide), the risk may be as high as 11/1,000 (Table 9.1). The Stratify JCV antibody test is available free of charge to health care providers, and we recommend testing for this prior to treatment initiation. Those who test negative should be rechecked periodically (e.g., every

6 to 12 months) due to the FDA's estimated false-negative rate of 3%, along with true conversion from seronegative to positive. Patients taking natalizumab should be informed of the above and alerted to typical symptoms of PML, which may be very difficult to distinguish from MS symptoms based on clinical grounds alone. Symptoms of PML are heterogeneous, progress over days to weeks, and include progressive weakness on one side of the body, clumsiness of limbs, disturbance of vision, and changes in thinking, memory, and orientation, which lead to confusion and personality changes. These progressive deficits can lead to death or severe disability over weeks or months.

In practice, we recommend Tysabri for patients who fail to respond to tier 1 medications, test negative for JCV, and have no history of chemotherapy exposure. We inform patients that we intend to monitor them. If their JCV tests turn positive, we inform them that the first 2 years of Tysabri treatment are relatively safe, after which PML risk increases. At the 2-year time point, we again offer patients the option of discontinuing the medication due to increased risk.

If patients remain negative for JCV, we recommend continuing medication. The current data indicate that less than 2% of patients who continued JCV-negative while taking Tysabri went on to develop PML. (Biogen continuously updates this information on its website.)

In the rare instances in which patients initially test positive for JCV, we have started Tysabri, with careful discussion of the risks, if the recurrence of disease activity (clinically or subclinically) is severe enough to indicate the use of tier 2 medications and if the properly educated patient with full understanding of the inherent risk prefers this option over the alternatives.

All of the above will be constantly modified as new treatment options and new data about the currently existing therapeutics become available.

FINGOLIMOD

Patients and physicians alike have long awaited oral therapies for MS. The first such treatment, fingolimod, was approved on September 21, 2010, at a cost of ~$4,000 a month per patient. This drug inhibits lymphocyte egress from secondary lymphoid tissues and the thymus by acting on the S1P1 receptor. In the pivotal fingolimod trial, 281 randomized patients received 1.25 mg, 5.0 mg, or placebo once a day. The primary endpoint of this 6-month study was MRI-based. Interestingly, the difference between the two doses was insignificant: the annualized relapse rate dropped from 0.77 to 0.35 in the lower-dose group versus 0.36 in the higher-dose group.[24] In the subsequent 24-month study of 1,272 patients receiving either 0.5 mg or 1.25 mg of fingolimod (FREEDOMS study), the annualized relapse rate was 0.18 with the lower dose versus 0.16 with the higher dose, compared to 0.4 in the placebo group. Both doses significantly and almost equally reduced the risk for disability progression. MRI outcome measures also showed a favorable response to fingolimod treatment.[25] In the comparative trial with weekly intramuscular interferon (TRANSFORMS study),[26] fingolimod was superior to interferon in terms of annualized RRR, and MRI results were also more favorable with fingolimod. Based on the FREEDOMS data, the evidence-based medicine calculations for fingolimod showed an RRR of approximately 50%, an ARR of 22%, and NNT of four over 2 years to increase the relapse-free proportion by one.

Both of these trials demonstrated the same adverse effects. Two fatal infections occurred (primary varicella zoster and herpes simplex encephalitis). Other adverse events among fingolimod recipients were nonfatal herpes virus infections, bradycardia and atrioventricular block, hypertension, macular edema, skin cancer, and elevated liver enzyme levels. Because of the risk of bradycardia, the original

Table 9–1 Estimated PML Incidence Stratified by Risk Factor

	Anti-JCV Antibody Positive	**Anti-JCV Antibody Positive**
Tysabri exposure	No prior immunosuppressant use	Prior immunosuppressant use
1–24 months	<1/1,000	2/1,000
25–48 months	4/1,000	11/1,000

approval of this drug required a 6-hour heart rate monitoring to assess the first-dose effect. After a cardiac death occurred several hours later than this window, new parameters were recommended. Fingolimod is now contraindicated (FDA advises against its use) in patients with certain preexisting or recent (within the past 6 months) heart conditions or stroke or if they take certain antiarrhythmic medications. In addition, the FDA now also recommends extending the time of cardiovascular monitoring past 6 hours in patients at higher risk for bradycardia. Extended monitoring should include continuous, overnight electrocardiographic monitoring. The official contraindications are as follows:

- Patients who experienced myocardial infarction, unstable angina, stroke, transient ischemic attack, decompensated heart failure requiring hospitalization or class III/IV heart failure in the previous 6 months
- History or presence of Mobitz type II second-degree or third-degree atrioventricular block or sick-sinus syndrome, unless patient has a functioning pacemaker
- Baseline QTc interval of 500 ms or more
- Treatment with class Ia or class III antiarrhythmic drugs

In addition, we recommend an eye examination prior to treatment, along with assessment of varicella zoster virus serum status and vaccination to seronegative patients. Liver function test results should also be reviewed prior to treatment.

Overall, fingolimod seems to be more effective than tier 1 medications but less so than Tysabri. Given the known side effects and the possibility of long-term, as-yet-unknown side effects, we reserve it as a tier 2 alternative to Tysabri.

Teriflunomide

Teriflunomide is the active metabolite of leflunomide, an oral isoxazole drug that inhibits *de novo* pyrimidine synthesis and is approved for the treatment of rheumatoid arthritis. Teriflunomide is a good example of drug development based on the EAE model, where it was found to be highly effective.[27] A placebo-controlled phase II trial clearly showed

benefits from the standpoint of inflammatory activity as detected by MRI.[28] The subsequent TEMSO phase III trial, in addition to lesional activity, revealed a positive impact on annualized relapse rate and on sustained disability.[29] The extensive rheumatology experience with leflunomide strongly suggests an overall benign safety profile, far more favorable than the currently approved single oral agent, fingolimod. In the MS trials, the most frequently reported adverse effects included elevated liver enzymes, neutropenia, trigeminal neuralgia, diarrhea, alopecia, nausea, and CK elevation.[30] There was no obvious increase in the rate of infections. This may represent a good tier 1 or tier 2 alternative. This drug was approved for use in MS by the FDA at the time of writing of this book (September 2012).

INTRAVENOUS IMMUNOGLOBULIN

Monthly treatment with low-dose (0.15–0.2 g/kg) intravenous immunoglobulin (IVIG) in RRMS patients resulted in fewer, less severe relapses and slower accumulation of disability in a single randomized trial. The outcome was similar to that of injectable interferons.[31] This therapy is not commonly prescribed in the United States. More studies with a larger number of patients and extended follow-up are needed to confirm these limited observations. We have failed to demonstrate that IVIG administration reverses established deficits from MS and optic neuritis.[32–34] IVIG also failed to demonstrate benefit on any of the outcome measures in acute optic neuritis.[35] One could, however, consider this as an adjunct treatment to tier 1 medications, but not as a sole choice.

COMBINED AZATHIOPRINE AND INTERFERON BETA-1B

A small NIH-based study showed significantly fewer contrast-enhancing lesions in six RRMS patients who received azathioprine in an average maintenance dose of 2 mg/kg/day in addition to interferon beta-1b; these patients were followed for a median period of 15 months. The addition of azathioprine as an adjunct may be considered in "treatment failure" patients who otherwise cannot use other tier 2 medications for various reasons. This study, however, was hampered by small number, no controls, and no blinding.[36]

Summary of RRMS Treatments

Several factors must be considered prior to starting MS patients on immunomodulators. Although there are several medications available for relapsing forms of MS, they are only partially effective. The most reliable data link short-term RRR and short-term reduced formation of MRI lesions, but these do not necessarily translate into reduction of future disability risk. Natural history data clearly suggest that a subset of MS patients do very well without treatment (see Chapter 1); this information can be very useful when deciding to treat patients with a 5- or 10-year disease history and minimal disability (Expanded Disability Severity Scale [EDSS] score of 2.0 or less). In such a stable patient group, a careful wait-and-see approach with appropriate monitoring is acceptable. Counseling of newly diagnosed MS patients is critical and should include family members as well as the patient. Most patients have easy access to abundant, frequently misleading, information on the Internet or from relatives and friends with MS. It is important to realize that every case is different. However, through the rational use of natural history data and clinical and MRI features of the specific case and through the clear understanding of the available clinical trial data, the clinician should be able to provide customized, individualized, and relevant advice to patients and their families. Because treatments are only partially effective, the wishes of an educated patient should play a major part in the decision-making process. In general, we consider interferon preparations as first-line treatment in most MS cases. Milder cases or patients at risk for potential interferon-related complications may be treated with glatiramer acetate. In some cases, when the inflammatory activity is very prominent and the future disability risk appears high, we may start natalizumab or fingolimod immediately from our current tier 2 choices. We follow the rationale of "stepped therapy"—in an "average" MS case (expected lesion load, relapse rate, moderate disability risk), we start with effective, well-tolerated agents with minimal side effects, such as interferons or glatiramer acetate. If "treatment failure," which includes both clear clinical and radiological worsening, is suspected, especially with significant new lesion formation, then the clinician should switch to a stronger agent. In addition to the official FDA-approved drugs, we may use the same in combination with monthly intravenous steroids. We may occasionally use cyclophosphamide or even mitoxantrone (discussed later) for very aggressive, hard-to-manage cases as our tier 3 choices.

The three interferon products and glatiramer acetate represent the most commonly used MS immunomodulators in the United States; therefore, it is important to draw some practical conclusions about these agents. By now, several class I studies demonstrate that these agents effectively reduce the relapse rate in RRMS over a 2- to 3-year period; the reduction is roughly 30% with the high-dose interferons and glatiramer acetate. The above-summarized NNT data also can assist the clinician and the well-informed patient in making treatment decisions. The EVIDENCE and INCOMIN studies offer evidence of a dose–response relationship among the interferon products. The double-dose intramuscular interferon beta-1a study did not show a dose–response relationship, perhaps because the increased dose was given with the same frequency as the standard dose. The injectable immunomodulators offer incomplete evidence for efficacy in disability-based outcome measures. Many long-term extension studies suffer from several drawbacks, including open-label unblinded design, significant dropout rates, and lack of controls. Overall, these agents remain partially effective in relapsing forms of MS; their long-term impact on disability remains largely unclear. As discussed further, based on currently available data, these medications do not alter the onset of a progressive disease course (as opposed to disability progression). Patients should be made aware of this fact to avoid any unrealistic expectations. This may reduce frustration on the part of the patient and physician.

ALTERING THE COURSE OF SECONDARY PROGRESSIVE MULTIPLE SCLEROSIS

Within 15 years of onset, almost 60% of RRMS patients enter the secondary progressive phase of the disease (SPMS). Treatment approaches that affect the natural course of disease are available for only a subset of these patients, while the secondary progressive course is the leading predictor of severe disability in MS (as extensively discussed in Chapter 1).

Interferons

Interferon beta-1b may have a beneficial effect on the overall outcome of SPMS and may also alter T1 "black hole" formation,[37,38] but the evidence is weak and equivocal. In the placebo-controlled European study[39] of interferon beta-1b in SPMS, the time to worsening was extended for treated patients. Treated patients were less likely to be wheelchair-bound and had fewer hospitalizations. Another analysis of this study confirmed the benefits, although the dropout rate in this study was high.[40] The patients who responded best to interferon therapy were those who experienced relapses during their disease course. T2 lesion load increased in the placebo-treated but not the interferon-treated patients in the first 2 years of treatment.[41]

Contrasting with these results, in another trial of SPMS patients,[42] both high-dose (44 mcg) and low-dose (22 mcg) interferon beta-1a failed to increase time to disability worsening. Positive effects were seen on relapse rate and reduction of MRI activity, but the disability effects did not replicate the European interferon beta-1b report. A more recent combined analysis of these trials concluded that continued relapse activity and more rapid progression over the preceding year (by more than 1 on the EDSS scale) are the best predictors of response in SPMS.[43] In our opinion, continued use of interferons or tier 2 medications as discussed earlier is justified during this overlap period of continued clinical or subclinical inflammatory activity. However, the clinician must make sure that the patient understands the goals and limitations of treatment—that is, to prevent further relapse-related disability progression. Patients must be made aware that the long-term progressive disease course, which determines disability, will not be altered with this approach.

Mitoxantrone

Mitoxantrone (Novantrone) is an anthracenedione chemotherapeutic agent licensed "for reducing neurologic disability and/or the frequency of clinical relapses in patients with secondary (chronic) progressive, progressive relapsing, or worsening relapsing–remitting multiple sclerosis (i.e. patients whose neurologic status is significantly abnormal between relapses)." It is not indicated in patients with primary progressive MS. A European phase III study of mitoxantrone[44-46] reported significant benefits in a group of early SPMS patients. It has also been used in combination with methylprednisolone.[47] Administration of this intravenous medication every 3 months appeared to stabilize or improve several clinical and functional outcome measures. The greatest concern regarding this medication is its cardiac toxicity: the cumulative lifetime maximum dose was established at 140 mg/m^2. Mitoxantrone can induce a seemingly dose-dependent cardiomyopathy, which leads to potentially fatal congestive heart failure. Conservatively, we generally avoid exceeding a total lifetime dose of 96 mg/m^2 (8 doses of 12 mg/m^2). Patients receiving mitoxantrone should also be monitored every 3 months with echocardiograms or MUGA scans to determine the ejection fraction. Reduction in the ejection fraction should prompt discontinuation of this therapy. Besides the cardiac side effects, mitoxantrone may cause menstrual irregularities or overall ablation of the menstrual cycle, which may be permanent. In a review of the literature, the authors[48] estimated the risk of mitoxantrone therapy-related acute leukemia in MS patients at 0.05% to 0.1%; in an international registry of MS patients on mitoxantrone, the risk of leukemia seems somewhat higher.

Overall, the limited evidence to date supports the conclusion that mitoxantrone reduces relapse frequency and MRI evidence for blood–brain barrier disruption in patients with very active MS. Indeed, in our practice, we reserve this agent as a tier 3 choice for patients with very active disease who either fail to respond to or cannot use tier 2 medications. The benefit for patients with relapse-independent progression is uncertain at best. From the MIMS results,[46] one would need to treat 11 patients with SPMS for 2 years to prevent one person from worsening by 1.0 EDSS point. This modest benefit must be carefully examined in light of the significant risk for toxicity.

Cyclophosphamide

As discussed in Chapter 8, induction and maintenance therapy with cyclophosphamide can be considered in selected cases of progressive MS. Much like the other available agents, the patients most likely to respond to this treatment are the ones with ongoing MRI-detectable inflammatory activity. The treatment protocols are the same as listed in Chapter 8.

IVIG

A recent European trial reported that IVIG did not have a significant impact on clinical and disability-related outcome measures. IVIG did reduce the accumulation of brain atrophy in SPMS but did not reduce the incidence of blood–brain barrier abnormalities. There was no statistically significant change on magnetization-transfer MRI measurements; however, IVIG did appear to conserve normal-appearing brain tissue.[49] This aspect is discussed here, since we still see patients under the impression that IVIG use will slow down their SPMS course.

Overall Recommendations for SPMS

Because the evidence that interferons alter long-term disability is limited and controversial, we generally do not start SPMS patients on interferon products. In the subset of patients still having disabling relapses or evidence of gadolinium enhancement and new lesion formation on MRI, interferon therapy may be offered specifically to reduce relapse rate, as we have previously discussed. Studies suggest that the EDSS score in populations of SPMS patients continues to progress independently of relapses[50] once a "fixed" baseline level of moderate disability has been reached. Interferons may reduce the relapse rate in SPMS as they do in RRMS with continued modest effects on attack-induced disability progression, but these treatments do not alter the progressive disease course significantly once it is established. In cases with rapid-onset progressive disease course and evidence of significant clinical or subclinical disease activity, mitoxantrone or cyclophosphamide may still play a role.

THERAPY OF PRIMARY PROGRESSIVE MULTIPLE SCLEROSIS

Unfortunately, none of the currently available treatments offers any clear benefit for patients with classical primary progressive MS (PPMS) who present with the insidious progression of myelopathic symptoms. The PROMISE trial, in which over 900 PPMS patients were treated with glatiramer acetate, was terminated early due to lack of effectiveness.[51] A potential benefit for male patients with more rapid progression was suggested.[52] A small study with intramuscular interferon beta-1a was also negative.[53] A large trial with rituximab in CSF oligoclonal band-positive PPMS patients also reported no clear benefit for the group as a whole but suggested that younger patients and those with active lesions on MRI may partially respond.[54] Some patients may respond to regular bolus intravenous methylprednisolone in the setting of more active disease. Until we clearly understand the pathophysiology of slow progression in MS, it is unlikely that we will find a treatment that has a meaningful impact on this form of MS. However, symptomatic treatment modalities, including physical and occupational therapy, are very important yet frequently overlooked in this patient population. This is a high-impact area in MS, as discussed extensively in the next chapter.

SUMMARY

While several treatment modalities are available mainly for relapsing and highly inflammatory forms of secondary progressive MS, all of these are only partially effective. We currently have no effective agent to address the most disabling feature of MS, the slow, insidious progressive stage. We also lack effective tissue-restorative strategies, although several promising agents are about to enter clinical trials (see Chapter 11).

REFERENCES

1. Pittock SJ, Weinshenker BG, Noseworthy JH, et al. Not every patient with multiple sclerosis should be treated at time of diagnosis. Arch Neurol; 63:611–614, 2006.

2. Frohman EM, Havrdova E, Lublin F, et al. Most patients with multiple sclerosis or a clinically isolated demyelinating syndrome should be treated at the time of diagnosis. Arch Neurol; 63:614–619, 2006.

3. Jacobs LD, Beck RW, Simon JH, et al. Intramuscular interferon beta-1a therapy initiated during a first demyelinating event in multiple sclerosis. CHAMPS Study Group. N Engl J Med; 343:898–904, 2000.

4. Beck RW, Chandler DL, Cole SR, et al. Interferon beta-1a for early multiple sclerosis: CHAMPS trial subgroup analyses. Ann Neurol; 51:481–490, 2002.

5. Comi G, Filippi M, Barkhof F, et al. Effect of early interferon treatment on conversion to definite multiple sclerosis: a randomised study. Lancet; 357:1576–1582, 2001.

6. Comi G, Martinelli V, Rodegher M, et al. Effect of glatiramer acetate on conversion to clinically definite multiple sclerosis in patients with clinically isolated syndrome (PreCISe study): a randomised, double-blind, placebo-controlled trial. Lancet; 374:1503–1511, 2009.

7. Paty DW, Li DK. Interferon beta-1b is effective in relapsing-remitting multiple sclerosis. II. MRI analysis results of a multicenter, randomized, double-blind, placebo-controlled trial. UBC MS/MRI Study Group and the IFNB Multiple Sclerosis Study Group. Neurology; 43:662–667, 1993.

8. Jacobs LD, Cookfair DL, Rudick RA, et al. Intramuscular interferon beta-1a for disease progression in relapsing multiple sclerosis. The Multiple Sclerosis Collaborative Research Group (MSCRG). Ann Neurol; 39:285–294, 1996.

9. Antonelli G, Simeoni E, Bagnato F, et al. Further study on the specificity and incidence of neutralizing antibodies to interferon (IFN) in relapsing remitting multiple sclerosis patients treated with IFN beta-1a or IFN beta-1b. J Neurol Sci; 168:131–136, 1999.

10. Randomised double-blind placebo-controlled study of interferon beta-1a in relapsing/remitting multiple sclerosis. PRISMS (Prevention of Relapses and Disability by Interferon beta-1a Subcutaneously in Multiple Sclerosis) Study Group. Lancet; 352:1498–1504, 1998.

11. Gold R, Rieckmann P, Chang P, Abdalla J. The long-term safety and tolerability of high-dose interferon beta-1a in relapsing-remitting multiple sclerosis: 4-year data from the PRISMS study. Eur J Neurol; 12:649–656, 2005.

12. Li DK, Paty DW. Magnetic resonance imaging results of the PRISMS trial: a randomized, double-blind, placebo-controlled study of interferon-beta1a in relapsing-remitting multiple sclerosis. Prevention of Relapses and Disability by Interferon-beta1a Subcutaneously in Multiple Sclerosis. Ann Neurol; 46:197–206, 1999.

13. Brod SA, Lindsey JW, Vriesendorp FS, et al. Ingested IFN-alpha: results of a pilot study in relapsing-remitting MS. Neurology; 57:845–852, 2001.

14. Waubant E, Vukusic S, Gignoux L, et al. Clinical characteristics of responders to interferon therapy for relapsing MS. Neurology; 61:184–189, 2003.

15. Bornstein MB, Miller A, Slagle S, et al. A pilot trial of Cop 1 in exacerbating-remitting multiple sclerosis. N Engl J Med; 317:408–414, 1987.

16. Johnson KP, Brooks BR, Cohen JA, et al. Copolymer 1 reduces relapse rate and improves disability in relapsing-remitting multiple sclerosis: results of a phase III multicenter, double-blind placebo-controlled trial. The Copolymer 1 Multiple Sclerosis Study Group. Neurology; 45:1268–1276, 1995.

17. Comi G, Filippi M, Wolinsky JS. European/Canadian multicenter, double-blind, randomized, placebo-controlled study of the effects of glatiramer acetate on magnetic resonance imaging—measured disease activity and burden in patients with relapsing multiple sclerosis. European/Canadian Glatiramer Acetate Study Group. Ann Neurol; 49:290–297, 2001.

18. Ge Y, Grossman RI, Udupa JK, et al. Glatiramer acetate (Copaxone) treatment in relapsing-remitting MS: quantitative MR assessment. Neurology; 54:813–817, 2000.

19. Wolinsky JS, Narayana PA, Johnson KP. United States open-label glatiramer acetate extension trial for relapsing multiple sclerosis: MRI and clinical correlates. Multiple Sclerosis Study Group and the MRI Analysis Center. Mult Scler; 7:33–41, 2001.

20. Noseworthy JH, Kirkpatrick P. Natalizumab. Nat Rev Drug Discov; 4:101–102, 2005.

21. Miller DH, Khan OA, Sheremata WA, et al. A controlled trial of natalizumab for relapsing multiple sclerosis. N Engl J Med; 348:15–23, 2003.

22. Langer-Gould A, Atlas SW, Green AJ, Bollen AW, Pelletier D. Progressive multifocal leukoencephalopathy in a patient treated with natalizumab. N Engl J Med; 353:375–381, 2005.

23. Kleinschmidt-DeMasters BK, Tyler KL. Progressive multifocal leukoencephalopathy complicating treatment with natalizumab and interferon beta-1a for multiple sclerosis. N Engl J Med; 353:369–374, 2005.

24. Kappos L, Antel J, Comi G, et al. Oral fingolimod (FTY720) for relapsing multiple sclerosis. N Engl J Med; 355:1124–1140, 2006.

25. Kappos L, Radue EW, O'Connor P, et al. A placebo-controlled trial of oral fingolimod in relapsing multiple sclerosis. N Engl J Med; 362:387–401, 2010.

26. Cohen JA, Barkhof F, Comi G, et al. Oral fingolimod or intramuscular interferon for relapsing multiple sclerosis. N Engl J Med; 362:402–415, 2010.

27. O'Connor PW, Li D, Freedman MS, et al. A phase II study of the safety and efficacy of teriflunomide in multiple sclerosis with relapses. Neurology; 66:894–900, 2006.

28. Noseworthy JH, Wolinsky JS, Lublin FD, et al. Linomide in relapsing and secondary progressive MS: part I: trial design and clinical results. North American Linomide Investigators. Neurology; 54:1726–1733, 2000.

29. Yang JS, Xu LY, Xiao BG, Hedlund G, Link H. Laquinimod (ABR-215062) suppresses the development of experimental autoimmune encephalomyelitis, modulates the Th1/Th2 balance and induces the Th3 cytokine TGF-beta in Lewis rats. J Neuroimmunol; 156:3–9, 2004.

30. Comi G, Jeffery D, Kappos L, et al. Placebo-controlled trial of oral laquinimod for multiple sclerosis. N Engl J Med; 366:1000–1009, 2012.

31. Strasser-Fuchs S, Fazekas F, Deisenhammer F, Nahler G, Mamoli B. The Austrian Immunoglobulin in MS (AIMS) study: final analysis. Mult Scler; 6 Suppl 2:S9–S13, 2000.

32. Noseworthy JH, O'Brien PC, Petterson TM, et al. A randomized trial of intravenous immunoglobulin in inflammatory demyelinating optic neuritis. Neurology; 56:1514–1522, 2001.

33. Noseworthy JH, O'Brien PC, van Engelen BG, Rodriguez M. Intravenous immunoglobulin therapy in multiple sclerosis: progress from remyelination in the Theiler's virus model to a randomised, double-blind, placebo-controlled clinical trial. J Neurol Neurosurg Psychiatry; 57 Suppl:11–14, 1994.
34. Noseworthy JH, O'Brien PC, Weinshenker BG, et al. IV immunoglobulin does not reverse established weakness in MS. Neurology; 55:1135–1143, 2000.
35. Stangel M, Boegner F, Klatt CH, Hofmeister C, Seyfert S. Placebo-controlled pilot trial to study the remyelinating potential of intravenous immunoglobulins in multiple sclerosis. J Neurol Neurosurg Psychiatry; 68:89–92, 2000.
36. Markovic-Plese S, Bielekova B, Kadom N, et al. Longitudinal MRI study: the effects of azathioprine in MS patients refractory to interferon beta-1b. Neurology; 60:1849–1851, 2003.
37. Barkhof F, van Waesberghe JH, Filippi M, et al. T(1) hypointense lesions in secondary progressive multiple sclerosis: effect of interferon beta-1b treatment. Brain; 124:1396–1402, 2001.
38. Placebo-controlled multicentre randomised trial of interferon beta-1b in treatment of secondary progressive multiple sclerosis. European Study Group on interferon beta-1b in secondary progressive MS. Lancet; 352:1491–1497, 1998.
39. Miller DH, Molyneux PD, Barker GJ, MacManus DG, Moseley IF, Wagner K. Effect of interferon-beta1b on magnetic resonance imaging outcomes in secondary progressive multiple sclerosis: results of a European multicenter, randomized, double-blind, placebo-controlled trial. European Study Group on Interferon-beta1b in secondary progressive multiple sclerosis. Ann Neurol; 46:850–859, 1999.
40. Kappos L, Polman C, Pozzilli C, Thompson A, Beckmann K, Dahlke F. Final analysis of the European multicenter trial on IFNbeta-1b in secondary-progressive MS. Neurology; 57:1969–1975, 2001.
41. Molyneux PD, Kappos L, Polman C, et al. The effect of interferon beta-1b treatment on MRI measures of cerebral atrophy in secondary progressive multiple sclerosis. European Study Group on Interferon beta-1b in secondary progressive multiple sclerosis. Brain; 123 (Pt 11):2256–2263, 2000.
42. Li DK, Zhao GJ, Paty DW. Randomized controlled trial of interferon-beta-1a in secondary progressive MS: MRI results. Neurology; 56:1505–1513, 2001.
43. Kappos L, Weinshenker B, Pozzilli C, et al. Interferon beta-1b in secondary progressive MS: a combined analysis of the two trials. Neurology; 63:1779–1787, 2004.
44. Gonsette RE. Mitoxantrone immunotherapy in multiple sclerosis. Mult Scler; 1:329–332, 1996.
45. Gonsette RE. Mitoxantrone in progressive multiple sclerosis: when and how to treat? J Neurol Sci; 206:203–208, 2003.
46. Hartung HP, Gonsette R, Konig N, et al. Mitoxantrone in progressive multiple sclerosis: a placebo-controlled, double-blind, randomised, multicentre trial. Lancet; 360:2018–2025, 2002.
47. Edan G, Miller D, Clanet M, et al. Therapeutic effect of mitoxantrone combined with methylprednisolone in multiple sclerosis: a randomised multicentre study of active disease using MRI and clinical criteria. J Neurol Neurosurg Psychiatry; 62:112–118, 1997.
48. Ghalie RG, Mauch E, Edan G, et al. A study of therapy-related acute leukaemia after mitoxantrone therapy for multiple sclerosis. Mult Scler; 8:441–445, 2002.
49. Filippi M, Rocca MA, Pagani E, et al. European study on intravenous immunoglobulin in multiple sclerosis: results of magnetization transfer magnetic resonance imaging analysis. Arch Neurol; 61:1409–1412, 2004.
50. Confavreux C, Vukusic S, Moreau T, Adeleine P. Relapses and progression of disability in multiple sclerosis. N Engl J Med; 343:1430–1438, 2000.
51. Wolinsky JS, Narayana PA, O'Connor P, et al. Glatiramer acetate in primary progressive multiple sclerosis: results of a multinational, multicenter, double-blind, placebo-controlled trial. Ann Neurol; 61:14–24, 2007.
52. Wolinsky JS, Shochat T, Weiss S, Ladkani D. Glatiramer acetate treatment in PPMS: why males appear to respond favorably. J Neurol Sci; 286:92–98, 2009.
53. Leary SM, Thompson AJ. Interferon beta-1a in primary progressive multiple sclerosis. J Neurol Sci; 206:215–216, 2003.
54. Hawker K, O'Connor P, Freedman MS, et al. Rituximab in patients with primary progressive multiple sclerosis: results of a randomized double-blind placebo-controlled multicenter trial. Ann Neurol; 66:460–471, 2009.

Managing Symptoms of Multiple Sclerosis

Abstract

Although MS is not currently a curable disease, management of day-to-day symptoms substantially improves patients' quality of life and general psychosocial functioning. Successful management requires a multidisciplinary integrated approach by all health care providers involved in the patient's care. While current treatment strategies focus primarily on preventing relapses and slowing disability, practicing physicians must not neglect helping patients find symptom-management strategies that improve the quality of their lives. In this chapter, we illustrate the interactive nature of symptomatic management of MS.

THE INTERACTIVE MATRIX OF SYMPTOMATIC MULTIPLE SCLEROSIS THERAPY

In previous chapters we described the pathophysiology of MS, which consists of bouts of inflammatory activity as well as a neurodegenerative process that afflicts the CNS. Symptoms

Table 10–1 **Complementary and Alternative Medicine Use by MS Patients[4]**

Therapy	% Use	% Improvement
Exercise	27	76
Vitamins	15	41
Minerals & other supplements	12	53
Herbal therapy	9	63
Relaxation techniques	9	86
Massage	5	83

of MS parallel these processes. As discussed in a previous chapter, most treatment approaches in MS focus on preventing or shortening relapses by modulation (e.g., interferons), suppression (e.g., steroids), or partial elimination (e.g., plasma exchange) of immunological insult. If the acute symptom relates directly to the relapse, then the above approaches achieve symptom relief or prevention. However, many MS symptoms correlate to the neurodegenerative component of the disease or are secondary to disease-associated lifestyle changes, and neither of these mechanisms responds to immunomediated strategies. Indeed, in several instances, commonly used immunomodulation strategies worsen symptoms of MS even while helping to prevent further relapses. In this chapter, we discuss how to control symptoms of MS and the evidence that supports the efficacy of these approaches. Extensive recent reviews have been written in this area.[1-3] We illustrate our own experience-based approaches as we discuss the subjects further with the available evidence.

Although information is limited by available publications and low response rates in surveys, it appears that at least one in four MS patients find complementary or alternative medicine strategies effective in treating their symptoms (Table 10.1).[4] The most commonly used modalities are exercise, vitamins, herbal and mineral supplements, relaxation techniques, acupuncture, cannabis, and massage.[4] The three most commonly cited symptoms are pain, fatigue, and stress.[4] For half of the respondents, the main reason for seeking complementary or alternative strategies is that conventional strategies have not worked for them.[4] This study effectively highlights the frustration associated with conventional medicine strategies for symptomatic relief.

At this point, we would like to introduce the "Interactive Matrix of Symptomatic MS Therapy" (Fig. 10.1). Many MS symptoms are so closely interrelated that it is difficult to treat one symptom without affecting another. This

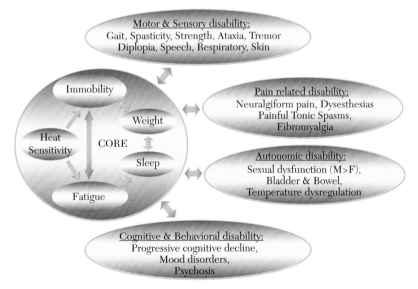

Figure 10–1. The interactive matrix of symptomatic MS therapy, illustrating the intimate relationship between management of core symptoms of MS and management of motor, sensory, pain, autonomic, cognitive, or behavioral disability.

close association often results in the patient accumulating a long list of medications, each addressing a specific symptom, from multiple providers. In separate sections of this chapter, we highlight the interaction between several symptoms and commonality of treatment approaches.

We have found several practical rules helpful in successfully managing symptoms of MS, as illustrated in Figure 10.2. These recommendations are a starting point for developing multidisciplinary treatment approaches for the patient.

We recommend initially assembling a multidisciplinary team consisting of consultants with specific interest in MS from neurology, physical medicine and rehabilitation, urology, psychology, speech therapy, sleep medicine, and pain rehabilitation; a nurse educator; and a social worker. While neurologists generally lead the care of patients with MS, especially regarding initial diagnosis, changes in diagnosis, choosing disease-modifying medications, and prognosis discussions, programs in integrative physical medicine and rehabilitation often provide more effective care in the area of symptom management.

We also recommend scheduled reassessments of the patient's needs as the disease evolves. While anticipation or prevention of relapses may take center stage early in the disease, reassurance, with imaging documentation of absence of disease activity, may be more important in relapse-free periods. These periods give the patient an opportunity to focus on lifestyle adjustments for sleep and weight control. Later in the disease, the primary focus can shift to chronic progressive worsening associated with neurodegeneration. Because many recommendations for symptomatic relief can be stage specific, it is important to prepare and reassure patients from the first interaction that their needs may change and there will be a team involved in their care. For chronic symptoms, it would make sense to focus on one or two problems at a time to prevent patient burnout associated with consultations with multiple providers on every visit to the medical center.

Finally, we recommend early recognition and treatment of the core complications of MS (immobility, fatigue, sleep problems, weight control, and heat sensitivity) to minimize their impact on future symptoms. In the next section we discuss these in detail.

THE CORE OF SYMPTOMATIC MULTIPLE SCLEROSIS THERAPY

At the core of symptomatic therapy for MS lies controlling fatigue, sleep, deconditioning, weight gain, and heat sensitivity. Because many of these factors physiologically induce or worsen each other, the first step in managing these symptoms is to explain the intimate and circular

1. Assemble a mulitidisciplinary "interest" team:
    -   PM&R, Neurology, nurse educator
    -   Urology, Psychology, Speech therapist, Sleep laboratory
    -   Pain rehabilitation program
    -   Social worker

2. Reassess patient needs that may shift dramatically throughout disease course with scheduled appointments even in the absence of ongoing relapses

3. Prioritize and focus on a few symptoms at a time rather than trying to address all symptoms at every visit to help prevent patient & physician exhaustion that may result from multiple visits to every specialty every time

4. Assess & prevent or treat core symptoms early:
    -   Immobility
    -   Weight control
    -   Fatigue
    -   Sleep problems
    -   Heat sensitivity

Figure 10–2. Practice recommendations for symptomatic therapy in MS.

relationship between them and try to highlight the importance of managing all of them in parallel for successful results. For example, it is difficult to control fatigue by medication alone in a patient with obesity and sleep apnea. These lead to daytime somnolence, which results in lack of energy and disincentives to exercise. The patient's ability to exercise may already be limited by heat sensitivity. The resulting deconditioning leads to further weight gain, which exacerbates sleep apnea and fatigue. A single-modality approach would clearly fail here. Although in the following sections we discuss individual treatment approaches to different symptoms of MS, we would like to reemphasize the need to treat core symptoms together.

Fatigue

Fatigue is common in chronic medical conditions. MS patients list fatigue as the worst symptom affecting their quality of life.[5,6] This is largely due to the chronic nature of fatigue but also because it affects cognitive efficiency, which affects day-to-day functioning more than most individual relapses. Fatigue is a core symptom of MS and is largely multifactorial. The time of day when fatigue peaks sometimes provides a clue to the predominant mechanism of fatigue in MS (Table 10.2).[7] Physical fatigue in MS is intimately associated with chronic pain and sleep problems, while cognitive fatigue intimately correlates with behavioral and psychosocial comorbidities that are modifiable in MS.[7]

MS-induced primary fatigue may be due to subtle ongoing inflammatory activity.[8] However, commonly used disease-modifying agents, such as interferon beta and glatiramer acetate, do not seem to affect fatigue levels.[9]

Indeed, in the case of interferon beta, patients often experience increased fatigue along with flu-like symptoms (albeit mostly intermittently and time-locked to the use of the medication). In another study, glatiramer acetate appeared to induce less fatigue than interferon beta.[10] It is unclear if this represents baseline fatigue in the case of glatiramer acetate and heightened fatigue in the case of interferon beta. Fatigue is a common reason to discontinue immunomodulatory treatment in MS.[11]

Natalizumab, with a stronger immune-mediated effect of blocking leukocyte migration through the blood–brain barrier, seemingly reduces severe fatigue by one third and moderate fatigue (both physical and cognitive) by one half. This means that it outperforms other immunomodulatory agents from this standpoint.[12] In an observational study, 1-year treatment with natalizumab led to a modest but significant reduction in both cognitive and physical fatigue in MS.[13] Several patients have anecdotally reported this in our practice as well. The individual benefits of immunomodulatory medications for MS-related fatigue are still open to debate. However, these studies have indicated that roughly two thirds of cases of severe fatigue in MS may be due to causes other than primary inflammatory mechanisms, and one should consider "other" modifiable mechanisms to control fatigue before citing severe fatigue as a reason to switch immunotherapy in MS.[7]

Treatment of MS-related fatigue should always include managing sleep, deconditioning, and heat sensitivity along with pharmacological and nonpharmacological approaches targeting fatigue itself. Table 10.3 illustrates some of the individual modalities with the strongest evidence used in management of fatigue alone in MS. Despite the prominence of fatigue in MS

Table 10–2 Proposed Mechanisms of Fatigue in MS

Potential Mechanism	Peak symptoms
Primary inflammation due to MS	Mostly p.m.
Immunomodulation	– Mostly time-locked to medication use
	– In some patients more persistent baseline
High or low core temperature	– Time-locked to overheating
	– In patients with low core temperature can follow the diurnal cycle *or* be paradoxically associated with infections
Immobility & deconditioning	Persistent throughout the day
Sleep problems	Mostly p.m. & associated with hypersomnolence
Depression	Predominantly cognitive fatigue & lack of motivation

Table 10–3 Treatment Options for Fatigue in MS

Pharmacological interventions

Prokarin[85]	Consists of 1.65 mg histamine & 100 mg caffeine in 0.2 mL cream on patch. When applied twice daily for 8 hours is moderately effective° & well tolerated. Impact of histamine is not clear and caffeine in this preparation equals about 1.5 shots of espresso, which some patients can casually use instead. Limiting caffeine use to before noon may be helpful in preventing any associated sleep disruption.
Amantadine[86,87]	100 mg twice daily is moderately effective° but 10–50% report significant side effects
Aspirin[88]	1,300 mg daily is modestly effective° and very well tolerated
Pemoline[89–91]	Probably modestly effective° in MS and other immune-mediated disorders such as HIV but is poorly tolerated and can induce autoimmune hepatitis
Modafinil[92–94]	200 mg daily is modestly effective,° but paradoxically 400 mg daily is ineffective.

Nonpharmacological interventions

Energy conservation education[95]	Moderately effective° in decreasing the impact of fatigue on quality of life
Yoga or exercise[31,32,34]	Regular weekly class with home practice of yoga or exercise continued for 6 months is modestly effective.° Only a program of 15 elliptical exercise sessions is associated with improvement in fatigue and quality of life. There is an obvious inverse relationship with disability and exercise capacity, so the exercise programs should be tailored to patient needs and disease stage.
Inpatient rehabilitation[96]	The 3-week intensive multidisciplinary inpatient program is moderately effective,° but more prominently so in patients with coexisting improvement in mood.

°Modest efficacy and moderate efficacy are defined as relative to each other.

patients, the evidence behind many treatment approaches is less than stellar, partly because of the limited sensitivity of tools available to measure fatigue objectively.[14] All the modalities listed in Table 10.3 have some evidence to support their use and do not seem to differ significantly from each other. To prevent insomnia, patients should try to avoid stimulants during the afternoon and evening, except in severe cases of fatigue. We advise the clinician to use sound judgment in limiting medication to choices that manage more than one symptom of MS while combining nonpharmacological techniques. This will avoid overmedicating patients.

Sleep Problems

While more than 50% of MS patients report some type of a sleep problem, sleep problems remain underdiagnosed in MS.[15–17] It is unclear whether sleep disorders are directly associated with a lesional pathology or due to any number of common sleep problems that coexist with MS.

Insomnia is the most common sleep complaint (40%) and is clearly multifactorial.[17] This is followed by periodic limb movements of sleep and restless leg syndrome, present in 15% of patients with MS, although iron deficiency has been associated with some cases, similar to the general population.[18–20] However, the restless leg syndrome frequency is about threefold higher than in the general population and specifically more so in women, suggesting a relationship to the primary lesional pathology in MS.[21–23] Indeed, imaging studies suggest a correlation with spinal cord disease in MS and restless leg syndrome.[24] Sleep-disordered breathing has been tightly linked to obesity and, as expected, varies by population but is

Table 10–4 Treatment Options for Sleep Problems in MS

Acute lesional pathology due to an MS attack leading to a sleep problem	
REM sleep behavior disorder[28,29]	Treatment approach should be like any other MS attack with corticosteroids, although counterintuitive initially. Usually done with methylprednisolone, daily 1-g intravenous infusions for 3–7 days, tailored to patient's needs.

Chronic persistent sleep problems	
Insomnia	Manage depression, pain, nocturia, interferon-induced symptoms; tricyclic antidepressants, zolpidem, benzodiazepines work equally; choose according to comorbidities
Narcolepsy[97]	Modafinil
REM sleep behavior disorder[28,29]	Clonazepam
Restless legs syndrome[98,99]	Specific evidence in MS is limited; however, based on the existing guidelines, our experience is that the treatment is the same as in the general population. Iron supplementation in select cases, if ferritin level is ≤45 mg/l. Dopamine agonists & levodopa have robust benefit/risk ratios. Anticonvulsants (e.g., gabapentin) have limited evidence. Choose according to comorbidities.
Sleep-disordered breathing[100,101]	Specific evidence in MS is limited; however, based on the existing guidelines, our experience is that the treatment is the same as in the general population. Lifestyle modifications and weight loss: common sense, but no real good trial to support. Continuous positive airway pressure (PAP) reduces apnea, increases O_2 saturation, reduces systolic and diastolic blood pressures, & is superior to oral appliances. Surgery (ENT) for appropriate cases, but no clear benefit over CPAP.

linked to increased fatigue even in the absence of increased daytime sleepiness.[25] However, patients with medullary lesions are more likely to develop central sleep apnea. Narcolepsy may accompany hypothalamic lesions with low CSF hypocretin.[26,27] REM sleep behavior disorder occurs in about 1% of MS patients and correlates with dorsal pontine lesions.[20,28,29]

Other comorbidities identified in MS patients may further enhance sleep problems. These include depression/anxiety, pain, nocturia, and medications commonly used for MS (interferons and steroids). In return, chronic sleep disruption leads to enhanced fatigue, refractory depression, cognitive inefficiency, and fibromyalgia. Unfortunately patients themselves underreport these problems unless specifically questioned. Therefore, sleep problems, whether primary or secondary to MS, are at the core of MS-related disability. It is critical to screen for and address any sleep issue early.

Individual treatment approaches to sleep problems in MS are not well studied, although they likely do not differ significantly from the treatment of other patients with sleep problems. Most evidence comes from small studies or individual case reports. Table 10.4 presents the common treatment approaches for sleep problems in MS.

Deconditioning and Exercise Therapy

Deconditioning and weight gain are core problems that need to be addressed initially, since they exacerbate many symptoms of MS. Weight gain is inversely related to fitness. Indeed, a recent study has suggested that a body mass index above 27 before age 20 doubles the risk of developing MS in the first place.[30]

Studies indicate that regular exercise and stretching therapy can mitigate many symptoms of MS (Fig. 10.3).[31–35] However, like the general population, most patients with MS struggle with balancing the daily requirements of life and staying reasonably fit. Although this is not a specific problem for MS, it seems to be enhanced by the chronic symptoms of MS that limit exercise potential later during the disease.

Exercise can help depression, although it is not superior to cognitive therapy.[36] Fibromyalgia is common in MS, although it is not a primary symptom of the MS disease process. Many other pain problems are also common in MS, as discussed later in this chapter. Fatigue in MS strongly correlates with chronic pain.[7] Aerobic exercise of slight to moderate intensity two or three times per week for at least 4 weeks alleviates symptoms of fibromyalgia and chronic fatigue syndrome.[37,38] However, the relationship between exercise and fatigue is complicated in MS and affected by many factors, such as age, stage of MS, and anxiety level.[39] Regardless, exercise is a core therapy to fight MS-related deconditioning and weight gain; improve sleep; mitigate depressive symptoms; lessen fatigue; improve pain, ataxia, and motor symptoms; and also regulate bladder and bowel function. Therefore, establishing a continued emphasis on exercise and fitness early in the disease course is necessary.

Temperature Dysregulation

Patients with MS develop temperature dysregulation, which is a core problem in MS because hypo- or hyperthermia increases fatigue, disrupts sleep, and increases pseudo-exacerbations.

The more common problem is the heat sensitivity or, in some patients, susceptibility to hyperthermia. These patients must avoid excessive heat if possible and hydrate well. Unfortunately this limits their exercise potential. We have anecdotally found it useful to recommend that patients exercise in a colder room or perform outdoor activities in cooler times of the day while performing warm-up routines in a warmer room. This seems to improve patient compliance with exercise and therapy recommendations. Water aerobics and swimming therefore seem to be optimal exercises for patients who are overtly heat-sensitive. In patients with mild to moderate disease severity, cooling garments are modestly effective in reducing fatigue and improving motor/visual functions.[40] Many patients create their own cooling garments consisting of pockets for cold packs or wear wet bandanas or hats. Some also purchase cooling vests.

Although less common, hypothermia in MS can contribute to unexplained intermittent confusion, worsening cognition, and increased fatigue and can be fatal. It is a paroxysmal symptom

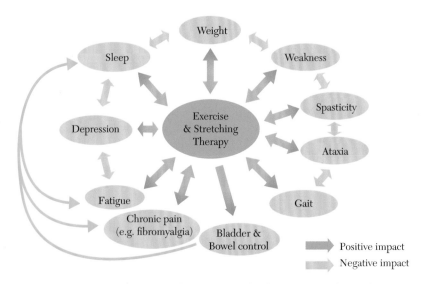

Figure 10–3. The interaction of exercise and stretching therapy with other symptoms of MS. Chronic symptoms of MS can interact with each other, emphasizing the central role of exercise and stretching therapy in managing these symptoms. Chronic symptoms of MS can limit the exercise and stretching therapy in MS.

that occurs most commonly during late MS with advanced disability.[41–43] Symptoms include coma, dysarthria, psychosis, meiosis, prolonged prothrombin time, and thrombopenia. MRI can show lesions in the preoptic hypothalamus. Acute exacerbations of hypothermia respond well to acute, short-duration (3-day) courses of 1,000 mg daily intravenous methylprednisolone treatment. Chronic recurrent patients seem to have worsening in early morning hours, following the diurnal pattern. Adjusting room temperature or using warming blankets during the times of the day with anticipated hypothermia symptoms has been helpful in our experience.

MOTOR DISABILITY

Motor symptoms are the strongest contributors to disability and reflect the disease course in MS. Exercise therapy is the mainstay for all chronic motor symptoms of MS (Fig. 10.3). However, additional specific treatment approaches can help individual symptoms.

Gait Impairment

Most motor and sensory deficits in MS that impair the lower extremities eventually culminate in complicated gait problems consisting of one or more of the following: apraxia, ataxia, weakness or spasticity, and, in some patients, additional psychogenic mechanisms. The success of any gait therapy relies on isolating each individual component contributing to the overall gait problem. Pharmacological approaches available for each of these problems are discussed in relevant sections later in the chapter.

Extensive discussion of gait therapy is beyond the scope of this book, but it suffices to say that a very structured and experienced gait rehabilitation program is needed (Fig. 10.4). Even though this seems to be a moving target, especially in patients with progressive MS, delayed intervention with gait mechanics seems to limit the benefits of any subsequent therapy. For safety, many patients may need a supportive device such as an ankle–foot orthosis, cane, walker, wheelchair, electric scooter, or, most recently, an electric personal assistive mobility devices such as a Segway. Use of these devices also limits energy expenditure, thereby alleviating fatigue and sleep disturbances, consistent with the interactive matrix of symptomatic MS therapy.

The decision to use a device or to switch from one device to another is a significant psychosocial decision for many patients. It is difficult to know when to recommend one of these devices unless patients actually report increased falls or unacceptable limitations

1. Gait problems in MS are multifactorial & dynamic:
    – Decreased mobility
       • Primary MS related
          – weakness, ataxia (sensory or motor), spasticity, pain or apraxia
       • Secondary
          – pain and limitations from osteoarthritis, osteoporosis and overuse injuries from gait compensation
    – Deconditioning
    – Vision problems
    – Other comorbid illnesses

2. Individualize rehabilitation programs through multidisciplinary approaches
    – Appropriately timing mobility aids to avoid worsening deconditioning or introducing overuse injuries
    – Considering psychosocial impact of mobility aids on patients

3. Pharmacological approaches to individual components of gait difficulty

Figure 10–4. Managing gait problems in MS.

to their life. While excessive use of a device can limit the long-term adaptation benefits of therapy and exercise, many patients also delay the use of devices that could help them walk or function better due to the social stigma associated with the use of the specific device. "I am not an old (wo)man" is a common remark when patients are first offered a cane. "It lets me stand tall" is a quote from one of our young patients with predominant but rather slowly progressive lower extremity ataxia who prefers a Segway device over an electric scooter. Both inappropriate and delayed use can also change gait mechanics, leading to secondary overuse injuries.

Tremor

Tremor is a debilitating symptom of MS that afflicts 25% to 60% of patients.[44] For early tremor, treatments include beta-blockers, primidone, isoniazid (high doses), carbamazepine, glutethimide, limb cooling, or an orthosis.[44] Any one of these approaches should be tried, but unfortunately no good general pharmacotherapy, stereotactic neurosurgery, or physical therapy efficacy has been established.[45] However, we have noted that thalamotomy provides up to 3 years of sustained benefit for refractory tremor, and deep brain stimulation can have sustained benefit for up to 5 years.[46] Unfortunately, the symptoms do return. The outcome is limited by the fact that these patients also had significant MS-related morbidity, and accompanying deaths limited complete long-term assessment.[46] An individualized, creative approach is needed in addition to what can be accomplished by physical therapy.

Weakness and Spasticity

The mainstay treatment for both weakness and spasticity is physical therapy, exercise, and stretching. However, for lower extremity weakness, especially 4-aminopyride (Dalfampridine SR), a broad-spectrum potassium-channel blocker, up to 20 mg daily, is helpful.[47] Specifically, this medicine improves walking speed by about 25% compared to 5% in placebo. However, when dosages exceed 20 mg/

day, common side effects include dizziness, insomnia, paresthesia, asthenia, nausea, headache, tremor, QT prolongation, and seizures.[48] In our practice, patients with ataxia may experience increased falls because they are unable to maintain balance with the more rapid walking that the drug allows. Balance retraining is essential prior to initiating this drug in ataxia patients. Many patients may experience only subjective improvement—or none. It is advisable to replicate the trial conditions in the examining room by conducting a 25-foot timed walk before and after starting the medicine in 1-week and 1-month intervals, coupled with ongoing therapy to assess the actual success of the drug. In the absence of documented benefit, medication can be stopped. Some patients have anecdotally reported upper-extremity functional improvement, although this was not documented in the original trial. The best candidates for this therapy are patients without significant ataxia with mild lower-extremity deficits, either with relapsing–remitting MS or early progressive MS.

Functional electrical stimulation to activate muscles on demand has been effective in overcoming some problems associated with unilateral foot drop-induced gait difficulty.[49] The concept utilizes a trigger (e.g., stepping on or releasing the foot from the ground) to initiate a targeted electrical stimulation to induce muscle contraction. Several FDA-approved devices are available. However, the use of these devices has significant drawbacks: the high cost and unbearable discomfort associated with the electrical shock. The current generation of devices administers shock nonselectively to motor nerves. However, we have had success in rare, selected patients.

Spasticity is a common problem in MS, especially in advanced disease. Some spasticity, especially in moderate-to-severe weakness, actually helps patients with supported gait and transfers. Overtreatment in this situation may increase weakness. Other patients whose spasticity (rather than weakness) causes impaired mobility, require aggressive treatment. As gait difficulties progress, it is important to assess whether the patient's primary issue is worsening ataxia/weakness or worsening spasticity, which can be modified. Severe spasticity may also be associated with a central pain syndrome (not to be confused with paroxysmal symptoms of painful flexion spasms).

Many pharmacological agents, such as oral baclofen, tizanidine, gabapentin, benzodiazepines, botulinum toxin, dantrolene sodium, vigabatrin, clonidine, mexiletine, ivermectin, and cannabinoids, have proven helpful in reducing spasticity when coupled with stretching therapy. While many of these agents have been accepted in practice following original studies with modest effects, absolute efficacy or head-to-head comparison of efficacy is not well documented.[50] Long-term efficacy and safety have been documented for intrathecal baclofen.[51–53] All of the above medications have been used by patients in our referral practice, and for each we have anecdotal evidence of benefit. However, our practical approach to patients with spasticity is illustrated in Figure 10.5. In addition to recommending stretching and massage therapy for every patient, we use oral baclofen or tizanidine[54] as our first-line approach. We use botulinum toxin (when oral medications lead to significant toxicity and absolute control of spasticity is needed) as our second-line treatment, followed by a baclofen pump (if we are not planning to do any further MRI studies). We use gabapentin or pregabalin as add-on treatments, especially in patients with additional pain problems.

Cannabis use for spasticity and associated pain has received significant attention in recent years. Indeed, there is some biological evidence that supports its efficacy.[55] Unfortunately, the mechanisms that contribute to the potential benefit of cannabis also contribute to side effects. As of this writing, a PubMed search using "cannabis and multiple sclerosis" terms leads to 194 entries. Most of the evidence supporting medicinal (as opposed to recreational) use of cannabis is anecdotal. In our practice, most patients report no benefit, while a few report significant benefit. A recent small study has documented a significant benefit of smoked cannabis over placebo in controlling spasticity and associated pain, without significant improvement in neurological function itself.[56] However, there were also increased side effects from the use of cannabis including a "too-high" feeling, dizziness, actual increase in fatigue, and nausea. The problem with such studies continues to be variation in the administration method and the subjective nature of patients' perceptions of intoxication levels. However, future work is needed. Currently there are many legal, social, and ethical aspects that complicate an open discussion of the use of cannabis in patients with MS.

PAIN AND PAROXYSMAL SYMPTOM-RELATED DISABILITY

The lifetime prevalence of pain in MS is about 40% in the original studies, and it correlates strongly with a progressive disease course.[57,58] Pain in MS can present in association with acute attacks (e.g., optic neuritis, painful dysesthesias). It can accompany paroxysmal sensory or motor symptoms due to ephaptic transmission (e.g., trigeminal neuralgia, Lhermitte's, migrating paresthesias, tonic spasms, paroxysmal dysarthria, or ataxia[59]), common in 10% to 20% of

1. Stretching & exercise followed by pharmacological interventions
2. First line pharmacological agents (usually in early MS):
    – Baclofen (up to 60 mg daily in 3 divided doses; doses as low as 20 mg increase risk of seizures, autonomic sx, hypothermia, withdrawal sx.),
    – Tizanidine (up to 36 mg daily in 3 divided doses; seems to be more sedating, interferes with oral contraception)
3. Second line pharmacological agents (usually in late MS):
    – Botulinium toxin (works best for focla spasticity)
    – Intrathecal baclofen (when daily dose requirements of oral baclofen cause significant side effects; however limits future MRI studies)
4. Add on pharmacological agents (helps spare side effects feom other medications):
    – Gabapentin or pregabalin (when there is also pain associated with spasticity)

Figure 10–5. Managing spasticity in MS.

MS patients, or can be persistent due to partial recovery of a lesion (e.g., chronic persistent dysesthesias). Pain can be related to spasticity or associated with injectable treatments such as interferons or glatiramer acetate. It may correlate with comorbidities of migraine[60] and fibromyalgia. While neither of these conditions is a primary MS symptom, both are common in MS patients due to the increased incidence in women and the direct association with sleep-, deconditioning-, and fatigue-related core symptoms of MS. Additionally, pain may result from immobility, overuse, and osteoarthritis (e.g., hip and knee pain, trochanteric bursitis) or from osteoporosis or vitamin D deficiency. This exhaustive list of likely pain mechanisms explains why pain occurs commonly in patients with MS.

Pain management depends on the mechanisms of pain. Indeed, most of these strategies are approaches that have been successful for treating different types of pain rather than specific for MS-related pain. This is further complicated by the fact that migraine with aura, fibromyalgia, and chronic fatigue syndromes are commonly misdiagnosed as MS in our referral practice.

Pain management in MS should be tailored to the individual patient.[61] Extensive management of pain is beyond the scope of this book; however, Table 10.5 summarizes the specific approaches commonly used for different pain problems and paroxysmal symptoms of MS. Nevertheless, given the chronicity of MS, some general principles should still be considered. The most important management strategy is to target core symptoms (Figs. 10.1 and 10.3), since sleep disruption, deconditioning, weight gain, and heat sensitivity can all exacerbate and, in return, be worsened by MS-related pain. The second therapeutic goal is to choose modalities that treat multiple problems simultaneously (e.g., tricyclic antidepressants that help incontinence, sleep, mood, migraines, and neurogenic pain). The third consideration is to avoid escalation of opioid use and other pain-related pharmaceuticals (e.g., increasing doses of oral baclofen) that disrupt sleep

Table 10–5 Treatment Options for Pain and Paroxysmal Symptoms in MS[61]

Acute pain associated with an MS attack: Optic neuritis Trigeminal neuralgia Painful dysesthesias Lhermitte's Tonic spasms Pelvic (bladder) spasms	If a pseudo-exacerbation is ruled out and the acute onset symptom can be localized to a new-onset lesional pathology by a change in the neurological examination, evoked potential studies, or MRI, the pain should be treated acutely as part of the attack with methylprednisolone, daily 1-gram intravenous infusions for 3–7 days, tailored to the patient's needs. In the case of first-time bladder spasms, a urinary tact infection needs to be ruled out before associating the pain directly with any spinal cord pathology.
Paroxysmal symptoms with or without pain:[102–107] Trigeminal neuralgia Migrating paresthesias Lhermitte's Tonic spasms Paroxysmal dysarthria/ataxia	When the paroxysmal symptoms are associated with a pseudo-exacerbation or associated with an acute attack but become persistent afterwards, regardless of the presence or absence of pain, carbamazepine (first choice), oxcarbazepine, lamotrigine, gabapentin, and pregabalin can be used. In the setting of recurrent and refractory symptoms (e.g., trigeminal neuralgia), standard surgical approaches (e.g., ablation, rhizotomy) for pain control can be used.
Persistent painful dysesthesias	Gabapentin (first choice), tricyclic antidepressants; lamotrigine, carbamazepine. Additionally, cold baths, topical anesthetics (e.g., lidocaine 4–5% 12 hours on/12 hours off) and intrathecal baclofen can be used
Pain due to subcutaneous injections	Local cooling ± topical anesthetic (e.g., lidocaine 4–5% 12 hours on/12 hours off) ± NSAIDs
Pain due to spasticity	See Figure 10.5 and spasticity discussion.
Fibromyalgia[108]	Exercise, stretching, muscle relaxation techniques, & sleep regulation ± gabapentin or pregabalin ± tricyclic antidepressants or duloxetine or milnacipran. A comprehensive fibromyalgia treatment program is needed.

patterns, substantially worsen cognitive and physical fatigue, and lead to habituation. Of course, exceptional situations, such as the setting of fractures or palliative care in patients with terminal or chronic progressive MS, will still require opioid use. Finally, local strategies, such as analgesic creams or injections, should be used whenever possible to complement other systemic pain management strategies.

AUTONOMIC DISABILITY

Autonomic dysfunction, including temperature dysregulation, bladder or bowel dyscontrol, and sexual dysfunction, is very common in MS; indeed, almost all MS patients have at least one form of autonomic dysfunction. Temperature dysregulation was discussed in a previous section. This section will focus on bladder/bowel dysfunction and sexual dysfunction in MS, both of which are multifactorial. However, given the extent of nervous system control needed to learn and execute bladder or bowel control and sexual function, it is not surprising that a lesional pathology easily disrupts these pathways. These autonomic systems are affected early in progressive MS, which predominantly affects the long tracts.

Neurogenic bladder affects 80% of patients with MS and is a major cause of morbidity.[57]

It can present either as overactive bladder (urgency, frequency, urge incontinence) or chronic urinary retention. Especially in men with MS, coexistent retention with overactive bladder ("bladder-sphincter dyssynergia") occurs in half of patients with bladder symptoms.[62,63] Complications of "neurogenic bladder" include recurrent urinary tract infections, which may lead to increased pseudo-exacerbations coupled with heat sensitivity or urosepsis, and vesicourethral dysfunction, which can lead to long-term upper urinary tract damage. The risk factors for the latter are age older than 50, male sex, longer duration of MS, indwelling catheter, high-amplitude neurogenic detrusor contractions, permanent high detrusor pressure, and detrusor–sphincter dyssynergia.[63] Therefore, timely management of bladder symptoms in MS is essential (Fig. 10.6).[64–69] Management strategies should be adjusted as the disease progresses. There has been extensive recent research into interventional strategies including various applications of botulinum toxin, electrical stimulation, and, generally as a last resort, permanent drainage conduits. Given the frequency of neurogenic bladder in patients with MS, urologists and women's health specialists need to be part of every multidisciplinary MS clinic.

In an earlier population-based study, 40% of MS patients have reported some level of sexual impairment, one in four reporting

1.   General management:
   –   *Initiation difficulty:* Suprapubic tapping, pressure, perineal stimulation
   –   *Retention:* Frequent and regular (e.g. q4hrs) voiding practice
   –   *Mild leakage:* pads
   –   *Nocturia:* Reduce fluid intake at night
   –   *Infection prevention:* Cranberry juice; avoid maintenance antibiotics if possible

2.   Specific first line interventions: (Customized to changes as disease progresses)
   –   *Overactive bladder:*
      •   Frequently check & treat urinary tract infections (avoid maintenance therapy)
      •   Urine residual < 100ml:
         –   pelvic floor exercises & intermittent use of detrusor inhibition agents (oxybutynin, tolterodine, propantheline; for midnight awakenings: oxybutynin SR, tolterodine SR)
      •   Urine residual > 100ml (coexisting incomplete emptying):
         –   add intermittent self catheterization to medication management
   –   *Isolated retention:*
      –   Intermittent self catheterization & detrusor stimulation agents (contraindicated in obstructions, e.g. prostatism (carbachol, bethanechol))

3.   Specific second line interventions:
   –   Botulinum toxin, electrical stimulation & surgery for permanent drainage conduits

Figure 10–6. Managing bladder symptoms in MS.

severe impairment.[70] However, as others have suggested, sexual dysfunction of some level remains a significantly underdiagnosed quality-of-life issue for young adults with MS, probably afflicting ~70% of MS patients.[71] The reasons for underreporting are likely due to patient discomfort in discussing sex-related topics, which, unfortunately, is an impediment to management. Significant work is required to obtain well-documented (vs. anecdotal) evidence-based approaches for managing MS-related sexual dysfunction. MS can induce all common sexual dysfunction problems including decreased libido, difficulty achieving orgasm, decreased genital sensation, decreased vaginal lubrication, erectile dysfunction, and ejaculation difficulty.[71] While all of these can be driven by MS lesional pathology, many psychosocial factors, as well as medications used to treat other facets of MS, contribute significantly to sexual dysfunction. A good starting point is to eliminate any medication that can be replaced with a nonpharmacological modality or another medication with lesser impact on sexual function. Sleep quality and fatigue play a significant role in sexual function, and these core symptoms have to be controlled aggressively. Depression, anxiety, weight-associated low self-esteem, and chronic illness also significantly affect MS-related sexual dysfunction. Therapy sessions with a rehabilitation psychologist that include the patient's partner are essential to managing the complex psychosocial problems surrounding sexual dysfunction in MS. Several alternative stimulation mechanisms, positional adaptations, medications for erectile and ejaculation dysfunction, and consultation with experienced sex therapists, urologists, and women's health specialists are all viable strategies. However, sexual dysfunction in MS remains a relatively uncharted territory, and every management strategy should be optimized within a holistic approach.[71]

COGNITIVE AND BEHAVIORAL DISABILITY

Some level of cognitive dysfunction affects 43% to 70% of patients with MS, and it affects every aspect of psychosocial functioning of MS patients.[72] It is generally subtle; overt dementia is rare except in later stages of the disease, although cortical lesions may occur more frequently than can be documented with conventional MRI techniques (see Chapter 4). Patients seldom present with significant symptomatic cortical lesions in the early stages. Cognitive impairment in MS depends on disease course, disease duration, and disease stage. *Primary cognitive impairment* is due to high brain lesion load, preferred gray-matter involvement, and atrophy. *Secondary cognitive impairment* is attributed to fatigue, sleep problems, depression, anxiety, medications, and visual problems. Given the chronicity of MS, comorbid additional neurodegenerative disease can also develop with more typical cognitive impairment reflecting these disorders.

Cognitive impairment in MS involves multiple domains; however, the core cognitive problems relate to processing speed, visual learning, and complex sustained attention difficulties.[73] These deficits present as early inability to multitask, difficulties with executive dysfunction, increased susceptibility to depression, long-term memory problems, and chronic frustration from "trying to keep up." As a result of these conditions, MS patients frequently experience increased psychosocial stress, withdrawal and dysfunction, and job loss or early retirement.[74–77]

Setting realistic life goals and expectations is a critical first step to managing cognitive impairment in MS. Simplifying lifestyle in both the work and home environment limits patient frustration and, more importantly, increases enjoyment of both work and leisure activities. While seemingly counterintuitive, since our modern lifestyle pushes patients to increased multitasking, our patients actually report increased productivity when they set realistic daily goals and focus on only one task at a time.

It is also critical to eliminate or minimize the causes of secondary cognitive impairment due to fatigue, sleep problems, depression and anxiety, medications, and visual problems in MS. Donepezil, 10 mg PO daily, modestly improves memory performance.[78] Cognitive rehabilitation programs are also helpful.[79] Specifically, the "story memory technique" improves learning in moderate-to-severe memory impairment, although not in mild impairment.[80] So far, immunomodulatory drugs used in MS have shown promise in slowing down the progressive cognitive impairment in MS, albeit

Table 10–6 **Treatment Options for Cognitive and Psychiatric Problems**

Cognitive problems in MS	
Long-term prevention[13,81–83]	– Primarily achieved by slowing down disease burden by primary immunomodulatory agents – Secondarily achieved by eliminating or minimizing contributing factors: depression, sleep problems, fatigue, as discussed in the core symptom control section
Symptomatic management[78–80]	– Donepezil 10 mg daily offers modest improvement in cognitive function in patients with mild to moderate MS – Cognitive rehabilitation programs are modestly helpful. "Story memory technique" is moderately helpful in severe but not mild memory impairment.

Psychiatric problems in MS	
Acute psychiatric attack	– Counterintuitive, but if the acute-onset symptom can be localized to a new-onset lesional pathology by a change in the neurological examination, evoked potential studies, or MRI, it can be treated with methylprednisolone, daily 1-g intravenous infusions for 3–7 days, tailored to patient's needs. – Due to the risk of increased anxiety, psychosis, mania, and self-harm, patients are best treated on an inpatient psychiatry floor. – Any additional acute psychiatric-management strategies can then be used while the patient is hospitalized. – Unless chronicity is established, antipsychotics and antidepressants can be discontinued in the future.
Chronic psychiatric disorders	– Very little MS-specific evidence for medications or psychotherapy, but can be managed like any other chronic psychiatric disorder – Try to eliminate or minimize the impact of contributing fatigue, pain, and sleep problems
Pseudobulbar affect[109,110]	– Dextromethorphan/quinidine: 30 mg/30 mg given orally twice daily decreases crying and laughing episodes, improves quality of life and relationships, and is well tolerated. Anecdotally, low-dose amitriptyline may also work in some patients, although evidence remains very limited.

as a secondary endpoint in short, open-label studies.[13,81–83] As these studies show, prevention of disease progression ultimately seems to be the key to long-term success in preventing primary cognitive impairment in MS.

Depression and anxiety are the most common psychiatric problems in 50% to 60% of MS patients, followed by a pseudobulbar affect in 10% and bipolar disorder and psychosis in 2% to 3%. Acute exacerbation-induced psychiatric problems are rare; chronic psychiatric problems are more typical in MS. The etiology is multifactorial and can be classified as *primary psychiatric problems* correlating with high lesion load and atrophy predominantly in frontal lobes and arcuate fasciculus, and *secondary psychiatric problems* associated with physical disability, fatigue, sleep problems, cognitive inefficiency, medications, and psychosocial

problems. Interferons used to treat MS may increase suicide risk and worsen depression but, unless there is premorbid depression, do not seem to induce depression.[84] Psychiatric problems in MS lead to psychosocial dysfunction and withdrawal, sleep problems, and increased fatigue as well as decreased rehabilitation and medication compliance. Table 10.6 summarizes the approaches for management of psychiatric and cognitive problems associated with MS.

SUMMARY

Although current treatment strategies in MS focus primarily on preventing relapses and disability progression through immunomodulatory agents, practicing physicians still need to focus on day-to-day management of patients' symptoms. In this chapter, we illustrate the interactive nature of symptomatic management of MS. Even though MS is not a curable disease, management of day-to-day symptoms substantially improves patients' quality of life and general psychosocial functioning. However, successful management requires a multidisciplinary integrated approach by a committed group of health care providers.

REFERENCES

1. Courtney AM, Castro-Borrero W, Davis SL, Frohman TC, Frohman EM. Functional treatments in multiple sclerosis. Curr Opin Neurol; 24:250–254, 2011.

2. Frohman TC, Castro W, Shah A, et al. Symptomatic therapy in multiple sclerosis. Ther Adv Neurol Disord; 4:83–98, 2011.

3. Samkoff LM, Goodman AD. Symptomatic management in multiple sclerosis. Neurol Clin; 29:449–463, 2011.

4. Olsen SA. A review of complementary and alternative medicine (CAM) by people with multiple sclerosis. Occup Ther Int; 16:57–70, 2009.

5. Fisk JD, Pontefract A, Ritvo PG, Archibald CJ, Murray TJ. The impact of fatigue on patients with multiple sclerosis. Can J Neurol Sci; 21:9–14, 1994.

6. Packer TL, Sauriol A, Brouwer B. Fatigue secondary to chronic illness: postpolio syndrome, chronic fatigue syndrome, and multiple sclerosis. Arch Phys Med Rehabil; 75:1122–1126, 1994.

7. Trojan DA, Arnold D, Collet JP, et al. Fatigue in multiple sclerosis: association with disease-related, behavioural and psychosocial factors. Mult Scler; 13:985–995, 2007.

8. Heesen C, Nawrath L, Reich C, Bauer N, Schulz KH, Gold SM: Fatigue in multiple sclerosis: an example of cytokine mediated sickness behaviour? J Neurol Neurosurg Psychiatry; 77:34–39, 2006.

9. Putzki N, Katsarava Z, Vago S, Diener HC, Limmroth V. Prevalence and severity of multiple-sclerosis-associated fatigue in treated and untreated patients. Eur Neurol; 59:136–142, 2008.

10. Metz LM, Patten SB, Archibald CJ, et al. The effect of immunomodulatory treatment on multiple sclerosis fatigue. J Neurol Neurosurg Psychiatry; 75:1045–1047, 2004.

11. Bischoff C, Schreiber H, Bergmann A. Background information on multiple sclerosis patients stopping ongoing immunomodulatory therapy: a multicenter study in a community-based environment. J Neurol; 259(11):2347–23–3, 2012.

12. Yildiz M, Tettenborn B, Putzki N. Multiple sclerosis-associated fatigue during disease-modifying treatment with natalizumab, interferon-beta and glatiramer acetate. Eur Neurol; 65:231–232, 2011.

13. Iaffaldano P, Viterbo RG, Paolicelli D, et al. Impact of natalizumab on cognitive performances and fatigue in relapsing multiple sclerosis: a prospective, open-label, two years observational study. PLoS One; 7:e35843, 2012.

14. Lee D, Newell R, Ziegler L, Topping A. Treatment of fatigue in multiple sclerosis: a systematic review of the literature. Int J Nurs Pract; 14:81–93, 2008.

15. Caminero A, Bartolome M. Sleep disturbances in multiple sclerosis. J Neurol Sci; 309:86–91, 2011.

16. Fleming WE, Pollak CP. Sleep disorders in multiple sclerosis. Semin Neurol; 25:64–68, 2005.

17. Tachibana N, Howard RS, Hirsch NP, Miller DH, Moseley IF, Fish D. Sleep problems in multiple sclerosis. Eur Neurol; 34:320–323, 1994.

18. Auger C, Montplaisir J, Duquette P. Increased frequency of restless legs syndrome in a French-Canadian population with multiple sclerosis. Neurology; 65:1652–1653, 2005.

19. Deriu M, Cossu G, Molari A, et al. Restless legs syndrome in multiple sclerosis: a case-control study. Mov Disord; 24:697–701, 2009.

20. Gomez-Choco MJ, Iranzo A, Blanco Y, Graus F, Santamaria J, Saiz A. Prevalence of restless legs syndrome and REM sleep behavior disorder in multiple sclerosis. Mult Scler; 13:805–808, 2007.

21. Aydar G, Kurt S, Karaer Unaldi H, Erkorkmaz U. Restless legs syndrome in multiple sclerosis. Eur Neurol; 65:302–306, 2011.

22. Li Y, Munger KL, Batool-Anwar S, De Vito K, Ascherio A, Gao X. Association of multiple sclerosis with restless legs syndrome and other sleep disorders in women. Neurology; 78:1500–1506, 2012.

23. Manconi M, Fabbrini M, Bonanni E, et al. High prevalence of restless legs syndrome in multiple sclerosis. Eur J Neurol; 14:534–539, 2007.

24. Manconi M, Rocca MA, Ferini-Strambi L, et al. Restless legs syndrome is a common finding in multiple sclerosis and correlates with cervical cord damage. Mult Scler; 14:86–93, 2008.

25. Kaminska M, Kimoff RJ, Benedetti A, et al. Obstructive sleep apnea is associated with fatigue in multiple sclerosis. Mult Scler; 18:1159–1169, 2012.

26. Iseki K, Mezaki T, Oka Y, et al. Hypersomnia in MS. Neurology; 59:2006–2007, 2002.

27. Vetrugno R, Stecchi S, Plazzi G, et al. Narcolepsy-like syndrome in multiple sclerosis. Sleep Med; 10:389–391, 2009.

28. Plazzi G, Montagna P. Remitting REM sleep behavior disorder as the initial sign of multiple sclerosis. Sleep Med; 3:437–439, 2002.

29. Tippmann-Peikert M, Boeve BF, Keegan BM. REM sleep behavior disorder initiated by acute brainstem multiple sclerosis. Neurology; 66:1277–1279, 2006.

30. Hedstrom AK, Olsson T, Alfredsson L. High body mass index before age 20 is associated with increased risk for multiple sclerosis in both men and women. Mult Scler; 18:1334–1336, 2012.

31. Huisinga JM, Filipi ML, Stergiou N. Elliptical exercise improves fatigue ratings and quality of life in patients with multiple sclerosis. J Rehabil Res Dev; 48:881–890, 2011.

32. Oken BS, Kishiyama S, Zajdel D, et al. Randomized controlled trial of yoga and exercise in multiple sclerosis. Neurology; 62:2058–2064, 2004.

33. Rietberg MB, Brooks D, Uitdehaag BM, Kwakkel G. Exercise therapy for multiple sclerosis. Cochrane Database of Reviews (Online); 1:CD003980, 2005.

34. Romberg A, Virtanen A, Aunola S, Karppi SL, Karanko H, Ruutiainen J. Exercise capacity, disability and leisure physical activity of subjects with multiple sclerosis. Mult Scler; 10:212–218, 2004.

35. White LJ, Dressendorfer RH. Exercise and multiple sclerosis. Sports Med; 34:1077–1100, 2004.

36. Mead GE, Morley W, Campbell P, Greig CA, McMurdo M, Lawlor DA. Exercise for depression. Cochrane Database of Reviews (Online); 3:CD004366, 2009.

37. Edmonds M, McGuire H, Price J. Exercise therapy for chronic fatigue syndrome. Cochrane Database of Reviews (Online); 3:CD003200, 2004.

38. Hauser W, Klose P, Langhorst J, et al. Efficacy of different types of aerobic exercise in fibromyalgia syndrome: a systematic review and meta-analysis of randomised controlled trials. Arthritis Res Ther; 12:R79, 2010.

39. Rietberg MB, van Wegen EE, Uitdehaag BM, Kwakkel G. The association between perceived fatigue and actual level of physical activity in multiple sclerosis. Mult Scler; 17:1231–1237, 2011.

40. Schwid SR, Petrie MD, Murray R, et al. A randomized controlled study of the acute and chronic effects of cooling therapy for MS. Neurology; 60:1955–1960, 2003.

41. Darlix A, Mathey G, Monin ML, et al. [Hypothalamic involvement in multiple sclerosis]. Rev Neurol (Paris); 168:434–443, 2012.

42. Darlix A, Mathey G, Sauvee M, Braun M, Debouverie M. Paroxysmal hypothermia in two patients with multiple sclerosis. Eur Neurol; 67:268–271, 2012.

43. Weiss N, Hasboun D, Demeret S, et al. Paroxysmal hypothermia as a clinical feature of multiple sclerosis. Neurology; 72:193–195, 2009.

44. Koch M, Mostert J, Heersema D, De Keyser J. Tremor in multiple sclerosis. J Neurol; 254:133–145, 2007.

45. Mills RJ, Yap L, Young CA. Treatment for ataxia in multiple sclerosis. Cochrane Database of Reviews (Online); 1:CD005029, 2007.

46. Hassan A, Ahlskog JE, Rodriguez M, Matsumoto JY. Surgical therapy for multiple sclerosis tremor: a 12-year follow-up study. Eur J Neurol; 19:764–768, 2012.

47. Goodman AD, Brown TR, Edwards KR, et al. A phase 3 trial of extended release oral dalfampridine in multiple sclerosis. Ann Neurol; 68:494–502, 2010.

48. Cornblath DR, Bienen EJ, Blight AR. The safety profile of dalfampridine extended release in multiple sclerosis clinical trials. Clin Ther; 34:1056–1069, 2012.

49. Paul L, Rafferty D, Young S, Miller L, Mattison P, McFadyen A. The effect of functional electrical stimulation on the physiological cost of gait in people with multiple sclerosis. Mult Scler; 14:954–961, 2008.

50. Shakespeare DT, Boggild M, Young CA. Anti-spasticity agents for multiple sclerosis. Cochrane Database of Reviews (Online); 4:CD001332, 2003.

51. Ben Smail D, Peskine A, Roche N, Mailhan L, Thiebaut I, Bussel B. Intrathecal baclofen for treatment of spasticity of multiple sclerosis patients. Mult Scler; 12:101–103, 2006.

52. Rekand T, Gronning M. Treatment of spasticity related to multiple sclerosis with intrathecal baclofen: a long-term follow-up. J Rehabil Med; 43:511–514, 2011.

53. Zahavi A, Geertzen JH, Middel B, Staal M, Rietman JS. Long-term effect (more than five years) of intrathecal baclofen on impairment, disability, and quality of life in patients with severe spasticity of spinal origin. J Neurol Neurosurg Psychiatry; 75:1553–1557, 2004.

54. Vakhapova V, Auriel E, Karni A. Nightly sublingual tizanidine HCl in multiple sclerosis: clinical efficacy and safety. Clin Neuropharmacol; 33:151–154, 2010.

55. Pryce G, Baker D. Control of spasticity in a multiple sclerosis model is mediated by CB1, not CB2, cannabinoid receptors. Br J Pharmacol; 150:519–525, 2007.

56. Corey-Bloom J, Wolfson T, Gamst A, et al. Smoked cannabis for spasticity in multiple sclerosis: a randomized, placebo-controlled trial. Canad Med Assoc J; 184:1143–1150, 2012.

57. Martinelli Boneschi F, Colombo B, Annovazzi P, et al. Lifetime and actual prevalence of pain and headache in multiple sclerosis. Mult Scler; 14:514–521, 2008.

58. Solaro C, Brichetto G, Amato MP, et al. The prevalence of pain in multiple sclerosis: a multicenter cross-sectional study. Neurology; 63:919–921, 2004.

59. Marcel C, Anheim M, Flamand-Rouviere C, et al. Symptomatic paroxysmal dysarthria-ataxia in demyelinating diseases. J Neurol; 257:1369–1372, 2010.

60. Putzki N, Pfriem A, Limmroth V, et al. Prevalence of migraine, tension-type headache and trigeminal neuralgia in multiple sclerosis. Eur J Neurol; 16:262–267, 2009.

61. Pollmann W, Feneberg W. Current management of pain associated with multiple sclerosis. CNS Drugs; 22:291–324, 2008.

62. Andrews KL, Husmann DA. Bladder dysfunction and management in multiple sclerosis. Mayo Clin Proc; 72:1176–1183, 1997.

63. de Seze M, Ruffion A, Denys P, Joseph PA, Perrouin-Verbe B. The neurogenic bladder in multiple sclerosis: review of the literature and proposal of management guidelines. Mult Scler; 13:915–928, 2007.

64. de Seze M, Raibaut P, Gallien P, et al. Transcutaneous posterior tibial nerve stimulation for treatment of the overactive bladder syndrome in multiple sclerosis: results of a multicenter prospective study. Neurourol Urodyn; 30:306–311, 2011.

65. Duthie JB, Vincent M, Herbison GP, Wilson DI. Botulinum toxin injections for adults with overactive bladder syndrome. Cochrane Database of Reviews (Online); 12:CD005493, 2012.

66. Herschorn S, Gajewski J, Ethans K, et al. Efficacy of botulinum toxin A injection for neurogenic detrusor overactivity and urinary incontinence: a randomized, double-blind trial. J Urol; 185:2229–2235, 2011.

67. Jepson RG, Miihaljevic L, Craig J. Cranberries for preventing urinary tract infections. Cochrane Database of Reviews (Online); 1:CD001321, 2004.

68. Shepherd JP, Lowder JL, Jones KA, Smith KJ. Retropubic and transobturator midurethral slings: a decision analysis to compare outcomes including efficacy and complications. Int Urogynecol J; 21:787–793, 2010.

69. Shepherd JP, Lowder JL, Leng WW, Smith KJ. InterStim sacral Neuromodulation and Botox botulinum-A toxin intradetrusor injections for refractory urge urinary incontinence: a decision analysis comparing outcomes including efficacy and complications. Female Pelvic Med Reconstr Surg; 17:199–203, 2011.

70. Rodriguez M, Siva A, Ward J, Stolp-Smith K, O'Brien P, Kurland L. Impairment, disability, and handicap in multiple sclerosis: a population-based study in Olmsted County, Minnesota. Neurology; 44:28–33, 1994.

71. Fletcher SG, Castro-Borrero W, Remington G, Treadaway K, Lemack GE, Frohman EM. Sexual dysfunction in patients with multiple sclerosis: a multidisciplinary approach to evaluation and management. Nat Clin Pract Urol; 6:96–107, 2009.

72. Chiaravalloti ND, DeLuca J. Cognitive impairment in multiple sclerosis. Lancet Neurol; 7:1139–1151, 2008.

73. Kalmar JH, Gaudino EA, Moore NB, Halper J, Deluca J. The relationship between cognitive deficits and everyday functional activities in multiple sclerosis. Neuropsychology; 22:442–449, 2008.

74. Julian LJ, Vella L, Vollmer T, Hadjimichael O, Mohr DC. Employment in multiple sclerosis. Exiting and re-entering the work force. J Neurol; 255:1354–1360, 2008.

75. Kornblith AB, La Rocca NG, Baum HM. Employment in individuals with multiple sclerosis. Int J Rehabil Res; 9:155–165, 1986.

76. Rao SM, Leo GJ, Bernardin L, Unverzagt F. Cognitive dysfunction in multiple sclerosis. I. Frequency, patterns, and prediction. Neurology; 41:685–691, 1991.

77. Rao SM, Leo GJ, Ellington L, Nauertz T, Bernardin L, Unverzagt F. Cognitive dysfunction in multiple sclerosis. II. Impact on employment and social functioning. Neurology; 41:692–696, 1991.

78. Krupp LB, Christodoulou C, Melville P, Scherl WF, MacAllister WS, Elkins LE. Donepezil improved memory in multiple sclerosis in a randomized clinical trial. Neurology; 63:1579–1585, 2004.

79. O'Brien AR, Chiaravalloti N, Goverover Y, Deluca J. Evidenced-based cognitive rehabilitation for persons with multiple sclerosis: a review of the literature. Arch Phys Med Rehabil; 89:761–769, 2008.

80. Chiaravalloti ND, DeLuca J, Moore NB, Ricker JH. Treating learning impairments improves memory performance in multiple sclerosis: a randomized clinical trial. Mult Scler; 11:58–68, 2005.

81. Barak Y, Achiron A. Effect of interferon-beta-1b on cognitive functions in multiple sclerosis. Eur Neurol; 47:11–14, 2002.

82. Fischer JS, Priore RL, Jacobs LD, etal. Neuropsychological effects of interferon beta-1a in relapsing multiple sclerosis. Multiple Sclerosis Collaborative Research Group. Ann Neurol; 48:885–892, 2000.

83. Pliskin NH, Hamer DP, Goldstein DS, et al. Improved delayed visual reproduction test performance in multiple sclerosis patients receiving interferon beta-1b. Neurology; 47:1463–1468, 1996.

84. Goeb JL, Even C, Nicolas G, Gohier B, Dubas F, Garre JB. Psychiatric side effects of interferon-beta in multiple sclerosis. Eur Psychiatry; 21:186–193, 2006.

85. Gillson G, Richard TL, Smith RB, Wright JV. A double-blind pilot study of the effect of Prokarin on fatigue in multiple sclerosis. Mult Scler; 8:30–35, 2002.

86. A randomized controlled trial of amantadine in fatigue associated with multiple sclerosis. The Canadian MS Research Group. Can J Neurol Sci; 14:273–278, 1987.

87. Pucci E, Branas P, D'Amico R, Giuliani G, Solari A, Taus C. Amantadine for fatigue in multiple sclerosis. Cochrane Database of Reviews (Online); 1:CD002818, 2007.

88. Wingerchuk DM, Benarroch EE, O'Brien PC, et al. A randomized controlled crossover trial of aspirin for fatigue in multiple sclerosis. Neurology; 64:1267–1269, 2005.

89. Breitbart W, Rosenfeld B, Kaim M, Funesti-Esch J. A randomized, double-blind, placebo-controlled trial of psychostimulants for the treatment of fatigue in ambulatory patients with human immunodeficiency virus disease. Arch Intern Med; 161:411–420, 2001.

90. Sterling MJ, Kane M, Grace ND. Pemoline-induced autoimmune hepatitis. Am J Gastroenterol; 91:2233–2234, 1996.

91. Weinshenker BG, Penman M, Bass B, Ebers GC, Rice GP. A double-blind, randomized, crossover trial of pemoline in fatigue associated with multiple sclerosis. Neurology; 42:1468–1471, 1992.

92. Rammohan KW, Rosenberg JH, Lynn DJ, Blumenfeld AM, Pollak CP, Nagaraja HN. Efficacy and safety of modafinil (Provigil) for the treatment of fatigue in multiple sclerosis: a two centre phase 2 study. J Neurol Neurosurg Psychiatry; 72:179–183, 2002.

93. Stankoff B, Waubant E, Confavreux C, et al. Modafinil for fatigue in MS: a randomized placebo-controlled double-blind study. Neurology; 64:1139–1143, 2005.

94. Zifko UA, Rupp M, Schwarz S, Zipko HT, Maida EM. Modafinil in treatment of fatigue in multiple sclerosis. Results of an open-label study. J Neurol; 249:983–987, 2002.

95. Mathiowetz VG, Finlayson ML, Matuska KM, Chen HY, Luo P. Randomized controlled trial of an energy conservation course for persons with multiple sclerosis. Mult Scler; 11:592–601, 2005.

96. Romberg A, Ruutiainen J, Puukka P, Poikkeus L. Fatigue in multiple sclerosis patients during inpatient rehabilitation. Disabil Rehabil; 30:1480–1485, 2008.

97. Kato T, Kanbayashi T, Yamamoto K, et al. Hypersomnia and low CSF hypocretin-1 (orexin-A) concentration in a patient with multiple sclerosis showing bilateral hypothalamic lesions. Intern Med; 42:743–745, 2003.

98. Hening WA. Restless legs syndrome. Curr Treat Options Neurol; 1:309–319, 1999.

99. Vignatelli L, Billiard M, Clarenbach P, et al. EFNS guidelines on management of restless legs syndrome and periodic limb movement disorder in sleep. Eur J Neurol; 13:1049–1065, 2006.

100. Smith I, Lasserson TJ. Pressure modification for improving usages of continuous positive airway pressure machines in adults with obstructive sleep apnoea. Cochrane Database of Reviews (Online); 4:CD003531, 2009.

101. Sundaram S, Bridgman SA, Lim J, Lasserson TJ. Surgery for obstructive sleep apnoea. Cochrane Database of Reviews (Online); 4:CD001004, 2005.

102. Solaro C, Boehmker M, Tanganelli P. Pregabalin for treating paroxysmal painful symptoms in multiple sclerosis: a pilot study. J Neurol; 256:1773–1774, 2009.

103. Solaro C, Brichetto G, Battaglia MA, Messmer Uccelli M, Mancardi GL. Antiepileptic medications in multiple sclerosis: adverse effects in a three-year follow-up study. Neurol Sci; 25:307–310, 2005.

104. Solaro C, Lunardi GL, Capello E, et al. An open-label trial of gabapentin treatment of paroxysmal symptoms in multiple sclerosis patients. Neurology; 51:609–611, 1998.

105. Solaro C, Restivo D, Mancardi GL, Tanganelli P. Oxcarbazepine for treating paroxysmal painful

symptoms in multiple sclerosis: a pilot study. *Neurol Sci*; 28:156–158, 2007.

106. Valentino P, Nistico R, Pirritano D, et al. Lamotrigine therapy for paroxysmal dysarthria caused by multiple sclerosis: a case report. J Neurol; 258:1349–1350, 2011.

107. Yetimalar Y, Gurgor N, Basoglu M. Clinical efficacy of gabapentin for paroxysmal symptoms in multiple sclerosis. Acta Neurol Scand; 109:430–431, 2004.

108. Arnold LM, Clauw DJ, Dunegan LJ, Turk DC. A framework for fibromyalgia management for primary care providers. Mayo Clin Proc; 87:488–496, 2012.

109. Panitch HS, Thisted RA, Smith RA, et al. Randomized, controlled trial of dextromethorphan/quinidine for pseudobulbar affect in multiple sclerosis. Ann Neurol; 59:780–787, 2006.

110. Szczudlik A, Slowik A, Tomik B. [The effect of amitriptyline on the pathological crying and other pseudobulbar signs]. Neurol Neurochir Pol; 29:663–674, 1995.

Chapter 11

Future Disease-Modifying Treatment Approaches in Multiple Sclerosis

CURRENT TREATMENT OUTLOOK
ANTICIPATED CLINICAL TRIALS
BG-12
Daclizumab

Alemtuzumab
Rituximab
Cladribine
Laquinimod

SUMMARY

Abstract

The currently available FDA-approved disease-modifying agents are only partially effective and are often inconvenient and expensive. Many have potentially life-threatening side effects. While some appear to prevent relapsing–remitting disease from evolving to a progressive disease, none meaningfully prevents the onset or worsening of progressive disease or addresses already ongoing insidious progression. This chapter discusses medications that may find their way to clinical practice as well as some of the medications that are in early clinical trials.

CURRENT TREATMENT OUTLOOK

While the seven currently available FDA-approved disease-modifying agents clearly have changed the horizon for MS patients, as discussed in Chapter 10, they remain partially effective and are sometimes inconvenient to use and extremely expensive; some have potentially life-threatening side effects. The most limiting and frustrating common characteristic of the current medications is that none can meaningfully address progressive forms or the progressive stage of MS. None appears to prevent relapsing–remitting MS (RRMS) from evolving to a progressive disease.

Several ongoing clinical trials with already approved or still-unapproved agents mainly address the active inflammatory component of MS, which results in blood–brain barrier disruption and new lesion formation. An excellent resource for clinical trials, in general, is the FDA-maintained website www.clinicaltrials.gov, where clinical trials being conducted for any condition must be listed by federal law. As of this writing (August 2012), there are 242 actively recruiting trials for MS listed on this website. Of note, this does not mean 242 new drugs are under investigation; these include observational studies, trials with symptom-control medications, extension trials of currently approved medications, and only 13 trials of as-yet-unapproved, experimental medications.

In this chapter, we will review several medications that may find their way to clinical practice as well as some of the medications that are in early clinical trials.

ANTICIPATED CLINICAL TRIALS

In general, medications reaching the clinical trial stage are either directly derived from animal model research, most commonly using the experimental autoimmune encephalomyelitis (EAE) model of MS, or from medications already approved or at least extensively studied to address other autoimmune conditions. There are problems with both of these approaches. First, it is well known that animal models often overestimate the response to medications (i.e., the sulfasalazine trial in MS). At times, clinical trials even lead to completely opposing results in mice versus humans; for example, the altered peptide ligand trial worked very efficiently in EAE but resulted in clinical and radiological worsening of MS. It may seem logical and convenient to consider MS as one of the many human autoimmune diseases, several of which respond to medications of the same mechanism of action, but clinical trials derived from these assumptions often fail. For example, the often extremely beneficial use of TNF-alpha blocking agents in a variety of systemic and other autoimmune conditions or cancer leads to radiological and often clinical worsening of MS, as discussed in earlier chapters. Among the patients receiving treatment with these agents for conditions other than MS, a low but definite proportion will develop a demyelinating disease.

BG-12

BG-12, also known as di-methyl fumaric acid, is a promising oral, disease-modifying agent in MS. Its mechanism of action is mainly related to the activation of nuclear factor-E2-related factor 2, resulting in anti-inflammatory, antioxidant, and, overall, neuroprotective effects.[1,2] In addition to demonstrating positive effects in EAE, it has also been used in psoriasis. In a phase II trial, BG-12 clearly demonstrated effects on MRI-related measures (enhancing lesions, overall T2 hyperintense lesions).[3] A phase III trial indicated sustained benefit on clinical and imaging endpoints.[4,5] Perhaps most importantly, this oral agent appears to be very safe, as demonstrated with similar agents in psoriasis.[6] In MS trials, the most common side effects were flushing, gastrointestinal symptoms, and headache.[7] No increase in the rate of infections has been reported. We believe that these agents will represent a viable tier 1 alternative to interferon or glatiramer acetate if long-term safety is established.

Daclizumab

Daclizumab is a humanized monoclonal antibody directed against IL-2Rα (CD25) that is currently approved by the FDA for the treatment of acute renal allograft rejection. The IL-2Rα–encoding gene was recently identified in a whole-genome screen as an MS risk allele,[8] as discussed in Chapter 3. Daclizumab blocks the binding of IL-2 to the high-affinity IL-2 receptor, thus inhibiting T-cell and B-cell proliferation; however, studies by other authors suggested that daclizumab's clinical effects in MS were mediated through the generation of CD56+ natural killer cells with immunoregulatory effects, mostly related to directly inhibiting CD8 T-cell functions.[9–13] In combination with maintained interferon treatment, daclizumab therapy resulted in a 72% reduction (p = .004) in the number of gadolinium-enhancing lesions on MRI scans during 6 months in the high-dose daclizumab group. Daclizumab was generally safe and well tolerated; long-term safety with chronic use is to be determined. Some centers already prescribe this as part of combination therapy, but it remains a nonapproved approach. New studies are under way to determine if official approval is warranted. We also think this may represent a good adjunct therapy for tier 1 medications in the near future once officially approved.

Alemtuzumab

Alemtuzumab, commonly known as CamPath (developed at the University of Cambridge), is a humanized monoclonal antibody directed against the surface antigen CD52, which is expressed by a variety of immune cells, including T, B, and NK cells, monocytes, macrophages, and eosinophils. Alemtuzumab is currently approved for the treatment of B-cell chronic lymphocytic leukemia. Intravenous administration produces prolonged and severe lymphopenia, where T cells typically recover over 14 to 16 months, whereas B cells recover within 6 months.

After the beneficial effects of MS relapse rate reduction and suppression of MRI activity were identified in a pilot trial at the University of Cambridge,[13] a multicenter, active-comparator, phase II active study in patients with RRMS was initiated. Randomized participants received 44 μg of subcutaneous interferon beta-1a three times a week or high-dose (24 mg per day) or low-dose (12 mg per day) intravenous alemtuzumab for 5 days at month 0, 3 days at month 12, and for some patients, 3 days at month 24. Alemtuzumab in both doses significantly and equally reduced the rate of sustained disability progression versus interferon beta-1a (9.0% vs. 26.2%; $p < .001$). Mean Expanded Disability Status Scale (EDSS) scores actually improved versus baseline scores by 0.39 points in the alemtuzumab group, while a reduction of 0.38 points was documented in the interferon beta-1a arm ($p < .001$). The annualized relapse rate was significantly reduced (0.10 vs. 0.36; $p < .001$). A significant benefit was demonstrated for proportion of relapse-free participants, T2-hyperintense MRI lesion volume change, and brain volume. A recent 5-year follow-up study established sustained benefits over interferon use in the studied cohort.[14] Potentially severe infusion reactions and cytokine-release syndrome may occur with alemtuzumab but can be prevented or at least reduced by antihistamines and corticosteroids.[15–17] Due to the lasting reduction of immune cell counts, infections and potentially cancer development are concerns. However, serious infection-related adverse effects have not been seen in the MS population. The most obvious and most concerning adverse effect of alemtuzumab is the onset of antibody-mediated autoimmunity syndromes.[18–20] Thyroid disorders, including Graves' disease, occurred in up to a third of alemtuzumab-treated patients. Potentially life-threatening idiopathic thrombocytopenic purpura, another antibody-mediated autoimmune disease, has developed in up to 2.8% of alemtuzumab-treated patients. Because of these severe adverse effects, it is unlikely that alemtuzumab will become a first-line agent, but it may be useful in the treatment of unusually aggressive or refractory cases as a tier 2 alternative to natalizumab.

Rituximab

Rituximab is a chimeric murine/human monoclonal antibody directed against CD20, a surface antigen expressed on pre-B cells and mature B cells. Intravenous rituximab leads to rapid and often complete elimination of circulating B cells. Rituximab is approved to treat non-Hodgkin's lymphoma and rheumatoid arthritis resistant to standard treatment. Although one could assume that the mechanism of action of rituximab should be related to reduced antibody production, CD20 is not expressed on plasma cells, and the rapid response to rituximab suggests that its effects are not mediated by decreasing antibody titers.[21,22] Initial rituximab infusions may produce potentially severe symptoms, including acute respiratory distress syndrome, myocardial infarction, or anaphylaxis. Commonly, only milder symptoms are experienced, such as fever, rigors, tachycardia, dyspnea, rashes, pruritus, and headache. Concomitant corticosteroid administration may reduce these symptoms. Another reported adverse outcome is related to cases of progressive multifocal leukoencephalopathy, similar to what was described with natalizumab, although the frequency of this complication appears to be lower.[23] In the phase II trial, rituximab correlated with rapid, circulating B-cell depletion that remained nearly complete (>95%) until week 24, followed by gradual recovery. While an increased risk of infection is a potential concern, most infections were mild and occurred equally in treatment groups.

In the phase II trial, ~25% of patients who received rituximab had human antichimeric antibodies at week 48, which may represent a challenge with repeated administration. A humanized anti-CD20 monoclonal antibody, ocrelizumab, may resolve this problem, as it is less likely that such antibodies would develop.[24,25]

Cladribine

Cladribine (2 chloro-2 deoxyadenosine) is a purine nucleoside analog that is resistant to adenosine deaminase, leading to a disruption of DNA synthesis and apoptosis.[26] In MS the medication targets lymphocytes due to their high level of expression of deoxycytidine kinase. Cladribine is currently approved in Australia and the Russian Federation; however, both the FDA and the European Medicines Agency declined to approve it because of safety concerns. As of this writing, further clinical development was reportedly discontinued. Subcutaneous cladribine reduced relapses and gadolinium-enhancing MRI lesions in a placebo-controlled phase II clinical trial in RRMS.[27] The phase III CLARITY clinical trial compared two doses of oral cladribine and demonstrated benefit in terms of relapses, disability progression, and MRI lesion activity in RRMS.[28] During the trials, one patient died of tuberculosis[29] reactivation, lymphocytopenia was relatively common, and herpes zoster was also encountered. Malignancies have also been documented in the treated group but none occurred in the placebo group; these included five cases of leiomyoma uteri and one case each of melanoma, ovarian cancer, and pancreatic cancer. We discuss it here as an example of a promising agent that did not become a treatment option for MS patients in the United States and the European Union due to its side effects.

Laquinimod

Laquinimod was developed from roquinimex, an immunomodulatory agent that worked very well in EAE and even in phase II trials (however, increased cardiac adverse effects and inflammatory activity halted its phase III trial).[30] Laquinimod was also effective in EAE,[31] has none of the problems reported with roquinimex, and was effective in phase II and III trials.[11] Elevated liver enzymes were observed but posed no significant risk.

In addition to the above therapies that may find their way to the practicing clinician's armamentarium, several others are undergoing various stages of clinical trials. These include idebenone, sunphenon EGCG, and polyphenon E for progressive forms of MS; abetecept, NU100, BAF312, and BG00002 for relapsing forms of MS; MEDI-551 and the above-mentioned ocrelizumab for targeting B-cell–derived mechanisms; and as a novel approach, even *Trichuris suis* (whipworm) ova have been tested to control relapsing forms of MS, based on their effects in other autoimmune conditions, related to the hygiene hypothesis of autoimmunity.

SUMMARY

There is no shortage of new medications developed in the hope of better controlling inflammation-mediated disease activity or of reaching current levels of efficacy with fewer side effects. Unfortunately, the pharmaceutical industry still focuses the bulk of its resources at the inflammatory phase in RRMS, and it is not yet clear whether controlling inflammation will lead to a "cure" in the sense of preventing further progression. Several new medications will surely become available over the next decade, and we may also see the advent of therapies to address the slow progressive stage and/or to possess tissue-restorative properties, as discussed elsewhere in this book.

REFERENCES

1. Schilling S, Goelz S, Linker R, Luehder F, Gold R. Fumaric acid esters are effective in chronic experimental autoimmune encephalomyelitis and suppress

macrophage infiltration. Clin Exp Immunol; 145:101–107, 2006.

2. Linker RA, Lee DH, Ryan S, et al. Fumaric acid esters exert neuroprotective effects in neuroinflammation via activation of the Nrf2 antioxidant pathway. Brain; 134:678–692, 2011.

3. Kappos L, Gold R, Miller DH, et al. Efficacy and safety of oral fumarate in patients with relapsing-remitting multiple sclerosis: a multicentre, randomised, double-blind, placebo-controlled phase IIb study. Lancet; 372:1463–1472, 2008.

4. Kappos L, Gold R, Miller DH, et al. Effect of BG-12 on contrast-enhanced lesions in patients with relapsing–remitting multiple sclerosis: subgroup analyses from the phase 2b study. Mult Scler; 18:314–321, 2012.

5. MacManus DG, Miller DH, Kappos L, et al. BG-12 reduces evolution of new enhancing lesions to T1-hypointense lesions in patients with multiple sclerosis. J Neurol; 258:449–456, 2011.

6. Hoefnagel JJ, Thio HB, Willemze R, Bouwes Bavinck JN. Long-term safety aspects of systemic therapy with fumaric acid esters in severe psoriasis. Br J Dermatol; 149:363–369, 2003.

7. Brousil JA, Roberts RJ, Schlein AL. Cladribine: an investigational immunomodulatory agent for multiple sclerosis. Ann Pharmacother; 40:1814–1821, 2006.

8. Wuest SC, Edwan JH, Martin JF, et al. A role for interleukin-2 trans-presentation in dendritic cell-mediated T cell activation in humans, as revealed by daclizumab therapy. Nat Med; 17:604–609, 2011.

9. Bielekova B, Catalfamo M, Reichert-Scrivner S, et al. Regulatory CD56(bright) natural killer cells mediate immunomodulatory effects of IL-2Ralpha-targeted therapy (daclizumab) in multiple sclerosis. Proc Natl Acad Sci USA; 103:5941–5946, 2006.

10. Bielekova B, Howard T, Packer AN, et al. Effect of anti-CD25 antibody daclizumab in the inhibition of inflammation and stabilization of disease progression in multiple sclerosis. Arch Neurol; 66:483–489, 2009.

11. Bielekova B, Richert N, Herman ML, et al. Intrathecal effects of daclizumab treatment of multiple sclerosis. Neurology; 77:1877–1886, 2011.

12. Bielekova B, Richert N, Howard T, et al. Humanized anti-CD25 (daclizumab) inhibits disease activity in multiple sclerosis patients failing to respond to interferon beta. Proc Natl Acad Sci USA; 101:8705–8708, 2004.

13. Paolillo A, Coles AJ, Molyneux PD, et al. Quantitative MRI in patients with secondary progressive MS treated with monoclonal antibody Campath 1H. Neurology; 53:751–757, 1999.

14. Coles AJ, Fox E, Vladic A, et al. Alemtuzumab more effective than interferon beta-1a at 5-year follow-up of CAMMS223 clinical trial. Neurology; 78:1069–1078, 2012.

15. Coles AJ, Compston DA, Selmaj KW, et al. Alemtuzumab vs. interferon beta-1a in early multiple sclerosis. N Engl J Med; 359:1786–1801, 2008.

16. Jones JL, Anderson JM, Phuah CL, et al. Improvement in disability after alemtuzumab treatment of multiple sclerosis is associated with neuroprotective autoimmunity. Brain; 133:2232–2247, 2010.

17. Jones JL, Coles AJ. Spotlight on alemtuzumab. Int MS J; 16:77–81, 2009.

18. Cossburn M, Pace AA, Jones J, et al. Autoimmune disease after alemtuzumab treatment for multiple sclerosis in a multicenter cohort. Neurology; 77:573–579, 2011.

19. Costelloe L, Jones J, Coles A. Secondary autoimmune diseases following alemtuzumab therapy for multiple sclerosis. Expert Rev Neurother; 12:335–341, 2012.

20. Cuker A, Coles AJ, Sullivan H, et al. A distinctive form of immune thrombocytopenia in a phase 2 study of alemtuzumab for the treatment of relapsing-remitting multiple sclerosis. Blood; 118:6299–6305, 2011.

21. Hawker K. B-cell-targeted treatment for multiple sclerosis: mechanism of action and clinical data. Curr Opin Neurol; 21 Suppl 1:S19–S25, 2008.

22. Ray A, Mann MK, Basu S, Dittel BN. A case for regulatory B cells in controlling the severity of autoimmune-mediated inflammation in experimental autoimmune encephalomyelitis and multiple sclerosis. J Neuroimmunol; 230:1–9, 2011.

23. Calabrese LH, Molloy ES, Huang D, Ransohoff RM. Progressive multifocal leukoencephalopathy in rheumatic diseases: evolving clinical and pathologic patterns of disease. Arthritis Rheum; 56:2116–2128, 2007.

24. Barun B, Bar-Or A. Treatment of multiple sclerosis with anti-CD20 antibodies. Clin Immunol; 142:31–37, 2012.

25. Hutas G. Ocrelizumab, a humanized monoclonal antibody against CD20 for inflammatory disorders and B-cell malignancies. Curr Opin Investig Drugs; 9:1206–1215, 2008.

26. Romine JS, Sipe JC, Koziol JA, Zyroff J, Beutler E. A double-blind, placebo-controlled, randomized trial of cladribine in relapsing-remitting multiple sclerosis. Proc Assoc Am Physicians; 111:35–44, 1999.

27. Giovannoni G, Comi G, Cook S, et al. A placebo-controlled trial of oral cladribine for relapsing multiple sclerosis. N Engl J Med; 362:416–426, 2010.

28. Miller AE, O'Connor P, Wolinsky JS, et al. Pre-specified subgroup analyses of a placebo-controlled phase III trial (TEMSO) of oral teriflunomide in relapsing multiple sclerosis. Mult Scler; 18(11):1625–1632, 2012.

29. Merrill JE, Hanak S, Pu SF, et al. Teriflunomide reduces behavioral, electrophysiological, and histopathological deficits in the Dark Agouti rat model of experimental autoimmune encephalomyelitis. J Neurol; 256:89–103, 2009.

30. Noseworthy JH, Wolinsky JS, Lublin FD, et al. Linomide in relapsing and secondary progressive MS: part I: trial design and clinical results. North American Linomide Investigators. Neurology; 54:1726–1733, 2000.

31. Hafler DA, Compston A, Sawcer S, et al. Risk alleles for multiple sclerosis identified by a genomewide study. N Engl J Med; 357:851–862, 2007.

Chapter 12

Treatment to Promote Remyelination

Abstract

Remyelination reinvests demyelinated axons with new myelin sheaths or internodes. Enhancing remyelination remains a major therapeutic goal of MS sclerosis research and appears possible because of the extensive spontaneous remyelination that occurs in areas of demyelination. Oligodendrocytes and Schwann cells demonstrate extensive remyelination. Schwann cell remyelination is easily distinguished from oligodendrocyte remyelination by the presence of a basement membrane and the one-to-one relationship between Schwann cells and axons. In contrast, remyelination by oligodendrocytes results in thinner myelin sheaths in relation to axon diameter, and one oligodendrocyte may remyelinate 50 to 100 axons. Spontaneous remyelination has been demonstrated in autoimmune, viral, and toxic models of demyelination. Experimental results have led to new hypotheses about the role of inflammatory cells in remyelination; they may, indeed, be necessary to facilitate the process. Investigators question

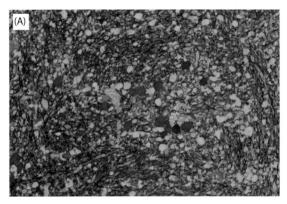 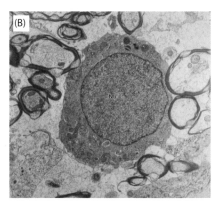

Figure 12–1. (**A**) Section from a patient undergoing cerebral biopsy for acute MS. This araldite-embedded section has been stained with toluidine blue. The purple-stained cells in this figure are oligodendrocytes. This rare abundance of oligodendrocytes in close contact suggests that the cells have recently divided as a result of the proliferative burst prior to remyelination. The entire field is made up of thinly myelinated axons, characteristic of the so-called "shadow plaques" of MS. This type of remyelination is quite common in pattern I lesions, in which oligodendrocytes appear relatively preserved and are not injured as the primary event in the pathological process. (**B**) Electron micrograph of an oligodendrocyte undergoing remyelination. This section is from a biopsy of an acute demyelinating lesion. The oligodendrocyte in this figure appears relatively normal; however, the oligodendrocyte is in contact with multiple thinly myelinated axons. Many of the axons show evidence of axonal swelling, typical in acute lesions with evidence of interstitial edema.

why remyelination, which appears in early MS, ultimately fails to repair the CNS. Possible explanations include the failure of oligodendrocyte recruitment or a failure of oligodendrocytes to receive and transmit appropriate signals to and from the axon. Also, theories vary about whether astrocytes help or hinder remyelination in demyelinated areas. Clearly, adoptive transfer of astrocytes, along with progenitor glial cells, results in the most robust, cell-based remyelination strategies in experimental animals. Finally, investigators have discovered that adoptive transfer of single polyclonal or monoclonal antibodies directed at antigens on the surface of oligodendrocytes promotes CNS remyelination and results in functional recovery.

Remyelination involves reinvesting demyelinated axons with new myelin sheaths or internodes. This has been described in MS[1,2] as well as in a number of experimental disease models. It occurs most notably in acute lesions of MS and becomes less prominent as the disease progresses (Fig. 12.1).[3] Remyelination is more commonly observed in acute lesions characterized by pattern I or pattern II MS pathology; it is virtually absent in acute lesions characterized by primary oligodendrogliopathy (patterns III and IV).[4] Remyelination allows the axon to transmit action potentials by saltatory conduction, a property consistently lost in demyelinating lesions. Although internode length may

actually be shorter in remyelinated lesions,[5] remyelinated lesions promote saltatory conduction at almost normal conduction velocity in both experimental animals and computer simulations. Even oligodendrocyte ensheathment, in which the glial cell wraps around the axon without actually forming compact myelin, may be sufficient to protect axons from injury and to allow saltatory conduction.[6] Current evidence indicates that remyelination significantly aids recovery of functional deficits arising from demyelinated lesions. In addition, remyelination may protect axons from atrophy and secondary inflammatory insult that features prominently in the disease process (secondary progression). Therefore, remyelination may be one of the most effective forms of neuroprotection.[7] Remyelination enhancement remains a major therapeutic goal of MS research because of its apparently positive impact on neurological function.[8] This appears possible because spontaneous remyelination occurs extensively in areas of MS demyelination in some acute lesions.

MORPHOLOGICAL FEATURES OF CNS REMYELINATION

The most characteristic feature of the morphology of remyelination is a thinner new myelin

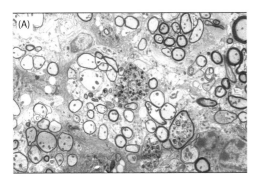
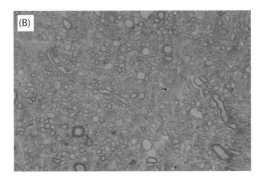

Figure 12–2. (**A**) Electron micrograph from an animal infected with Theiler's virus and treated with antibodies that promote remyelination in the CNS. As can be seen from this electron micrograph, most of the axons in this figure have very thin myelin sheaths in reference to axon diameter. A number of the axons, however, show axonal degeneration. Possibly some of the axons undergoing degeneration have been remyelinated. The degenerated axons are characterized by the presence of multiple dark osmophilic profiles, which represent accumulated mitochondria that degenerate as a result of the axonal injury. The remaining axons in these figures, however, have normal-appearing mitochondria. Many of the inflammatory cells seen in the figure are macrophages in the process of consuming myelin debris. Many astrocytes are present in the context of remyelinated axons. Clearly, inflammatory cells and astrocytes are necessary for remyelination to occur. (**B**) Araldite-embedded section from a patient with acute MS. This section comes from a biopsied acute cerebral lesion. The edge of the lesion presents evidence of new myelin formation characterized by thin myelin sheaths in reference to axon diameter. A number of axons in this figure, however, have a normal ratio of myelin sheath to axon diameter for comparison. In addition, the lightly stained oligodendrocytes throughout the field are probably cells contributing to CNS remyelination.

sheath and shorter internodes than would be expected from the diameter of the axon (Fig. 12.2). The degree of thinning is approximately two thirds of what would be expected from the axon diameter. This results in paler staining in the quality of the myelin with various myelin stains, especially Luxol fast blue, paraphenylenedianine, toluidine blue, and others that stain the myelin sheath. As a result, these plaques are known as *shadow plaques* because of their apparently paler staining with traditional dyes. In normal myelination, axon diameter and myelin internode length and thickness correlate more closely: both increase with increasing axonal diameter. In remyelination this relationship becomes less distinct: internodal dimensions decrease considerably with increasing axonal diameter. Demonstration of the abnormally thin myelin sheath remains by far the most unequivocal means of demonstrating remyelination by oligodendrocytes in the pathological samples. This is especially notable with plastic-embedded sections; however, it is easily observed also with routine formaldehyde-fixed, paraffin-embedded sections stained with Luxol fast blue. In addition, specific approaches document remyelination more precisely. Myelin basic protein, exon 2,[9] appears to express primarily during early myelin development.[10] Since the process of

remyelination may be similar to the process of myelination during early development, exon 2 expression appears reflected in areas of remyelination. Unfortunately, there are no other well-established reliable surrogate markers to distinguish remyelinated tissues from normal myelinated tissues. Therefore, the identification of remyelination is difficult in sections in which myelin thickness begins to approach that of normal myelination. The reason why the myelin sheath of the remyelinated axon differs from the myelin sheath of the normal axon has never been satisfactorily explained. Most hypotheses conclude that the myelinating oligodendrocytes associated with axons prevalent in adults have a different dynamic phase of growth in comparison to those observed during early development. In developmental myelination, the oligodendrocyte responds to the increasing area of expanding axon thickness by appropriately regulating the generated myelin, resulting in a close association between axonal diameter beneath the myelin sheath and the length of the internode. In contrast, remyelinating oligodendrocytes, which occur primarily in the adult nervous system after the process of developmental myelination is complete, engage axons with a largely static diameter, thus representing a sheath of default dimensions that are similar regardless of axon diameter. Unique relationships exist in the cerebrum between oligodendrocytes of the optic nerve, spinal cord, and white matter that may be distinct in relationship to their corresponding axons. This may explain the propensity for remyelination to occur in the optic nerves and the white matter of the cerebrum but to be less prominent in some cases of spinal cord disease, especially during the chronic phases of the demyelinating process.

OLIGODENDROCYTE REMYELINATION IN MULTIPLE SCLEROSIS

As early as 1906, investigators demonstrated the presence of myelin regeneration.[11] Groups in the 1970s demonstrated clearly that remyelination could occur in MS based on observations obtained from two MS patients who exhibited thin fibers from the abnormal central myelin sheath at the margins of most of the plaques studied.[12] The most common were the presence of bare stretches of axon between contiguous internodes. However, thin paranodes as well as internodes changed markedly in thickness along their length due to premature termination of myelin that ended in a hypertrophic lateral loop. In addition, abnormally thin internodes were present; these were of uniform thickness along the length but were shorter than normal and terminated in the form of normal nodal complexes. The findings were among the first to demonstrate morphological evidence of remyelination in MS lesions.

SCHWANN CELL REMYELINATION IN MULTIPLE SCLEROSIS

Other investigators have clearly corroborated the remyelination process in MS. It is also important to note that Schwann cells[13] as well as oligodendrocytes play an important role in remyelination in MS. These investigators examined remyelination in MS lesions and primarily stained these sections with the antisera to P0 protein, which is one of the constituents of peripheral nervous system myelin. They studied eight patients with evidence of neurological disease and found that P0 staining was confined

exclusively to peripheral nerve sheaths and was not present within the CNS.[13] In contrast, MS patients provided multiple examples of remyelination in the CNS that were stained for the P0 antigen, specifically indicating Schwann cell remyelination. Schwann cell remyelination can be easily distinguished from oligodendrocyte remyelination by the presence of the basement membrane that is a essential component of the Schwann cell. In addition, the myelin from the Schwann cell is uniformly thicker than that in the CNS. There is also a one-to-one association between individual Schwann cells and axons, whereas oligodendrocytes may remyelinate up to 70 to 100 axons. Electron microscopy can be used to observe and distinguish the lesions. It is clear that Schwann cell remyelination in MS occurs primarily in areas of the root entry zone. Apparently, the Schwann cells enter the CNS via the spinal cord as a consequence of the destruction of the glia limitans. However, there is also evidence of Schwann cell remyelination in areas remote from the root entry zone; for example, in the center of the centrum semiovale. In these situations, Schwann cells may arise from peripheral nerve terminals present on the surface of blood vessels to migrate into the CNS and remyelinate the areas of interest. Clearly, Schwann cell remyelination is more extensive than previously thought, particularly in the spinal cord. However, it is not known whether the functional improvements following Schwann cell remyelination are similar to oligodendrocyte remyelination.

EXPERIMENTAL MODELS OF REMYELINATION

Most experimental work focused on the issue of cell-mediated remyelination derives from experimental models. The classical experimental model, in which remyelination follows demyelination, is induced by immunization of myelin antigens in experimental autoimmune encephalomyelitis (EAE).[2] In the 1960s, investigators were able to show spontaneous remyelination in EAE.[14] There is increased interest in demonstrating that transfer of glial lineage cells remyelinates areas of previously demyelinated lesions. Some of these studies have even shown functional improvement correlated with areas of remyelination in animals.

Remyelination may fail in EAE due to an inflammatory response that either attacks the oligodendrocyte progenitor or disrupts the interaction between oligodendrocytes and the axon membrane.

Remyelination in Viral Models of Multiple Sclerosis

Other animal models of MS are induced by the Theiler's murine encephalomyelitis virus (TMEV) or the mouse hepatitis virus.[15,16] Both models offer strong evidence for spontaneous remyelination. Both models demonstrate remyelination in the early and chronic phases of disease. Of interest, in contrast to MS, the spontaneous remyelination in Theiler's virus primarily occurs in what is clearly the chronic demyelinating phase of the disease (6–9 months after infection with the virus). It is unclear why remyelination occurs at this very late stage in the disease process; one possibility is that oligodendrocytes in the early phase of the disease may be damaged or dysfunctional as a result of a dying-back oligodendrogliopathy.[17,18] Then, remyelination takes place only after the virus titers begin to decrease and the oligodendrocyte progenitors are healthier.

The mouse hepatitis virus model of MS has a more acute disease course, with demyelination occurring within weeks of infection. This is followed by almost complete remyelination, primarily in the spinal cord, in association with clearance of virus infection. Depending on the mouse strain and the viral strain, chronic forms of demyelination have been observed following infection with mouse hepatitis virus. In this situation, remyelination also occurs but not as consistently, since persistence of virus is needed in all the models for the demyelinating disease to continue for the life of the animal. The mouse hepatitis virus model implies that if virus infection were the cause of MS, then control of the virus infection should result in almost complete remyelination of demyelinated plaques in humans.

Remyelination in Toxic Models of Demyelination

In the oral toxic models of demyelination (i.e., cuprizone) and the models of direct injury to the spinal cord with (i.e., lysolecithin or ethidium bromide), there is also evidence of spontaneous remyelination. In the cuprizone model, removing cuprizone from the drinking water results in spontaneous remyelination within 2 to 3 weeks. In these situations, remyelination may be complete, and all the demyelinated lesions may be repaired.[19] This is similarly the case with lysolecithin injection to the spinal cord. Lysolecithin acts as a mild detergent to destroy the myelin sheath but leaves the oligodendrocyte relatively intact. About 2 to 3 weeks following lysolecithin administration, a progenitor-based burst of glial cells enters the demyelinated lesion to form thin myelin sheaths around the axons.[20] This remyelination process appears almost complete by 5 weeks.[21]

ROLE OF INFLAMMATION IN REMYELINATION

The role of inflammatory cells in the remyelinating process has become the focus of intense interest. Previously inflammation was considered to be generally injurious to remyelination, and inflammatory cells presumably presented major obstacles to remyelination in diseases such as MS and EAE. However, exactly the opposite has been observed experimentally. Innovative use of the lysolecithin model demonstrated clearly that efficient CNS remyelination by oligodendrocytes requires T cells.[22] In these experiments, the investigators used rag-1-deficient mice to block the presence of both T and B cells. They induced lysolecithin demyelination in these mice in the absence of inflammatory cells, but the animals showed significantly less spontaneous remyelination than immune-competent animals that were matched for genetic background. Normal mice depleted of either CD4+ or CD8+ T cells with monoclonal antibodies also had reduced remyelination. In contrast, when immune cells were adoptively transferred into these rag-1-deficient mice, remyelination then returned to normal levels. This provides the strongest evidence that T and B cells or, possibly, other inflammatory cells or factors recruited by these cells are necessary for the process of remyelination to be complete. Even in MS, remyelinated lesions are frequently associated within an inflammatory milieu. Other investigators have also proposed that microglial cells or macrophages affect the process of remyelination.[23] The general conceptual idea is that these inflammatory cells secrete specific regenerative factors.[24] These factors, recently cloned and sequenced, have been the source of increasing numbers of experiments that have attempted to deliver specific growth factors in toxic models of demyelination. Unfortunately, many experiments have not proven effective, probably due to delivery problems of the specific growth factors.[25] The specific growth factors of greatest interest are those that prevent the death or enhance the proliferation of progenitor cells, such as insulin growth factors (IGF), platelet-derived growth factors (PDGF), basic fibroblast growth factor, and others.[26,27]

CELLULAR BASIS OF REMYELINATION

An attractive approach to enhance remyelination is the adoptive transfer of CNS glial cells to demyelinated lesions.[28] The cellular basis of CNS remyelination has generated intense interest as the result of experiments in toxic models of demyelination using lysolecithin or ethidium bromide. The general approach is to use radiation-ionizing barriers in the toxic models of demyelination to prevent normal progenitor cells from dividing in an effort to prevent the occurrence of normal spontaneous remyelination. This allows investigators to transfer adoptively different combinations of astrocytes, oligodendrocytes, and progenitor cells to determine the specific cell types most likely to induce remyelination.

Similar experiments have also been done in myelin-mutant models in which there is a defect in one of the myelin proteins;[28,29] specifically, in the *jimpy* myelin mutant, which has a deficiency in proteolipid protein, and in the *shiverer* mouse mutant, which has a deficiency in myelin basic protein. Early classic experiments clearly demonstrated that adoptive transfer of progenitor glial cells induces remyelination in mouse-model mutants and in toxic models of demyelination.[30] Of interest, purified remyelination-inducing oligodendrocytes apparently do not remyelinate as extensively or robustly without a glial-cell population consisting of mixtures of astrocytes, microglial cells, and oligodendrocytes. The

oligodendrocytes themselves are apparently the remyelination-inducing cells; however, factors secreted by astrocytes, microglial cells, and immune cells are critical for extensive remyelination. These factors may promote the survival of oligodendrocytes in the lesions and may also support migration and proliferation of the progenitor oligodendrocytes to the site of the lesion.

In all likelihood, a burst of proliferation by progenitor glial cells precedes remyelination by 1 to 2 weeks. Following this burst, the progenitor cells then migrate to the center of the lesion to remyelinate the entire plaque. The extent of migration of these progenitor cells is somewhat limited and, in most models, may be as small as 1 to 3 millimeters. However, this may be sufficient to remyelinate small structures such as the optic nerve or even small spinal cord lesions in MS. Clearly, a strong relationship exists between the size of the lesion and the extent of remyelination, with smaller lesions having the greatest potential for complete remyelination. This may be the result of the limited migration of the progenitor glial cells. Therefore, the more heterogeneous the population of cells that is used in the adoptive transfer experiments, the more effective the process of remyelination is likely to be. This is important for any future transplantation experiment proposed in humans.

A number of investigators have proposed using Schwann cells obtained from the sural nerve of individual patients as the source of remyelinating cells in the CNS. Unfortunately, despite some positive results in animals, a definite correlation between adoptive transfer of Schwann cells and functional improvement remains to be established. Despite this, phase I trials have begun to determine the safety of this approach.

A more effective approach would be adoptive transfer of a combination of glial cells from human neonatal tissue. This obviously has ethical implications, since this tissue would likely have to be obtained from fresh aborted fetuses. Because of the ethical issues, none of these experiments have yet been attempted in humans. However, human fetal cells have been implanted into experimental animals induced with either toxic models of demyelination or genetic models of dysmyelination.[31] The results appear positive and suggest that this approach may be quite effective.

WHY DOES REMYELINATION FAIL IN MULTIPLE SCLEROSIS?

The major question in MS is why remyelination is incomplete. Despite our increased understanding of the biology of glial cells and remyelination, there is still no clear explanation of why remyelination occurs but ultimately fails in MS. Remyelination occurs in the early phases of the disease but then appears much less prominent as the disease progresses. The extent of remyelination in older animals also appears less pronounced.[32] For example, experiments with lysolecithin in young versus old animals have shown that older animals have much less spontaneous remyelination than the younger ones. One obvious cause may be aging oligodendrocytes, which have a very low turnover rate in the nervous system. This is, of course, highly probable in MS, since onset of progressive disease seems to be age-dependent, as discussed in Chapter 1.[33] The other possibility is that axonal injury increases as MS disease progresses. In addition to axon loss, remaining dysfunctional axons may lose specific molecular signals that tell oligodendrocytes to wrap and form myelin sheaths. Remyelination failure may also be related to failures of oligodendrocyte recruitment.[34] Remyelination may fail because oligodendrocyte progenitor numbers are depleted as part of the disease process.[15] These cells may be particularly targeted as the disease progresses. Providing support for this hypothesis are experiments in which specific antibodies that label oligodendrocyte progenitor cells are used in MS tissue to determine the number of progenitor cells as a function of length of disease. These experiments demonstrate the loss of oligodendrocyte progenitors in many cases of MS. Similar phenomena occur in the adult rat. However, there is also evidence that oligodendrocyte progenitor cells have very robust ability to repopulate areas from which they are missing.[35]

The other concern is that areas of remyelination are very susceptible to the second "hit" of demyelination. This second-hit hypothesis may account for many cases of failed remyelination as well as failed remyelination-enhancing attempts in humans. One interesting possibility is that not only is there a failure to recruit progenitor oligodendrocytes, but there may also be a failure to differentiate these cells.

Chronic demyelinating lesions have a deficiency of oligodendrocyte progenitor cells, and these cells may not be able to differentiate into remyelinating oligodendrocytes. The cells may need specific factors secreted by astrocytes or inflammatory cells to become functional remyelinating cells. However, when these oligodendrocytes do receive the appropriate signals in experimental models, the disruption can be overcome. This suggests that overcoming obstacles to proliferation or differentiation may be quite effective in promoting remyelination.

Another possibility is that the signals between oligodendrocytes and axons become dysregulated.[36] Signals sent from oligodendrocytes to axons may be either inappropriate or inappropriately regulated. However, it is difficult to discern whether the specific villain is the axon or the oligodendrocyte progenitor cell; both may likely be part of the problem. In some situations, the axons are missing or dysfunctional, whereas in others, the axons may be normal in number and function but missing progenitor cells. Both components (axons and progenitor cells) must be intact and able to accept "remyelination signals" for the process to ensue.

Clearly, if oligodendrocyte progenitor cells are recruited from outside the site of demyelination, the lesion size will determine how many oligodendrocyte progenitors are needed to promote remyelination. Large lesions require more protracted recruitment phases of progenitor cells and more viable axons to be able to remyelinate the area completely.[37] Based on the rate of oligodendrocyte migration, an average-sized (~2 cm) lesion in MS may require up to 5 months to remyelinate completely. This provides an opportunity for other beneficial factors, including those secreted by inflammation, which could be useful in the remyelination process, to allow remyelination to occur. If demyelination is complete, then the resulting lesion could remain chronically demyelinated; thus, there appears to be a critical balance between the inflammatory response participating in the injury and the inflammatory response participating in the repair.

Finally, the issue of the glial scar needs to be considered. Many view this to be a component of remyelination failure in MS.[38] This is based primarily on pathology studies in which astrocytic processes appear in areas of chronic demyelination. However, the alternative view is also feasible because remyelination seldom occurs in experimental models or in human MS in the absence of astrocytes. In addition, in adoptive transfer experiments, some astrocytes are required in the transferred cells to allow maximal remyelination.[39] Astrocytes may aid rather than impair the process of remyelination.[40] Astrocytes secrete a wide range of signaling molecules (PDGF, FGF, IGF)[41–43] that support recruitment and survival of oligodendrocytes.[44] However, in relatively quiescent, burnt-out plaques in which scarring astrocytes predominate, the likelihood of remyelination is relatively small, possibly due to the absence of inflammation in many of these lesions.

CAN THE IMMUNE SYSTEM BE HARNESSED TO ENHANCE REMYELINATION?

A much-considered approach to enhance remyelination is the use of natural factors to promote spontaneous remyelination. Based on the observation that immune cells, including B and T cells, are necessary for the reparative process, investigators tested the possibility that the immunoglobulin germline repertoire affects remyelination. These experiments resulted from immunization studies using spinal cord homogenate in animals chronically infected

with Theiler's virus.[45] Instead of these animals showing increased demyelination as would be observed with EAE, they showed extensive remyelination. Adoptive transfer experiments followed in which purified immunoglobulins or T cells were taken from animals immunized with spinal cord homogenate and then adoptively transferred into animals chronically infected with Theiler's virus with demyelination but no remyelination.[46,47] These experiments demonstrated that adoptive transfer of immunoglobulins enhanced spontaneous remyelination (Fig. 12.3). Later experiments showed that adoptive transfer of single polyclonal or monoclonal antibodies directed to antigens at the surface of oligodendrocytes or oligodendrocyte progenitor cells could promote remyelination.[48,49] The remyelination-promoting monoclonal antibodies were all directed against surface antigens on oligodendrocytes (Fig. 12.4).[50] Molecular sequencing of these antibodies showed minimal somatic mutations in the DNA sequence.[48] Therefore, these antibodies were made directly from the germline, likely from a special subset of B cells identified with the marker CD5.

These findings support the hypothesis that these antibodies are part of the natural autoantibody pool present in both rodents and humans.[51,52] Based on these observations, investigators attempted to determine whether protective, natural autoantibodies were

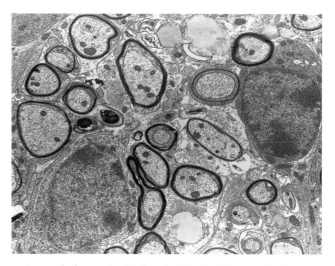

Figure 12–3. Electron micrograph from animal infected with Theiler's virus for 6 months, then treated with a remyelination-promoting antibody. The figure shows multiple remyelinated axons characterized by thinly myelinated axons. The figure also offers a rare view of two oligodendrocytes in close proximity. These oligodendrocytes may have recently divided as a result of the proliferative burst of oligodendrocyte progenitors necessary for remyelination to occur.

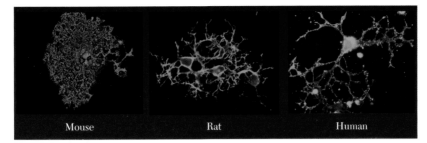

Figure 12–4. Confocal immunofluorescence microscopy with oligodendrocytes obtained from mouse, rat, and human. Mouse and rat oligodendrocytes were obtained from neonatal tissue. The human oligodendrocyte was obtained from cerebral tissue of a patient undergoing temporal lobectomy for intractable seizures. These oligodendrocytes have been stained with human monoclonal recombinant antibody 22, which has been shown to promote remyelination. Note that the recombinant human antibody is able to label oligodendrocytes from multiple tissue including mouse, rat, and human. Primate tissue (not shown) is also positive for the antibody. This provides strong evidence that the antibody may be useful in human clinical trials, since it shows affinity to human and primate tissue.

present in the human population. As a source of monoclonal immunoglobulins, investigators used serum proteins from patients with monoclonal gammopathies. Screening of a large number of samples (200–300) revealed only two or three monoclonal proteins that could bind to live oligodendrocytes or myelin in slices and in culture. These antibodies were then adoptively transferred into animals with either Theiler's virus-induced or lysolecithin-induced demyelination, where they were shown to promote extensive remyelination, with approximately 50% to 70% of the lesions completely repaired (Figs. 12.2A and 12.5).[53,54] Remarkably, only a single dose of antibody was necessary to start the process.[55] Because a human protein was transferred to a mouse, multiple injections of the

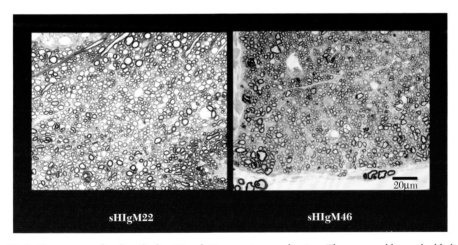

Figure 12–5. Human monoclonal antibodies 22 and 46 promote remyelination. These are araldite-embedded sections stained with paraphenylenediamine from spinal cords of animals infected with Theiler's murine encephalomyelitis virus (TMEV). Six months after infection, the animals received human monoclonal antibodies (mAbs) directed against oligodendrocytes. Two human mAbs were shown to promote extensive CNS remyelination, antibodies 22 and 46 shown in the figures. Note the presence of very thinly myelinated axons in the center of the figure in 22 and in the bottom of the figure of 46. Thinly myelinated axons stain less brown than normally myelinated axons, and as a result such lesions were described as *shadow plaques* in the old neuropathological literature. Further analysis of such lesions demonstrates that the axons showing remyelination have fewer myelin wraps than axons in the normal-appearing white matter. In the bottom of the figure of Ab 46 is an example of peripheral nervous system remyelination, which comes from the root entry zone and demonstrates very large, thick myelin compared to the thin myelin of CNS-type remyelination by oligodendrocytes. (Adapted from Warrington AE, Asakura K, Bieber AJ, et al. Human monoclonal antibodies reactive to oligodendrocytes promote remyelination in a model of multiple sclerosis. Proc Natl Acad Sci USA; 97:6820–6825, 2000.[54])

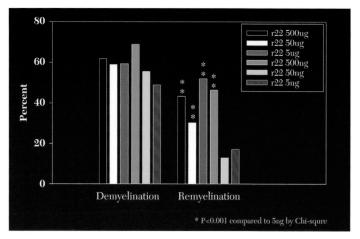

Figure 12–6. Dose response of recombinant antibody 22 shown to promote remyelination. In this experiment, animals were infected with Theiler's virus, and 6 months after infection, when the animals had extensive demyelination, they were treated with a single dose of recombinant 22 antibody. The dose of recombinant 22 antibody ranged from 5,000 ng to 5 ng. The experiment shows that a single dose of 500 ng of antibody induces extensive remyelination of 40% to 60% of the lesions. Statistically significant values are shown by the asterisks. A comparative analysis per weight (assuming that a mouse weighs ~20 g and a human weighs ~70 kg) estimates that the comparable dose of antibody necessary to induce remyelination in humans would be in the 2-mg range. (Adapted from Warrington AE, Bieber AJ, Ciric B, Pease LR, Van Keulen V, Rodriguez M. A recombinant human IgM promotes myelin repair after a single, very low dose. J Neurosci Res; 85:967–976, 2007.[56])

human protein would have resulted in anaphylactic shock. In addition, dose-titration experiments showed that only a small amount of antibody is necessary to induce the remyelinating process (Fig. 12.6).[56] Based on a weight-per-weight calculation of mice versus humans, it is estimated that the total dose of antibody necessary to induce remyelination in a human would be approximately 2 mg. As a result of these experiments, a monoclonal antibody, designated rHIgM22, has been synthesized and cloned in an expression vector. The recombinant (r) antibody has been generated in a GMP facility,[55] and experiments were undertaken to test the toxicity of the antibody in both mice and primates with the goal of beginning a phase I clinical trial to enhance spontaneous remyelination in patients with viable axons. These antibodies promote remyelination by mobilizing calcium (Ca^{++}) stores in oligodendrocytes (Fig. 12.7).[57] In addition, the antibodies cross the blood–brain barrier and target the demyelinated lesions (Fig. 12.8).[58] The proposed mechanism is that they stimulate progenitor oligodendrocytes to proliferate (Fig. 12.9) as a result of antibodies binding to the lipid rafts on the surface of oligodendrocytes and bringing molecules

together to make a signaling complex (Fig. 12.10).[59] Other recently discovered antibodies promote neurite extension (Fig. 12.11).[60] Thus, it is possible to target either oligodendrocytes or neurons (axons) to promote CNS repair. We provide this example to highlight a future vision of MS therapeutics that go beyond prevention of relapses to actual restoration of previous levels of well-being and function.

SUMMARY

CNS remyelination of oligodendrocytes and peripheral nervous system-type remyelination by Schwann cells occur in MS. Remyelination occurs early in the disease course but then becomes less frequent as the disease progresses. Possible reasons for the failure of remyelination in MS include absence of progenitor glial cells, absence of critical factors needed for glial cell survival and proliferation, lack of appropriate signals between oligodendrocytes and surviving axons, and even the absence of an inflammatory milieu consisting of T cells, B cells, and microglia/macrophages. Recent

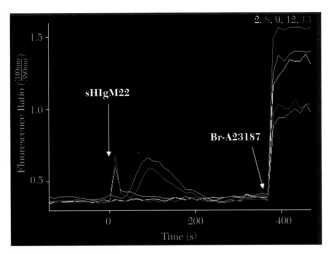

Figure 12–7. Fluorometric ratio analysis of calcium from a tracing of glial cells treated with a monoclonal remyelination-promoting antibody (Ab22). Ab22 results in two clear calcium spikes, the first of which is a very quick spike mediated exclusively by astrocytes and coming from internal stores. The second spike is mediated exclusively by oligodendrocytes. This slower response takes ~200 seconds to return to normal. This response comes from external sources and can be blocked by EDTA. This response by oligodendrocytes is mediated by an AMPA receptor, which can be blocked by molecule CNQX. Each response is independent, such that blocking the astrocyte response does not alter the oligodendrocyte response, nor does the oligodendrocyte response block the astrocyte response. These responses return to normal as is characteristic of a response beneficial to the cell. However, these cells are still able to respond to a calcium ionophore, BR83187. As can be seen, all the cells respond to calcium ionophores. Following the ionophore, the cells die and do not return to baseline. (Adapted from Paz Soldan MM, Warrington AE, Bieber AJ, et al. Remyelination-promoting antibodies activate distinct Ca2+ influx pathways in astrocytes and oligodendrocytes: relationship to the mechanism of myelin repair. Mol Cell Neurosci; 22:14–24, 2003.[57])

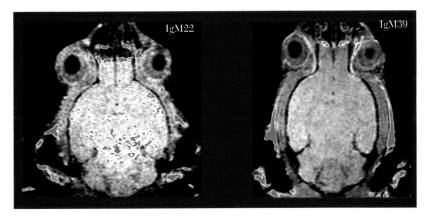

Figure 12–8. MRIs taken with 7-Tesla magnet from animals infected with Theiler's virus and treated with recombinant antibody 22 or control antibody 39. These animals show evidence of disease in the brain and the spinal cord. The treatment with the biotinylated antibody followed by streptavidin USPIO complexes shows that the recombinant 22 antibodies localize to areas of demyelination. In contrast, a similar treatment with animals infected with Theiler's virus but treated with control antibody 39, which does not label CNS cells, shows no binding to the CNS. These experiments prove definitively that recombinant human pentameric antibodies cross the blood–brain barrier in animals with inflammatory demyelinating lesions and that these antibodies bind to areas of injury within the lesion. In contrast, antibodies do not enter the normal-appearing white matter, where the blood–brain barrier remains intact. (Adapted from Pirko I, Ciric B, Gamez J, et al. A human antibody that promotes remyelination enters the CNS and decreases lesion load as detected by T2-weighted spinal cord MRI in a virus-induced murine model of MS. FASEB J; 18:1577–1579, 2004.[58])

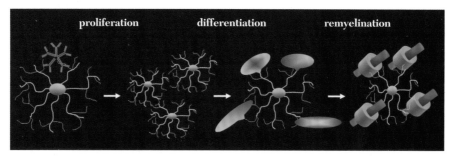

Figure 12–9. How antibodies (pentameric structure, labeled in orange) bind to the surface of progenitor oligodendrocytes. The antibodies bind to the surface of progenitor oligodendrocytes to induce proliferation of cells. This proliferative burst is necessary to initiate remyelination and occurs approximately 2 weeks prior to the completion of remyelination. The proliferative cells need to migrate into the demyelinated area and then differentiate into very large sheets of myelin. Finally, the oligodendrocytes wrap demyelinated axons. The number of wraps produced in this way is less than expected from the size of axon diameter. Thinly wrapped axons are characteristic of CNS remyelination in adults.

experiments have shown the importance of inflammatory cells for CNS remyelination to be extensive and complete. Even astrocytes, frequently considered a remyelination-inhibiting cell via the glial scar, have now been shown to secrete important factors for the health of oligodendrocytes. Adoptive transplantation experiments have shown that a mixture of oligodendrocytes, astrocytes, and macrophages results in more robust remyelination than do pure, highly enriched oligodendrocytes. There is also support for the concept that natural immunoglobulins from humans or mice have the potential to enhance CNS remyelination with functional improvements. Thus, treatment to enhance remyelination will soon be tested in humans, providing the possibility of a curative therapy.

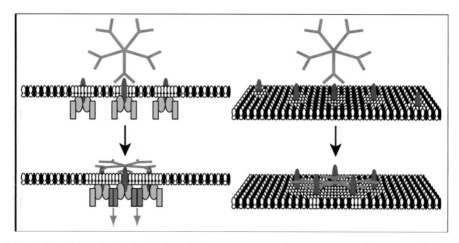

Figure 12–10. Potential mechanism by which antibodies promote remyelination or neuronal extension. All the antibodies with reparative functions have a pentameric structure. In this figure, they are depicted as pink pentameric antibodies. The five potential binding sites allow binding of multiple antigens as is characteristic of natural autoantibodies. Molecules on the cell surface are cross-linked to interact with each other. As a result, they phosphorylate specific proteins on the cytoplasmic side of the cell membrane (as shown by the *red arrows*) and induce signaling events within the cell. All antibodies that promote CNS repair bind to lipid rafts, which are on the surface of oligodendrocytes or neurons. These antibodies also cause the influx of calcium, which is critical to initiate the repair process. (Adapted from Howe CL, Rodriguez M. Remyelination as neuroprotection. In: Watman S, ed. Multiple Sclerosis as a Neuronal Disease. New York: Elsevier Academic Press; 2005:389–419.[61])

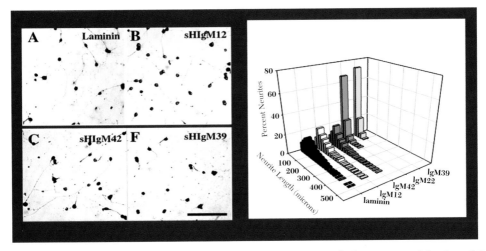

Figure 12–11. Example of axonal extension by human antibodies. Human antibodies were tested for their ability to promote CNS neurite extension and, in particular, axon extension. The human antibodies were placed on a tissue culture plate along with neurons from the cerebellum or the hippocampus, and neurite length was measured. As a positive control, neurons were placed on laminin, which promotes neural extension. Antibody 12 and antibody 42 promote neural extension, as shown in the bar graph, with some neurites extending up to 500 microns. In contrast, control antibodies 22 and 39, which do not bind neurons, extend neurites up to 100 microns. Treatment of mice with neuron-binding recombinant antibodies prevents axonal death and neuronal death. Animals show improvement in neurological function following the axonal phase of Theiler's virus-induced demyelinating disease. Antibody 12 has been cloned and sequenced, and recombinant forms replicate the findings of the serum-derived antibody. (Adapted from Warrington AE, Bieber AJ, Van Keulen V, Ciric B, Pease LR, Rodriguez M. Neuron-binding human monoclonal antibodies support central nervous system neurite extension. J Neuropathol Exp Neurol; 63:461–473, 2004.[60])

REFERENCES

1. Prineas JW, Kwon EE, Goldenberg PZ, et al. Multiple sclerosis. Oligodendrocyte proliferation and differentiation in fresh lesions. Lab Invest; 61:489–503, 1989.
2. Raine CS, Traugott U. Chronic relapsing experimental autoimmune encephalomyelitis. Ultrastructure of the central nervous system of animals treated with combinations of myelin components. Lab Invest; 48:275–284, 1983.
3. Ghatak NR, Leshner RT, Price AC, Felton WL 3rd. Remyelination in the human central nervous system. J Neuropathol Exp Neurol; 48:507–518, 1989.
4. Lucchinetti C, Bruck W, Parisi J, Scheithauer B, Rodriguez M, Lassmann H. A quantitative analysis of oligodendrocytes in multiple sclerosis lesions. A study of 113 cases. Brain; 122 (Pt 12):2279–2295, 1999.
5. Weiner LP, Waxman SG, Stohlman SA, Kwan A. Remyelination following viral-induced demyelination: ferric ion-ferrocyanide staining of nodes of Ranvier within the CNS. Ann Neurol; 8:580–583, 1980.
6. Talbott JF, Loy DN, Liu Y, et al. Endogenous Nkx2.2+/Olig2+ oligodendrocyte precursor cells fail to remyelinate the demyelinated adult rat spinal cord in the absence of astrocytes. Exp Neurol; 192:11–24, 2005.
7. Rodriguez M. A function of myelin is to protect axons from subsequent injury: implications for deficits in multiple sclerosis. Brain; 126:751–752, 2003.
8. Murray PD, McGavern DB, Sathornsumetee S, Rodriguez M. Spontaneous remyelination following extensive demyelination is associated with improved neurological function in a viral model of multiple sclerosis. Brain; 124:1403–1416, 2001.
9. Jordan CA, Friedrich VL, Jr., de Ferra F, Weismiller DG, Holmes KV, Dubois-Dalcq M. Differential exon expression in myelin basic protein transcripts during central nervous system (CNS) remyelination. Cell Mol Neurobiol; 10:3–18, 1990.
10. Capello E, Voskuhl RR, McFarland HF, Raine CS. Multiple sclerosis: re-expression of a developmental gene in chronic lesions correlates with remyelination. Ann Neurol; 41:797–805, 1997.
11. Marburg O. Die sogenannt "akute multiple sklerose" (Encephalomyelitis periaxialis scleroticans). Jhrd Psychiatr Neurol; 27:211–312, 1906.
12. Prineas JW, Connell F. Remyelination in multiple sclerosis. Ann Neurol; 5:22–31, 1979.
13. Itoyama Y, Webster HD, Richardson EP, Jr., Trapp BD. Schwann cell remyelination of demyelinated axons in spinal cord multiple sclerosis lesions. Ann Neurol; 14:339–346, 1983.
14. Lampert PW, Kies MW. Mechanism of demyelination in allergic encephalomyelitis of guinea pigs. An electron microscopic study. Exp Neurol; 18:210–223, 1967.
15. Armstrong R, Friedrich VL, Jr., Holmes KV, Dubois-Dalcq M. In vitro analysis of the oligodendrocyte lineage in mice during demyelination and remyelination. J Cell Biol; 111:1183–1195, 1990.
16. Godfraind C, Friedrich VL, Holmes KV, Dubois-Dalcq M. In vivo analysis of glial cell phenotypes during a viral demyelinating disease in mice. J Cell Biol; 109:2405–2416, 1989.

17. Rodriguez M. Virus-induced demyelination in mice: "dying back" of oligodendrocytes. Mayo Clin Proc; 60:433–438, 1985.

18. Rodriguez M, Leibowitz JL, Lampert PW. Persistent infection of oligodendrocytes in Theiler's virus-induced encephalomyelitis. Ann Neurol; 13:426–433, 1983.

19. Ludwin SK. Chronic demyelination inhibits remyelination in the central nervous system. An analysis of contributing factors. Lab Invest; 43:382–387, 1980.

20. Blakemore WF. Observations on remyelination in the rabbit spinal cord following demyelination induced by lysolecithin. Neuropathol Appl Neurobiol; 4:47–59, 1978.

21. Jeffery ND, Blakemore WF. Remyelination of mouse spinal cord axons demyelinated by local injection of lysolecithin. J Neurocytol; 24:775–781, 1995.

22. Bieber AJ, Kerr S, Rodriguez M. Efficient central nervous system remyelination requires T cells. Ann Neurol; 53:680–684, 2003.

23. Kotter MR, Setzu A, Sim FJ, Van Rooijen N, Franklin RJ. Macrophage depletion impairs oligodendrocyte remyelination following lysolecithin-induced demyelination. Glia; 35:204–212, 2001.

24. Yamamura T, Sun D, Aloisi F, Klinkert WE, Wekerle H. Interaction between oligodendroglia and immune cells: mitogenic effect of an oligodendrocyte precursor cell line on syngeneic T lymphocytes. J Neurosci Res; 32:178–189, 1992.

25. Franklin RJ. Why does remyelination fail in multiple sclerosis? Nature Reviews; 3:705–714, 2002.

26. Liu X, Yao DL, Webster H. Insulin-like growth factor I treatment reduces clinical deficits and lesion severity in acute demyelinating experimental autoimmune encephalomyelitis. Mult Scler; 1:2–9, 1995.

27. McMorris FA, Smith TM, DeSalvo S, Furlanetto RW. Insulin-like growth factor I/somatomedin C: a potent inducer of oligodendrocyte development. Proc Natl Acad Sci USA; 83:822–826, 1986.

28. Duncan ID. Glial cell transplantation and remyelination of the central nervous system. Neuropathol Appl Neurobiol; 22:87–100, 1996.

29. Tontsch U, Archer DR, Dubois-Dalcq M, Duncan ID. Transplantation of an oligodendrocyte cell line leading to extensive myelination. Proc Natl Acad Sci USA; 91:11616–11620, 1994.

30. Gumpel M, Gout O, Lubetzki C, Gansmuller A, Baumann N. Myelination and remyelination in the central nervous system by transplanted oligodendrocytes using the shiverer model. Discussion on the remyelinating cell population in adult mammals. Dev Neurosci; 11:132–139, 1989.

31. Kondo Y, Duncan ID. Transplantation of oligodendrocyte progenitor cells in animal models of leukodystrophies. Meth Mol Biol; 549:175–185, 2009.

32. Shields SA, Gilson JM, Blakemore WF, Franklin RJ. Remyelination occurs as extensively but more slowly in old rats compared to young rats following gliotoxin-induced CNS demyelination. Glia; 28:77–83, 1999.

33. Tutuncu M, Tang J, Zeid NA, et al. Onset of progressive phase is an age-dependent clinical milestone in multiple sclerosis. Mult Scler; 2012 June 26 [E-pub ahead of print].

34. Barres BA, Hart IK, Coles HS, et al. Cell death and control of cell survival in the oligodendrocyte lineage. Cell; 70:31–46, 1992.

35. Scolding N, Franklin R, Stevens S, Heldin CH, Compston A, Newcombe J. Oligodendrocyte progenitors are present in the normal adult human CNS and in the lesions of multiple sclerosis. Brain; 121 (Pt 12):2221–2228, 1998.

36. Wood PM, Bunge RP. Evidence that axons are mitogenic for oligodendrocytes isolated from adult animals. Nature; 320:756–758, 1986.

37. Blakemore WF, Chari DM, Gilson JM, Crang AJ. Modelling large areas of demyelination in the rat reveals the potential and possible limitations of transplanted glial cells for remyelination in the CNS. Glia; 38:155–168, 2002.

38. Rosen CL, Bunge RP, Ard MD, Wood PM. Type 1 astrocytes inhibit myelination by adult rat oligodendrocytes in vitro. J Neurosci; 9:3371–3379, 1989.

39. Imaizumi T, Lankford KL, Waxman SG, Greer CA, Kocsis JD. Transplanted olfactory ensheathing cells remyelinate and enhance axonal conduction in the demyelinated dorsal columns of the rat spinal cord. J Neurosci; 18:6176–6185, 1998.

40. Keilhauer G, Meier DH, Kuhlmann-Krieg S, Nieke J, Schachner M. Astrocytes support incomplete differentiation of an oligodendrocyte precursor cell. EMBO J; 4:2499–2504, 1985.

41. Bogler O, Wren D, Barnett SC, Land H, Noble M. Cooperation between two growth factors promotes extended self-renewal and inhibits differentiation of oligodendrocyte-type-2 astrocyte (O-2A) progenitor cells. Proc Natl Acad Sci USA; 87:6368–6372, 1990.

42. Hart IK, Richardson WD, Bolsover SR, Raff MC. PDGF and intracellular signaling in the timing of oligodendrocyte differentiation. J Cell Biol; 109:3411–3417, 1989.

43. McKinnon RD, Matsui T, Dubois-Dalcq M, Aaronson SA. FGF modulates the PDGF-driven pathway of oligodendrocyte development. Neuron; 5:603–614, 1990.

44. Bhat S, Pfeiffer SE. Stimulation of oligodendrocytes by extracts from astrocyte-enriched cultures. J Neurosci Res; 15:19–27, 1986.

45. Rodriguez M, Lennon VA, Benveniste EN, Merrill JE. Remyelination by oligodendrocytes stimulated by antiserum to spinal cord. J Neuropathol Exp Neurol; 46:84–95, 1987.

46. Rodriguez M. Immunoglobulins stimulate central nervous system remyelination: electron microscopic and morphometric analysis of proliferating cells. Lab Invest; 64:358–370, 1991.

47. Rodriguez M, Lennon VA. Immunoglobulins promote remyelination in the central nervous system. Ann Neurol; 27:12–17, 1990.

48. Miller DJ, Rodriguez M. A monoclonal autoantibody that promotes central nervous system remyelination in a model of multiple sclerosis is a natural autoantibody encoded by germline immunoglobulin genes. J Immunol; 154:2460–2469, 1995.

49. Miller DJ, Sanborn KS, Katzmann JA, Rodriguez M. Monoclonal autoantibodies promote central nervous system repair in an animal model of multiple sclerosis. J Neurosci; 14:6230–6238, 1994.

50. Asakura K, Miller DJ, Murray K, Bansal R, Pfeiffer SE, Rodriguez M. Monoclonal autoantibody SCH94.03, which promotes central nervous system remyelination, recognizes an antigen on the surface of oligodendrocytes. J Neurosci Res; 43:273–281, 1996.

51. Asakura K, Miller DJ, Pease LR, Rodriguez M. Targeting of IgMkappa antibodies to oligodendrocytes promotes CNS remyelination. J Neurosci; 18:7700–7708, 1998.

52. Miller DJ, Bright JJ, Sriram S, Rodriguez M. Successful treatment of established relapsing experimental autoimmune encephalomyelitis in mice with a monoclonal natural autoantibody. J Neuroimmunol; 75:204–209, 1997.

53. Ciric B, VanKeulen V, Rodriguez M, Kyle RA, Gertz MA, Pease LR. Clonal evolution in Waldenstrom macroglobulinemia highlights functional role of B-cell receptor. Blood; 97:321–323, 2001.

54. Warrington AE, Asakura K, Bieber AJ, et al. Human monoclonal antibodies reactive to oligodendrocytes promote remyelination in a model of multiple sclerosis. Proc Natl Acad Sci USA; 97:6820–6825, 2000.

55. Mitsunaga Y, Ciric B, Van Keulen V, et al. Direct evidence that a human antibody derived from patient serum can promote myelin repair in a mouse model of chronic-progressive demyelinating disease. FASEB J; 16:1325–1327, 2002.

56. Warrington AE, Bieber AJ, Ciric B, Pease LR, Van Keulen V, Rodriguez M. A recombinant human IgM promotes myelin repair after a single, very low dose. J Neurosci Res; 85:967–976, 2007.

57. Paz Soldan MM, Warrington AE, Bieber AJ, et al. Remyelination-promoting antibodies activate distinct Ca2+ influx pathways in astrocytes and oligodendrocytes: relationship to the mechanism of myelin repair. Mol Cell Neurosci; 22:14–24, 2003.

58. Pirko I, Ciric B, Gamez J, et al. A human antibody that promotes remyelination enters the CNS and decreases lesion load as detected by T2-weighted spinal cord MRI in a virus-induced murine model of MS. FASEB J; 18:1577–1579, 2004.

59. Watzlawik J, Holicky E, Edberg DD, et al. Human remyelination promoting antibody inhibits apoptotic signaling and differentiation through Lyn kinase in primary rat oligodendrocytes. Glia; 58:1782–1793, 2010.

60. Warrington AE, Bieber AJ, Van Keulen V, Ciric B, Pease LR, Rodriguez M. Neuron-binding human monoclonal antibodies support central nervous system neurite extension. J Neuropathol Exp Neurol; 63:461–473, 2004.

61. Howe CL, Rodriguez M. Remyelination as neuroprotection. In: Watman S, ed. *Multiple Sclerosis as a Neuronal Disase.* New York: Elsevier Academic Press; 2005:389–419.

Index